Clinical Psychiatry

Clinical Psychiatry

Editor: John Dalvi

FOSTER ACADEMICS
www.fosteracademics.com

www.fosteracademics.com

FOSTER ACADEMICS

Cataloging-in-Publication Data

Clinical psychiatry / edited by John Dalvi.
p. cm.
Includes bibliographical references and index.
ISBN 978-1-63242-535-5
1. Psychiatry. 2. Clinical psychology. I. Dalvi, John.
RC454 .C55 2018
616.89--dc23

Foster Academics,
118-35 Queens Blvd., Suite 400,
Forest Hills, NY 11375, USA

ISBN 978-1-63242-535-5 (Hardback)

Printed and bound in China.

Contents

Preface

I am honored to present to you this unique book which encompasses the most up-to-date data in the field. I was extremely pleased to get this opportunity of editing the work of experts from across the globe. I have also written papers in this field and researched the various aspects revolving around the progress of the discipline. I have tried to unify my knowledge along with that of stalwarts from every corner of the world, to produce a text which not only benefits the readers but also facilitates the growth of the field.

The study focused on diagnosis, treatment, and prevention of mental disorders is known as psychiatry. As a field of medical science, it includes studying the problems occurring due to mood, perception, behavior, and cognition changes or mood swings. The treatments of such diseases includes psychotherapy and psychiatric medication. This book consists of contributions made by international experts. It includes some of the vital pieces of work being conducted across the world, on various topics related to psychiatry. This book is a valuable compilation of topics, ranging from the basic to the most complex advancements in the field. It will serve as a reference to a broad spectrum of readers.

Finally, I would like to thank all the contributing authors for their valuable time and contributions. This book would not have been possible without their efforts. I would also like to thank my friends and family for their constant support.

Editor

1

The Use of Physical Restraint in Norwegian Adult Psychiatric Hospitals

Rolf Wynn[1,2]

[1] *Department of Clinical Medicine, Faculty of Health Sciences, UiT The Arctic University of Norway, 9037 Tromsø, Norway*
[2] *Department of Psychogeriatric Services, Division of Mental Health and Addictions, University Hospital of North Norway, 9291 Tromsø, Norway*

Correspondence should be addressed to Rolf Wynn; rolf.wynn@gmail.com

Academic Editor: Yvonne Forsell

Background. The use of coercion within the psychiatric services is problematic and raises a range of ethical, legal, and clinical questions. "Physical restraint" is an emergency procedure used in psychiatric hospitals to control patients that pose an imminent physical danger. We wished to review the literature published in scientific peer-reviewed journals describing studies on the use of physical restraint in Norway, in order to identify the current state of knowledge and directions for future research. *Design.* The databases PubMed, PsycINFO, CINAHL, Web of Science, and Embase were searched for studies relating to physical restraint (including holding) in Norwegian psychiatric hospitals, supplemented with hand searches. *Results.* 28 studies were included. Most of the studies were on rates of restraint, but there were also some studies on perceptions of patients and staff, case studies, and ethnographic studies. There was only one intervention study. There are differences in use between wards and institutions, which in part may be explained by differences in patient populations. Staff appear to be less negative to the use of restraint than patients. *Conclusions.* The studies that were identified were primarily concerned with rates of use and with patients' and staff's perspectives. More interventional studies are needed to move the field forward.

1. Introduction

The use of coercion within the psychiatric services is problematic and raises a range of ethical, legal, and clinical questions [1, 2]. Physical restraint, also referred to as "mechanical restraint," is a technique whereby a patient is physically restrained so that the range of movement is restricted. Typically, the patient is restrained to a bed, with a belt over the chest area and four belts restraining each limb ("five-point fixation") [3–5]. Other types of physical restraints, such as walking restraints and special clothing, are rarely used in Norway. Staff that physically hold a patient against the patient's will might also be considered as carrying out a type of physical restraint ("holding").

In Norway, physical restraint (including holding) may be used as an emergency intervention, with the purpose of increasing the safety of the patient in question and/or fellow patients and staff or avoiding significant damage to buildings and objects [6, 7]. The intervention is typically used when patients are violent or self-harming [3, 8, 9]. It is in Norway not permitted to use physical restraint for therapeutic purposes (i.e., "behavioural treatment") or as punishment, and the use of physical restraint within the psychiatric hospitals is strictly regulated and monitored [6].

The use of physical restraint is challenging from both a clinical viewpoint and an ethical viewpoint. Subjecting patients to physical restraint carries a risk of physical and psychological harm to patients; staff may be physically harmed when restraining patients, and it may harm the provider-patient relationship and further treatment [10, 11]. Moreover, it is a goal to base psychiatric treatment—to the extent possible—on voluntary cooperation and to subject patients to as little coercion as possible [6].

In recent years, there has in Europe and the US, as well as in other parts of the world, been an increasing focus on the need to reduce coercion within the psychiatric services [2, 11], and more research has been carried out in this area. The purpose of this review was to search and

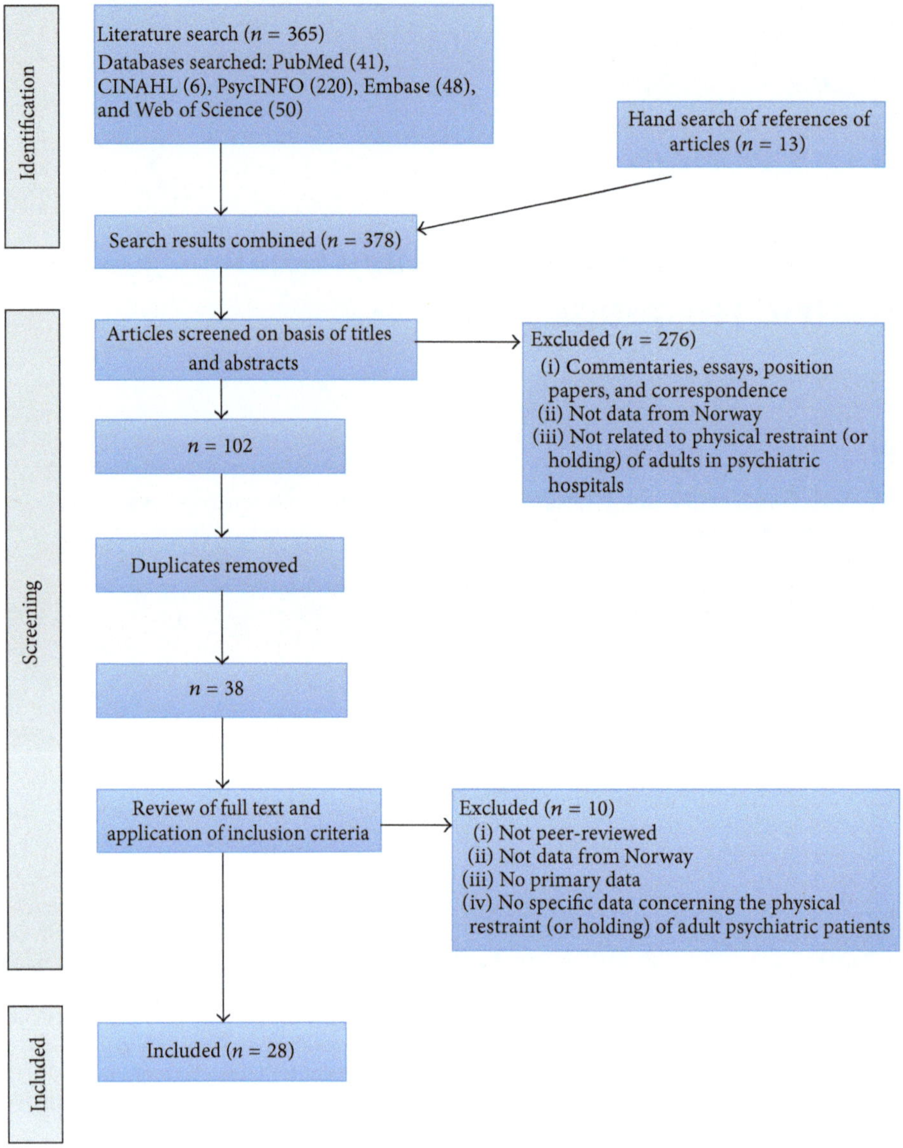

FIGURE 1: Process for selection of studies included in the review.

appraise peer-reviewed scientific publications documenting the use of physical restraint in Norwegian hospital-based adult psychiatric services.

2. Material and Methods

2.1. Strategy for Database Search. A literature search of relevant electronic databases, including PubMed, PsycINFO (Ovid), Embase (Ovid), Web of Science, and CINAHL (EBSCO), was performed to identify relevant articles. The search was carried out in September 2015. The search terms used were various combinations of psychiatry, Norway, physical restraint, mechanical restraint, and holding. The search terms were in English, as Norwegian scientists typically publish in English to reach a wider audience. There are a very small number of Norwegian scientific peer-reviewed journals that might publish relevant articles in the Norwegian language, such as the Journal of the Norwegian Medical Association. However, these journals typically provide English abstracts that are indexed in one or more of the databases that were searched. Hand searches were done of the reference lists of those articles that were identified as relevant to the study. The details of the search process can be found in Figure 1.

2.2. Inclusion and Exclusion of Studies. A total of 365 articles were identified in the initial electronic search. Hand searching of the references of articles gave an additional 13 potentially relevant articles. The titles and abstracts of the publications were screened for relevance, reducing the number to 102. When duplicates were removed, 38 articles remained, and these were read in full and considered against the inclusion and exclusion criteria (see below). This gave the final 28 articles that were included in the review (see Table 1 and Figure 1).

2.3. Inclusion and Exclusion Criteria. All articles published in peer-reviewed journals carried out with data from Norway and involving the use of physical restraint (including physical holding by staff) within adult psychiatric hospitals were considered for inclusion. Articles not specifically mentioning restraint or that examined coercion only as a general concept were excluded. Studies only involving municipal services, nursing homes, and services for the intellectually disabled were excluded. Studies without data from Norway were excluded, as were studies that did not include primary empirical data (i.e., literature reviews, etc.). Surveys on rates of use of restraint in Norway that had not been published in peer-reviewed journals were not included in the review, but some have nevertheless been mentioned in Discussion.

2.4. Data Synthesis and Analysis. The 28 included articles were grouped into five different categories according to their study purposes and methods used. The key findings in each article in the different categories were condensed and the common findings in the various categories were identified.

3. Results

The 28 articles were categorized according to their study purposes and methods used (see Table 1). 27 articles described observational studies and only one article [31] described an interventional study.

21 of the studies followed a quantitative methodology. Seven articles had a qualitative design, that is, in-depth interviews [13], case studies [32–34], and ethnographic designs [35–37].

The following categorization was devised: (1) studies examining patients' perceptions of physical restraint, (2) studies examining staff's perceptions of physical restraint by means of questionnaires, (3) studies examining the rates of use of physical restraint and factors that influence such rates; these studies were typically reviews of protocols and/or medical records at one or more departments at one or more hospitals, (4) studies examining the effects of interventions on reducing physical restraint, (5) case studies of individual patients subjected to physical restraint, and (6) ethnographic studies.

3.1. Studies Examining Patients' Perceptions of Physical Restraint. Three studies were identified [12–14] that treated the topic of patients' perceptions of physical restraint. One study used only questionnaires filled in by patients [12]; one study used questionnaires filled in partly by patients and partly by researchers as well as data from medical records [14], while one study used in-depth interviews with patients [13].

3.1.1. Main Findings. In one study [12], 19 patients subjected to coercive interventions were matched to controls. There was no significant difference in satisfaction between coerced and matched noncoerced patients; however only three of the included patients had been subjected to physical restraint. An interview study of 12 patients following physical restraint [13] found that patients gave refusal of medication, refusal to follow staff directions, or their own aggression as reasons for restraint. Many felt that restraint could have been avoided, and some felt angry and distrustful of staff after restraint. Iversen et al. [14], drawing on data from 173 patients, found that objective coercion (including mechanical restraint) had a significant negative effect on overall patient satisfaction.

3.2. Studies Examining Staff's Perceptions of Physical Restraint by means of Questionnaires. Four studies [15–18] examined the topic of staff's perceptions of physical restraint by means of questionnaires. Two studies used a traditional questionnaire format [15, 16], while two studies used simulated cases, where staff responded to vignettes describing typical situations where restraint was believed to be an option [17, 18].

3.2.1. Main Findings. A study based on questionnaires from 85 staff at one psychiatric hospital found that patients' assault, acting-out, and self-harming were given as most important reasons for physical restraint. 80% of staff believed that physical restraint was used appropriately, and 94% believed that it did not influence patients' recovery [15]. In a study involving questionnaires to 267 staff at a hospital, a majority of staff believed that the interventions were used correctly. Male staff, highly educated staff, and staff at high-use wards were most critical to use. 70% had been assaulted in connection with the interventions [16]. The same questionnaire also included simulated cases, and staff preferred informal interventions above physical restraint [17]. Such informal interventions were typically not recorded and their importance may therefore have been overlooked. A study involving 180 staff at two adult psychiatric units found that there was a limited degree of variance in staff's responses with respect to degree of restrictiveness. The study supported the idea that a range of different interventions are used in emergency situations [18].

3.3. Studies Examining Rates of Use of Physical Restraint and Factors That Influence Such Rates. These studies were typically reviews of protocols and/or medical records at one or more departments at one or more hospitals. With one exception [9], all the studies in this category had a retrospective design.

3.3.1. Main Findings. One study from 1983 of a forensic psychiatric hospital found that the use of restraint had been reduced dramatically from more than 15,000 patient days in 1977 to only 1.5 patient days in the first third of 1981 [19]. Høyer and Drange [20], in an examination of protocols of restraint, found that, during the first six months of 1988, 203 patients had been mechanically restrained for 10,767 hours. In a similar study in 1994 [21], they found that 9402 hours of mechanical restraint was recorded in the first half of 1990. Single patients created large variations in use. There was no correlation between size of ward or staff ratio and use of coercion and no difference in levels from the previous study.

Linaker et al. [22], examining the use of restraint in Norwegian security units, found that 25% had been subjected to physical restraint during a six-month period in 1993. Wynn [23], reviewing protocols and medical records from a psychiatric hospital during a 5.5-year period, found that there

Table 1: Included articles ($n = 28$).

Number	Category	Articles [reference]	Methods/participants (n)	Key findings
1	Patients' perceptions (1)	Patients' satisfaction and self-rated improvement following coercive interventions [12]	Questionnaire to adult psychiatric patients (total sample $n = 410$, of which 19 subjected to coercion were matched to other patients) (only 3 had been physically restrained)	No significant difference in satisfaction between coerced and matched noncoerced patients
2	Patients' perceptions (1)	Psychiatric inpatients' experiences with restraint [13]	Interviews with adult psychiatric patients ($n = 12$) following physical restraint	(i) Patients gave refusal of medication, refusal to follow staff directions, or their own aggression as reasons for restraint (ii) Many felt that restraint could have been avoided (iii) Some felt angry and distrustful of staff after restraint
3	Patients' perceptions (1)	Coercion and patient satisfaction on psychiatric acute wards [14]	173 interviews and questionnaires with patients, data from medical records	Objective coercion (including mechanical restraint) had a significant negative effect on overall patient satisfaction
4	Staff's perceptions (2)	Staff's experiences with patients' assaults in a Norwegian psychiatric university hospital [15]	Questionnaire to staff at one adult psychiatric hospital ($n = 85$)	(i) Patients' assault, acting-out, and self-harming were given as most important reasons for physical restraint (ii) 80% of staff believed that physical restraint was used appropriately, and 94% believed it did not influence patients' recovery
5	Staff's perceptions (2)	Staff's attitudes to the use of restraint and seclusion in a Norwegian university psychiatric hospital [16]	Questionnaire to staff at one adult psychiatric hospital ($n = 267$)	(i) A majority of staff believed that the interventions were used correctly (ii) Male staff, highly educated staff, and staff at high-use wards were most critical to use (iii) 70% had been assaulted in connection with the interventions
6	Staff's perceptions (2)	Staff's choice of formal and informal coercive interventions in psychiatric emergencies [17]	Questionnaire with simulated cases to staff at one adult psychiatric hospital ($n = 267$)	(i) Informal interventions are preferred by staff (ii) Such interventions are typically not recorded and their importance may therefore be overlooked
7	Staff's perceptions (2)	Attitudes to coercion at two Norwegian psychiatric units [18]	Questionnaire with simulated cases to staff at two adult psychiatric units ($n = 180$)	There was a limited degree of variance in staff's responses with respect to degree of restrictiveness The study supported the idea that a range of different interventions are used in emergency situations
8	Rates, characteristics (3)	The care conditions for especially dangerous psychotic patients [19]	Review of records at one institution (Reitgjerdet)	(i) In 1977, physical restraint was used 15 444 days (22.4% of all patient days) (ii) In 1980, it was used 566 patient days (iii) In the first third of 1981, it was used only 1,5 patient days
9	Rates, characteristics (3)	Use of coercive measures in Norwegian psychiatric institutions [20]	Examination of records of mechanical restraint ("screening")	During the first six months of 1988, 203 patients had been mechanically restrained for 10,767 hours

Table 1: Continued.

Number	Category	Articles [reference]	Methods/participants (n)	Key findings
10	Rates, characteristics (3)	Changes in the use of coercive measures in Norwegian psychiatric institutions [21]	Examination of records of mechanical restraint ("screening")	(i) 9402 hours of mechanical restraint were recorded in the first half of 1990 (ii) Single patients create large variations in use (iii) No correlation between size of ward or staff ratio and use of coercion (iv) No difference in levels from previous study (1986–1988)
11	Rates, characteristics (3)	Psychiatric security units in Norway; patients and activity [22]	Review of medical records of patients in Norwegian security units ($n = 123$)	25% had been subjected to physical restraint during a six-month period in 1993
12	Rates, characteristics (3)	Polar day and polar night: month of year and time of day and the use of physical and pharmacological restraint in a north Norwegian university psychiatric hospital [23]	Review of protocols and medical records regarding restraint during a 5.5-year period	(i) There was a daily peak with most use of restraint in the afternoon and early evening and a seasonal peak—with the most use of restraint in autumn (ii) Patterns of use might be caused by light-dark cycles, variations in life-events, and variations in the ward environment
13	Rates, characteristics (3)	Medicate, restrain, or seclude? Strategies for dealing with violent and threatening behaviour in a Norwegian university psychiatric hospital [24]	Review of protocols and medical records from a 5.5-year period at a psychiatric hospital	(i) 797 episodes of physical restraint were identified (ii) Patients' sex, age group, and diagnostic group were of importance to use (more use with male, younger, and nonpsychotic patients)
14	Rates, characteristics (3)	Association between patients' gender, age, and immigrant background and use of restraint—a 2-year retrospective study at a department of emergency psychiatry [25]	The study retrospectively examined routinely collected data and data from restraint protocols in a department of acute psychiatry over a 2-year period	(i) 14% of the patients were subjected to physical and/or pharmacological restraint (ii) The rate was significantly higher among patients with immigrant background, especially in the younger age groups
15	Rates, characteristics (3)	Staff injuries after patient-staff incidences in psychiatric acute wards [26]	507 patient-staff incidents in a psychiatric acute ward	Holding the patient with force was more frequent in incidents where more than one body part was injured
16	Rates, characteristics (3)	A cross-sectional prospective study of seclusion, restraint, and involuntary medication in acute psychiatric wards [9]	Medical records data from 1014 involuntarily admitted patients in acute psychiatric wards, of which 117 had been physically restrained	(i) Increased risk of restraint for patients that were aggressive or had tendency to self-injury (ii) Lower risk for patients from other ethnic groups (iii) Increased risk in urban areas
17	Rates, characteristics (3)	Characteristics of psychiatric inpatients who experienced restraint and those who did not: a case-control study [27]	Retrospective case-control study of records' data from three acute wards, two-year sample	Restrained patients (mechanically and pharmacologically) were more likely to be male, reside outside catchment area, have immigrant background, have longer stays, be involuntarily admitted, and have specific diagnoses (substance use, schizophrenia, psychoses, and bipolar disorder)

Table 1: Continued.

Number	Category	Articles [reference]	Methods/participants (n)	Key findings
18	Rates, characteristics (3)	Mechanical and pharmacological restraints in acute psychiatric wards—why and how are they used? [8]	Data from records of patients ($n = 306$) that had been subjected to mechanical restraint in three acute wards during a two-year period	(i) Occurring or imminent assault was most frequent reason for restraint (ii) Diagnoses, age, and reason for restraint increased the likelihood of being subjected to specific types of restraint
19	Rates, characteristics (3)	Characteristics of patients frequently subjected to pharmacological and mechanical restraint—a register study in three Norwegian acute psychiatric wards [28]	Retrospective study of records' data from three acute wards	9.1% of those restrained (either mechanically or pharmacologically) had been so 6 or more times, accounting for 39.2% of all restraint episodes
20	Rates, characteristics (3)	Mechanical restraint in psychiatry: preventive factors in theory and practice [29]	Different data sources, including questionnaire to clinical nurse managers in Norway ($n = 47$)	Mandatory review, patient involvement, and no crowding were identified as preventive factors
21	Rates, characteristics (3)	Comparing the effect of nonmedical mechanical restraint preventive factors between psychiatric units in Denmark and Norway [30]	Cross-sectional survey of psychiatric units	The following factors were found to partly explain differences in restraint levels: staff education, substitute staff, acceptable work environment, separation of acutely disturbed patients, patient-staff ratio, and identification of the patients' crises triggers
22	Intervention studies (5)	Patients' perception of coercion in acute psychiatric wards: an intervention study [31]	Three interventions were used: patients' engagement in the formulation of treatment plans, patient and staff evaluations, and renegotiations of treatment plans. Data were obtained on self-rating scales	(i) The interventions resulted in marginal changes (in the staff's respect and understanding and total satisfaction) (ii) Actions taken to control behaviour (i.e., seclusion) were more strongly related to perceived coercion than aspects of compulsory treatment
23	Case studies (6)	Venous thromboembolism in connection with physical restraint [32]	Case report	Venous thromboembolism may occur in connection with physical restraint
24	Case studies (6)	Thrombosis associated with physical restraints [33]	Literature review and two cases	Immobilization and trauma to the legs while restraining a patient may lead to thrombosis
25	Case studies (6)	Physical restraint and near death of a psychiatric patient [34]	Literature review and case report	Physically restraining (holding) a patient in the prone position with a significant weight load on the torso can lead to asphyxiation
26	Ethnographic studies (7)	Creating trust in an acute psychiatric ward [35]	Ethnographic study (observation and interviews with five patients and six nurses) of an open seclusion unit	Distrust is prevalent, but trust can be created Regarding themselves as potential causes of distrust can contribute to nurses' developing a realistic view of their practice
27	Ethnographic studies (7)	Coercion in a locked psychiatric ward: perspectives of patients and staff [36]	Ethnographic study	Description of one patient's negative perceptions of physical restraint
28	Ethnographic studies (7)	Fear, danger, and aggression in a Norwegian locked psychiatric ward [37]	Ethnographic study	Physical restraint seen as a threat and means of control and as a reminder of danger

was a daily peak with most use of restraint in the afternoon and early evening and a seasonal peak—with the most use of restraint in autumn. Patterns of use might be caused by light-dark cycles, variations in life events, and variations in the ward environment. A different article from the same study [24] also demonstrated that there had been 797 episodes of physical restraint and that male, younger, and nonpsychotic patients more often were subjected to physical restraint.

Knutzen et al. [25], in a retrospective study of routinely collected data at one emergency psychiatric department, found that 14% of the patients were subjected to physical and/or pharmacological restraint. The rate of restraint was significantly higher among patients with immigrant background, especially in the younger age groups. Langsrud et al. [26] found that holding the patient with force was more frequent in those incidents where more than one body part had been injured. Husum et al. [9], in a study of 1014 involuntarily admitted patients, found that 117 had been physically restrained and that there was an increased risk of restraint for patients that were aggressive or had a tendency to self-harm. There was a lower risk for patients from other ethnic groups, but an increased risk in urban areas. In a case-control study of patients in three acute wards, Knutzen et al. [27] found that those who had been restrained (mechanically and pharmacologically) were more likely to be male, reside outside the catchment area, have an immigrant background, have longer stays, be involuntarily admitted, and have specific diagnoses (substance use, schizophrenia, psychoses, and bipolar disorder).

In a study of records of 306 patients who had been subjected to physical restraint, Knutzen et al. [8] found that occurring or imminent assault was the most frequent reason for restraint. Moreover, they found that diagnoses, age, and reason for restraint increased the likelihood of being subjected to specific types of restraint, that is, physical or pharmacological. Knutzen et al. [28], in a retrospective study of records data from three acute wards, found that 9.1% of those restrained (either mechanically or pharmacologically) had been so 6 or more times, accounting for 39.2% of all restraint episodes. In a cross-sectional survey of psychiatric units in Norway and Denmark, Bak et al. [29] found that mandatory review, patient involvement, and no crowding were preventive factors. Bak et al. [30] found that the following factors were found to partly explain differences in restraint levels: staff education, substitute staff, acceptable work environment, separation of acutely disturbed patients, patient-staff ratio, and the identification of the patients' crises triggers.

3.4. Studies Examining the Effects of Various Interventions on Reducing Rates of Physical Restraint. The only intervention study identified was by Sørgaard, who used three interventions: patients' engagement in the formulation of treatment plans, patient and staff evaluations, and renegotiations of treatment plans [31].

3.4.1. Main Findings. Sørgaard [31] found that the interventions resulted in marginal changes (i.e., in the staff's respect and understanding and total satisfaction). Actions taken to control behaviour (i.e., seclusion) were more strongly related to perceived coercion than aspects of compulsory treatment.

3.5. Case Studies of Individual Patients Subjected to Physical Restraint. Three case studies were identified [32–34]. These studies combined literature reviews of the topics discussed with presentation and discussion of cases involving patients that had been subjected or attempted subjected to physical restraint.

3.5.1. Main Findings. All of the studies warned against physical complications that may arise as a consequence of attempting to restrain a patient or actually restraining a patient. Hem and coworkers [32, 33] found that immobilization and trauma to the legs while restraining a patient may lead to thrombosis. Nissen et al. [34] found that physically restraining (holding) a patient in the prone position with a significant weight load on the torso can lead to asphyxiation.

3.6. Ethnographic Studies. Three studies had an ethnographic approach. One involved observation and interviews with five patients and six nurses of an open seclusion unit [35], while two other articles [36, 37] were from the same study involving 12 patients and 22 professionals.

3.6.1. Main Findings. A central finding in the study by Hem et al. [35] was that distrust is prevalent, but trust can be created. Regarding themselves as potential causes of distrust can contribute to nurses' developing a realistic view of their practice. Larsen and Terkelsen [36] described the negative experiences of one patient subjected to physical restraint. Terkelsen and Larsen [37] described how physical restraint could be seen as a threat, as a means of control, and as a reminder of potential danger.

4. Discussion

A main finding of this review was that half of the included articles (14 of 28) were on rates and factors that influenced rates, especially patient-related factors, such as patients' sex, age, ethnicity, diagnoses, level of aggression, legal status, and duration of stay. A few studies described the importance of organizational or staff-related factors on rates of restraint, including staff-patient ratios, ward size, and staff education levels. Despite this being the category with the highest number of articles, the differences in samples, study designs, and outcomes make it challenging to aggregate the findings. Methodological challenges of this kind have also been highlighted by researchers assessing data from other countries [38–40].

In the present review, one study [25] found that 14% of the patients at an emergency ward had been physically and/or pharmacologically restrained, while another study [9] found that 10% of the involuntarily admitted patients had been physically restrained. These figures are higher than the aggregated numbers reported in the most recent national surveys (2012) [41], where 4.6% were reported to have been physically restrained (and 4.9% had been held). National surveys have also suggested that there are substantial differences in rates between different institutions and possibly also in how different hospitals register and report the use of physical restraint [42]. Routine reporting of physical restraint may be incomplete [43]. However, differences in patient populations may explain some of the differences found in use, with more use in emergency and forensic wards, with involuntarily admitted patients, and with patients with certain diagnoses [3, 27, 44]. Two of the older studies included, examining forensic populations [19, 22], found even higher rates of physical restraint. From 2007, the regulations were revised and holding was also subject to registration. These and other changes in regulations make it difficult to compare older and newer studies on the use of restraint. While one older study included in the review [19] described a dramatic reduction in use of restraint at a single institution at the beginning of the 1980s, studies and surveys with data from the late 1980s and the 1990s showed a lower and more stable use [20, 21, 45]. Several more recent national surveys have found that rates have remained relatively stable [38, 46] and comparable to the rates in other Western European countries [47].

Four studies were concerned with staff perceptions. Overall, the studies suggested that staff believed that restraint was carried out correctly, although there were some differences in opinion between different groups of staff. There were also some differences in opinion as to when physical restraint should be used. Three studies dealt with patients' perceptions. The studies suggested that the patients felt that restraint could have been avoided and most patients reacted negatively to the experience. There were also three ethnographic studies, in part describing staff and patient perceptions, underlining the negative experience of patients to this intervention. Three articles presented cases discussed in the relevant literature, emphasizing physical complications that may arise in connection with the use of restraints or holding [10].

A main finding in this review was that nearly all the identified studies on restraint in Norwegian adult psychiatric hospitals were observational, with only one exception. While there have been several interventional projects with the aim to reduce restraint, these appear not to have been published in peer-reviewed and indexed journals. A next step in the development of the research in this field of research in Norway would be increasing the number of interventional studies and ensuring that they follow needed scientific rigour in order to allow their publication in scientific journals. Researchers in other countries have also pointed to the need to increase the number of high quality intervention studies in this field [48, 49], and some such studies have been carried out in other countries [48, 50, 51]. Studies examining the effects of early identification protocols, deescalation protocols/teams, implementation of the least restrictive alternative model, or systematic debriefing [5, 50] would be examples that would contribute substantially to the field.

The present review showed that there was some variation in the quality of the identified studies, and intervention studies were almost nonexistent. While it might be challenging to carry out intervention studies in this field [2], there is in Norway as in many other countries a need for more studies with a design that will further increase the quality of the evidence and move the field forward [48–51].

The number of studies used in the present review is relatively small as the number of studies in this field is still quite limited. While it is likely that the search captured nearly all the relevant studies that have been published in peer-reviewed journals, there is a possibility that some studies published in journals not indexed by the databases might have been missed.

5. Conclusions

The studies that were identified were primarily concerned with patients' and staff's perspectives and rates of use. There is a need for interventional studies with stronger designs.

Disclosure

This study did not receive external funding.

Conflict of Interests

The author declares that there is no conflict of interests.

References

[1] W. K. Mohr, "Restraints and the code of ethics: an uneasy fit," *Archives of Psychiatric Nursing*, vol. 24, no. 1, pp. 3–14, 2010.

[2] R. Wynn, "Coercion in psychiatric care: clinical, legal, and ethical controversies," *International Journal of Psychiatry in Clinical Practice*, vol. 10, no. 4, pp. 247–251, 2006.

[3] W. A. Fisher, "Restraint and seclusion: a review of the literature," *The American Journal of Psychiatry*, vol. 151, no. 11, pp. 1584–1591, 1994.

[4] K. Lanthén, M. Rask, and C. Sunnqvist, "Psychiatric patients experiences with mechanical restraints: an interview study," *Psychiatry Journal*, vol. 2015, Article ID 748392, 8 pages, 2015.

[5] R. Wynn, *Restraint and Seclusion in a Norwegian University Psychiatric Hospital*, University Hospital of North Norway, 2004.

[6] The Mental Health Care Act, Act number 62, relating to the provision and implementation of mental health care, with later amendments, 1999.

[7] R. Wynn, L.-H. Myklebust, and T. Bratlid, "Psychologists and coercion: decisions regarding involuntary psychiatric admission and treatment in a group of Norwegian psychologists," *Nordic Journal of Psychiatry*, vol. 61, no. 6, pp. 433–437, 2007.

[8] M. Knutzen, S. Bjørkly, G. Eidhammer et al., "Mechanical and pharmacological restraints in acute psychiatric wards-why and how are they used?" *Psychiatry Research*, vol. 209, no. 1, pp. 91–97, 2013.

[9] T. L. Husum, J. H. Bjørngaard, A. Finset, and T. Ruud, "A cross-sectional prospective study of seclusion, restraint and involuntary medication in acute psychiatric wards: patient, staff and ward characteristics," *BMC Health Services Research*, vol. 10, article 89, 2010.

[10] M. Rakhmatullina, A. Taub, and T. Jacob, "Morbidity and mortality associated with the utilization of restraints: a review of literature," *Psychiatric Quarterly*, vol. 84, no. 4, pp. 499–512, 2013.

[11] T. D. Strout, "Perspectives on the experience of being physically restrained: an integrative review of the qualitative literature," *International Journal of Mental Health Nursing*, vol. 19, no. 6, pp. 416–427, 2010.

[12] R. Wynn and L.-H. Myklebust, "Patients' satisfaction and self-rated improvement following coercive interventions," *Psychiatry, Psychology and Law*, vol. 13, no. 2, pp. 199–202, 2006.

[13] R. Wynn, "Psychiatric inpatients' experiences with restraint," *Journal of Forensic Psychiatry and Psychology*, vol. 15, no. 1, pp. 124–144, 2004.

[14] K. I. Iversen, G. Høyer, and H. C. Sexton, "Coercion and patient satisfaction on psychiatric acute wards," *International Journal of Law and Psychiatry*, vol. 30, no. 6, pp. 504–511, 2007.

[15] R. Wynn and T. Bratlid, "Staff's experiences with patients' assaults in a norwegian psychiatric university hospital," *Scandinavian Journal of Caring Sciences*, vol. 12, no. 2, pp. 89–93, 1998.

[16] R. Wynn, "Staff's attitudes to the use of restraint and seclusion in a Norwegian university psychiatric hospital," *Nordic Journal of Psychiatry*, vol. 57, no. 6, pp. 453–459, 2003.

[17] R. Wynn, "Staff's choice of formal and informal coercive interventions in psychiatric emergencies," *International Journal of Forensic Mental Health*, vol. 2, no. 2, pp. 157–164, 2003.

[18] R. Wynn, A.-M. Kvalvik, and T. Hynnekleiv, "Attitudes to coercion at two Norwegian psychiatric units," *Nordic Journal of Psychiatry*, vol. 65, no. 2, pp. 133–137, 2011.

[19] O. H. Robak, "The care conditions for especially dangerous psychotic patients," *Nordisk Psykiatrisk Tidsskrift*, vol. 37, no. 4, pp. 311–314, 1983 (Norwegian).

[20] G. Høyer and H. Drange, "Use of coercive measures in Norwegian psychiatric institutions," *Tidsskrift for den Norske Laegeforening*, vol. 111, no. 14, pp. 1709-1713, 1991.

[21] G. Høyer and H. Drange, "Changes in the use of compulsory measures in Norwegian psychiatric institutions," *Tidsskrift for Den Norske Laegeforening*, vol. 114, no. 5, pp. 585–588, 1994 (Norwegian).

[22] O. M. Linaker, R. Thoresen, L. Figenschou, H. Sølvberg, U. Refsnes, and D. Jakobsen, "Psychiatric security units in Norway. Patients and activity," *Tidsskrift for Den Norske Laegeforening*, vol. 114, no. 13, pp. 1520–1523, 1994 (Norwegian).

[23] R. Wynn, "Polar day and polar night: month of year and time of day and the use of physical and pharmacological restraint in a north Norwegian university psychiatric hospital," *Arctic Medical Research*, vol. 55, no. 4, pp. 174–181, 1996.

[24] R. Wynn, "Medicate, restrain or seclude? Strategies for dealing with violent and threatening behaviour in a Norwegian university psychiatric hospital," *Scandinavian Journal of Caring Sciences*, vol. 16, no. 3, pp. 287–291, 2002.

[25] M. Knutzen, L. Sandvik, E. Hauff, S. Opjordsmoen, and S. Friis, "Association between patients' gender, age and immigrant background and use of restraint—a 2-year retrospective study at a department of emergency psychiatry," *Nordic Journal of Psychiatry*, vol. 61, no. 3, pp. 201–206, 2007.

[26] K. Langsrud, O. M. Linaker, and G. Morken, "Staff injuries after patient—staff incidences in psychiatric acute wards," *Nordic Journal of Psychiatry*, vol. 61, no. 2, pp. 121–125, 2007.

[27] M. Knutzen, N. H. Mjosund, G. Eidhammer et al., "Characteristics of psychiatric inpatients who experienced restraint and those who did not: a case-control study," *Psychiatric Services*, vol. 62, no. 5, pp. 492–497, 2011.

[28] M. Knutzen, S. Bjørkly, G. Eidhammer et al., "Characteristics of patients frequently subjected to pharmacological and mechanical restraint—a register study in three Norwegian acute psychiatric wards," *Psychiatry Research*, vol. 215, no. 1, pp. 127–133, 2014.

[29] J. Bak, V. Zoffmann, D. M. Sestoft, R. Almvik, and M. Brandt-Christensen, "Mechanical restraint in psychiatry: preventive Factors in theory and practice. A Danish-Norwegian association study," *Perspectives in Psychiatric Care*, vol. 50, no. 3, pp. 155–166, 2014.

[30] J. Bak, V. Zoffmann, D. M. Sestoft, R. Almvik, V. D. Siersma, and M. Brandt-Christensen, "Comparing the effect of non-medical mechanical restraint preventive factors between psychiatric units in Denmark and Norway," *Nordic Journal of Psychiatry*, vol. 69, no. 6, pp. 433–443, 2015.

[31] K. W. Sørgaard, "Patients' perception of coercion in acute psychiatric wards. An intervention study," *Nordic Journal of Psychiatry*, vol. 58, no. 4, pp. 299–304, 2004.

[32] E. Hem, S. Opjordsmoen, and P. M. Sandset, "Venous thromboembolism in connection with physical restraint," *Tidsskrift for den Norske Laegeforening*, vol. 118, no. 14, pp. 2156–2157, 1998.

[33] E. Hem, O. Steen, and S. Opjordsmoen, "Thrombosis associated with physical restraints," *Acta Psychiatrica Scandinavica*, vol. 103, no. 1, pp. 73–75, 2001.

[34] T. Nissen, P. Rørvik, L. Haugslett, and R. Wynn, "Physical restraint and near death of a psychiatric patient," *Journal of Forensic Sciences*, vol. 58, no. 1, pp. 259–262, 2013.

[35] M. H. Hem, K. Heggen, and K. W. Ruyter, "Creating trust in an acute psychiatric ward," *Nursing Ethics*, vol. 15, no. 6, pp. 777–788, 2008.

[36] I. B. Larsen and T. B. Terkelsen, "Coercion in a locked psychiatric ward: perspectives of patients and staff," *Nursing Ethics*, vol. 21, no. 4, pp. 426–436, 2014.

[37] T. B. Terkelsen and I. B. Larsen, "Fear, danger and aggression in a Norwegian locked psychiatric ward: dialogue and ethics of care as contributions to combating difficult situations," *Nursing Ethics*, 2014.

[38] W. A. Janssen, R. van de Sande, E. O. Noorthoorn et al., "Methodological issues in monitoring the use of coercive measures," *International Journal of Law and Psychiatry*, vol. 34, no. 6, pp. 429–438, 2011.

[39] V. Martin, W. Kuster, M. Baur et al., "Incidence of coercive measures as an indicator of quality in psychiatric hospitals. Problems of data recording and processing, preliminary results of a benchmarking study," *Psychiatrische Praxis*, vol. 34, no. 1, pp. 26–33, 2007 (German).

[40] T. Steinert, P. Lepping, R. Bernhardsgrütter et al., "Incidence of seclusion and restraint in psychiatric hospitals: a literature review and survey of international trends," *Social Psychiatry and Psychiatric Epidemiology*, vol. 45, no. 9, pp. 889–897, 2010.

[41] S. O. Ose and I. Pettersen, *Inpatients in Adult Psychiatric Services 20 November 2012*, SINTEF, Oslo, Norway, 2014 (Norwegian).

[42] R. Bremnes, T. Hatling, and J. H. Bjørngaard, *The Use of Coercive Measures in Mental Health Care in 2001, 2003, 2005, and 2007*, SINTEF, Oslo, Norway, 2008 (Norwegian).

[43] S. Bjørkly, M. Knutzen, A. Furre, and L. Sandvik, "Sampling and analysis of data regarding restraint and seclusion in adult psychiatric services in 2009," Kompetansesenter for sikkerhets-, fengsels- og rettspsykiatri for Helseregion Sør-Øst, 2011 (Norwegian).

[44] R. Wynn, M. H. Høiseth, and G. Pettersen, "Psychopathy in women: theoretical and clinical perspectives," *International Journal of Women's Health*, vol. 4, no. 1, pp. 257–263, 2012.

[45] T. Hatling and T. Krogen, *Use of Coercion in Norwegian Psychiatric Services—An Empirical Review*, SINTEF Unimed Nis, Trondheim, Norway, 1998 (Norwegian).

[46] R. Bremnes, S. E. Lilleeng, P. B. Pedersen, V. Hellevik, and F. Bergesen, *Use of Coercion in Mental Health Services for Adults in 2013*, Directorate of Health, 2014 (Norwegian).

[47] J. Bak and H. Aggernæs, "Coercion within Danish psychiatry compared with 10 other European countries," *Nordic Journal of Psychiatry*, vol. 66, no. 5, pp. 297–302, 2012.

[48] J. N. Scanlan, "Interventions to reduce the use of seclusion and restraint in inpatient psychiatric settings: what we know so far a review of the literature," *International Journal of Social Psychiatry*, vol. 56, no. 4, pp. 412–423, 2010.

[49] E. Sailas and M. Fenton, "Seclusion and restraint for people with serious mental illnesses," *Cochrane Database of Systematic Reviews*, no. 1, Article ID CD001163, 2000.

[50] C. Abderhalden, I. Needham, T. Dassen, R. Halfens, H.-J. Haug, and J. E. Fischer, "Structured risk assessment and violence in acute psychiatric wards: randomised controlled trial," *The British Journal of Psychiatry*, vol. 193, no. 1, pp. 44–50, 2008.

[51] J. Bergk, B. Einsiedler, E. Flammer, and T. Steinert, "A randomized controlled comparison of seclusion and mechanical restraint in inpatient settings," *Psychiatric Services*, vol. 62, no. 11, pp. 1310–1317, 2011.

2

Near-Infrared Transcranial Radiation for Major Depressive Disorder: Proof of Concept Study

Paolo Cassano,[1] Cristina Cusin,[1] David Mischoulon,[1] Michael R. Hamblin,[2] Luis De Taboada,[3] Angela Pisoni,[1] Trina Chang,[1] Albert Yeung,[1] Dawn F. Ionescu,[1] Samuel R. Petrie,[1] Andrew A. Nierenberg,[1] Maurizio Fava,[1] and Dan V. Iosifescu[1,4]

[1]*Depression Clinical & Research Program, Massachusetts General Hospital, Boston, MA 02114, USA*
[2]*Wellman Center for Photomedicine, Massachusetts General Hospital, Boston, MA 02114, USA*
[3]*LiteCure LLC, Newark, DE 19702, USA*
[4]*Department of Psychiatry, The Mount Sinai Hospital, New York, NY 10029, USA*

Correspondence should be addressed to Paolo Cassano; pcassano@mgh.harvard.edu

Academic Editor: Antonio Vita

Transcranial near-infrared radiation (NIR) is an innovative treatment for major depressive disorder (MDD), but clinical evidence for its efficacy is limited. Our objective was to investigate the tolerability and efficacy of NIR in patients with MDD. We conducted a proof of concept, prospective, double-blind, randomized study of 6 sessions of NIR versus sham treatment for patients with MDD, using a crossover design. Four patients with MDD with mean age 47 ± 14 (SD) years (1 woman and 3 men) were exposed to irradiance of 700 mW/cm^2 and a fluence of 84 J/cm^2 for a total NIR energy of 2.40 kJ delivered per session for 6 sessions. Baseline mean HAM-D_{17} scores decreased from 19.8 ± 4.4 (SD) to 13 ± 5.35 (SD) after treatment ($t = 7.905$; $df = 3$; $P = 0.004$). Patients tolerated the treatment well without any serious adverse events. These findings confirm and extend the preliminary data on NIR as a novel intervention for patients with MDD, but further clinical trials are needed to better understand the efficacy of this new treatment. This trial is registered with ClinicalTrials.gov NCT01538199.

1. Introduction

Near-Infrared Radiation: Mechanism of Action. In experimental and animal models, laser near-infrared radiation (NIR) noninvasively delivers energy to cytochrome c oxidase and by stimulating this key mitochondrial respiratory chain enzyme (COMPLEX IV, electron transfer chain) leads to increased adenosine triphosphate (ATP) production [1–3]. While several NIR wavelengths have been shown to benefit neuronal cell cultures, the most effective ones (830 nm, 670 nm) paralleled the NIR and red action spectra of oxidized cytochrome c oxidase [4]. Data suggest that coherent red light (670 nm diode laser) protects the viability of cell culture after oxidative stress, as indicated by increased mitochondrial membrane potentials [5]. NIR also stimulates neurite outgrowth mediated by nerve growth factor, and this effect could also have positive implications for axonal protection [5]. Neuroprotective effects of incoherent red light, 670 nm light emitting diode (LED) and 630 nm narrow angle LED, have been documented in *in vivo* models of mitochondrial optic neuropathy [6, 7]. *In vivo* bioenergetic changes with coherent NIR (810 nm diode laser) were observed at McLean Hospital (Belmont, MA) in beagle dogs, where a shift towards greater bioenergetic efficiency (PCr/β-NTP ratio) occurred in the anterior cingulate cortex after transcranial NIR exposure (3 times/week for 2 weeks) (Mintzopoulos et al., unpublished). In animal models of traumatic brain injury (TBI), coherent NIR (810 nm diode laser) appears to be an effective treatment [8–10] and improves neurogenesis [11]. In addition, incoherent NIR exposure (1072 nm LED) has been shown to improve memory performance in middle-aged mice [12].

Near-Infrared Radiation for Depression and Cognition. In a double-blind randomized study in healthy volunteers, exposure to coherent NIR (1064 nm laser) significantly improved overall affect, sustained attention, and visual memory [13].

A report of two individual cases and a case series of eleven patients with TBI suggested that exposure to incoherent NIR and red light (870 nm/633 nm LEDs) positively affected sustained attention, memory and executive functions, and self-awareness, self-regulation, sleep, and depressed mood [14, 15]. These benefits in TBI patients were confirmed in a cohort of ten, treated with coherent NIR light (810 nm/980 nm laser) [16]. A preliminary open study in ten depressed subjects has shown that NIR (810 nm LED) may be effective and well tolerated for depression and anxiety despite a history of treatment resistance [17].

Our pilot study aimed at confirming and extending these findings by including a ^{31}P-MRS assessment of brain metabolism, as well as safety and efficacy data on repeated administrations of transcranial NIR with a high power laser diode. As an explanatory note to the readers, the authors would like to clarify the circumstances under which our controlled clinical trial (https://www.clinicaltrials.gov/: NCT01538199) only yielded preliminary uncontrolled data on repeated NIR sessions for MDD. The present study was in fact prematurely interrupted by its sponsor, the PhotoThera Inc. PhotoThera had largely invested in three clinical trials (NEST 1, NEST 2, and NEST 3), testing the same NIR device (NeuroThera Laser) used in our study for the treatment of ischemic stroke. NEST 3, the largest of the NEST trials, was stopped due to an interim analysis revealing futility [18]. PhotoThera, financed by venture capitalists, revoked the funding for all its clinical trials, including investigator initiated studies such as ours. PhotoThera closed down in October 2012 and filed for bankruptcy in May 2013.

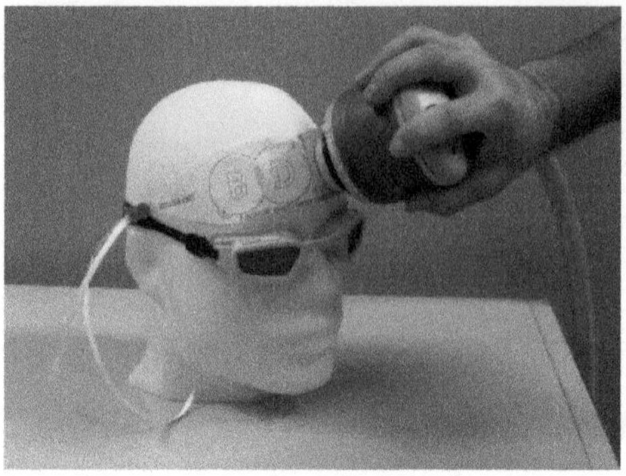

FIGURE 1: The picture shows the handheld portion of the NeuroThera device, which is pressed against the forehead of the subject. A paper band is used to locate the sites of irradiation across the forehead. Prior to irradiation on each site, the corresponding area of skin is exposed by peeling off the overlying circle of paper from the band.

2. Methods

This single-site study was approved by the Massachusetts General Hospital (MGH) institutional review board (IRB); the Food and Drug Administration (FDA) confirmed that an Investigational Device Exemption (IDE) was not required, as the investigation entailed nonsignificant risks. The Harvard Psychiatry Department (Dupont-Warren Fellowship and Livingston Award), the Brain and Behavior Research Foundation (NARSAD Young Investigator Award), and PhotoThera Inc. sponsored this investigation. Subjects meeting the Diagnostic Statistical Manual-IV (DSM-IV) criteria for MDD, with at least moderate depression (Hamilton depression rating scale, HAM-D_{17} total score between 14 and 24), were included in the study after providing written informed consent. Subjects had failed at most one antidepressant medication and psychotherapy course (stable treatment for at least 6 and 8 weeks, resp.) during the current episode. Active substance use disorders (within prior 6 months), lifetime psychotic episodes, unstable medical illness, and active suicidal or homicidal ideation were exclusionary criteria. Subjects with head-implants, taking light-activated drugs, or having forehead skin conditions (e.g., rash or tattoo) were also excluded. In addition, subjects with implanted metal devices, severe claustrophobia, or weight above 275 lbs were excluded for MRI contraindications. Subjects were randomized to a 7-week double-blind sham-controlled treatment, involving three weeks of either NIR or sham exposures twice a week followed by crossover to three more weeks of the alternate exposure; that is, patients that were exposed to NIR during the first three weeks of the study were exposed to sham, after a washout week, and vice versa. At each treatment session, NIR light (NeuroThera, continuously emitting GaAlAs-laser, manufactured by PhotoThera Inc., with 808 ± 10 nm wavelength (or the same device acting as a sham), with active cooling, total power output 5 W, and verified with a power meter attached to a photodiode detector, Ophir NOVA, prior to the experimental sessions) was administered to the forehead bilaterally at four sites total (2 min per site, 3.3 cm lens piece aperture, 3 cm spot diameter, and 7.1 cm^2 spot area). We decided to cover the forehead widely (4 sites) to extensively irradiate the prefrontal cortex without overlaps; the data on safety from the NEST 1, NEST 2, and NEST 3 studies on stroke for our same instrument showed that irradiation of up to 20 sites on the scalp was safe (2 min each) [18–21]. Our parameters (including the localization to the forehead) were somewhat consistent with those of Schiffer and colleagues [17], which had demonstrated clinical efficacy of a single session of NIR in depression. NIR was administered with an irradiance of approximately 700 mW/cm^2 and a fluence of 84 J/cm^2 (same parameters as in NEST 1, NEST 2, and NEST 3) for a total NIR energy of 2.40 kJ delivered per session with the devices' actively cooled sapphire output lens in direct skin contact. See Table 1 for a summary of the NIR parameters used for this study and comparable studies of transcranial laser therapy (TLT). See Figure 1 for the picture of the handheld portion of the NeuroThera device. No additional information was provided by the manufacturer.

The NeuroThera device was programmed with a list of subjects' treatment codes randomly assigning patients to either NIR or sham exposure for the first three weeks of the crossover study; the device program kept track of the initial assignment and switched the patient's exposure, NIR to sham and vice versa, for the second three weeks of the study treatment. Since the study from Schiffer and colleagues [17] demonstrated that one treatment with NIR was insufficient

TABLE 1: Summary of the NIR parameters used for this study (Cassano et al.) and other comparison studies.

	Cassano et al. (this study)	Schiffer et al., 2009 [17]	Barrett and Gonzalez-Lima, 2013 [13]	Naeser et al., 2014 [15]
Study design	Pilot, open	Open	Double-blind randomized NIR versus sham	Open
Subjects enrolled	4 MDD completers	10 resistant MDD	40 psychology undergraduates	11 chronic TBI (8 cases with depression; 5 with at least moderate severity)
Number of treatment sessions	2/week for 3 weeks	1	1	3/week for 6 weeks
Duration of clinical follow-up	8 weeks	4 weeks	2 weeks	14 weeks
Clinical outcome(s)	50% remission of MDD at weeks 6-7 (HAM-D_{17} ≤7)	60% remission of MDD at week 2 (HAM-D-21 <10)	Maintained positive affect at 2 weeks compared to decline of control group (PANAS)	37% response of depression at week 7 (decrease of BDI-II total score ≥50% from baseline)
Device specifications				
Manufacturer/model/type	PhotoThera/NeuroThera/laser diode	Custom device/Marubeni America Corp./LED	Cell Gen Therapeutics/Model CG-5000/laser diode	MedX Health/Model 1100/LED
Wavelength (nm)	808	810	1064	870 and 633
Spot diameter (cm)	3	—	4	5.35
Spot area (cm^2)	7.1	~1	12.6	22.5
Site exposure parameters				
Time (sec)	120	240	240	585
Irradiance (mW/cm^2)	700	250	250	22.2
Fluence (J/cm^2)	84	60	60	13
Treatment exposure parameters				
Number of exposed sites	Four	Two	Two	Eleven
Site locations, transcranial treatments	Bilateral (R and L forehead center at 20 and 40 mm from sagittal line)	Bilateral (R and L forehead at EEG map sites: F3, F4)	Unilateral (R, frontal pole on 4 cm medial and lateral)	Midline and bilateral (forehead (prefrontal) and temporal, parietal, and occipital area)
Total area exposed ("treatment window," cm^2)	28.4 (7.1 × 4 sites)	2 (1 × 2 sites)	25.2 (12.6 × 2 sites)	247 (22.5 × 11 sites)
Total energy delivered, per session (kJ)	2.4 (0.6 × 4 sites)	0.12 (0.06 × 2 sites)	1.51 (0.76 × 2 sites)	3.21 (0.29 × 11 sites)
Total energy delivered, per treatment (kJ)	14.4 (total energy per session × 2 sessions/week × 3 weeks)	0.12 (total energy per session × 1 session)	1.51 (total energy per session × 1 session)	57.87 (total energy per session × 3 sessions/week × 6 weeks)

to determine a durable antidepressant response, we then decided to deliver a course of 6 treatments within 3 weeks. The relatively short timeframe of 3 weeks was decided to allow crossover within an overall 8-week length of trial. The double-blinding was ensured by carrying out identical procedures, identical device interface, including prompts and sounds, and actively cooling the skin surface at the treatment area during both NIR and sham exposures. PhotoThera Inc., the company that manufactured the device, produced data showing that active cooling of the sapphire lenses ensured blinding by preventing skin warming. A specific semistructured scale, the Transcranial Light Therapy Self-Report Questionnaire (T-SR-Q) was completed by participants after the first 6 sessions. The scale explored any discomfort and inconvenience related to the treatment sessions, to detect potential unblinding due to warming effect or to other phenomena. None of the subjects reported skin warming (on the contrary one reported excessive cooling), which validated our blinding. The NIR light is otherwise invisible. All subjects remained on stable antidepressant treatment during the trial. There were no restrictions on class of concomitant antidepressant medications or other concomitant medications, except for photosensitive medications which were exclusionary. Tolerability was assessed with the Systematic Assessment for Treatment Emergent Events (SAFTEE) scale [22]. The primary outcome measures were both change in depressive symptoms (HAM-D_{17}) at endpoint and remission from depressive symptoms, defined as HAM-$D_{17} \leq 7$. A recent assessment of the interrater reliability among clinicians at our group (MGH Depression Clinical and Research Program) in diagnosing MDD and in measuring the severity of depression has yielded a kappa >0.75. The assessment of interrater reliability was established through live, independent interviews of patients with the use of the HAM-D and SCID-I/P, indicating satisfactory agreement.

We present analysis of four subjects from a sample of eight adults who met study criteria and were initially enrolled in the study. The four subjects excluded from analysis either did not complete the study or, upon review of final study results, failed to meet the study's inclusion/exclusion criteria. One subject dropped out before the first treatment session and two shortly after the first session. These patients could not commit to the full treatment course. One of the patients that dropped out after the first treatment session experienced a headache and left hand paresthesias during the MRS scan, possibly related to preexisting carpal tunnel syndrome. Upon unblinding the device's preprogrammed treatment codes, it was determined that none of the dropouts received active NIR. Data from one more subject were subsequently excluded as her urine repeatedly tested positive for cannabinoids. This latter subject's exclusion was based on her meeting criteria for substance use disorder, which was determined towards the end of her participation. The unblinded treatment codes also showed that all four subjects who completed the 7-week treatment phase and were analyzed received NIR exposures in their first 3 weeks. By means of a paired t-test we tested the significance of the change in the mean HAM-D_{17} total score (from baseline) to week 8. Although the primary comparison was with the last assessment (week 8), exploratory analyses were conducted for change from baseline to weeks 4, 5, 6, and 7. A last observation carried forward (LOCF) was also performed to account for one missing value at week 8. We decided not to present the available ^{31}P-MRS data since our lack of adequate comparison and our small sample size limited scientific inferences.

3. Results

The four completers had a mean age of 47 ± 14 (SD) years (1 woman and 3 men). Their length of depressive episode was at least 18 months. Baseline HAM-D_{17} scores averaged 19.75 ± 4.35 (SD). None of them was taking antidepressant medications at the time of the trial and only one was receiving (long-standing) counseling; however, the counseling was not a proven effective form of psychotherapy for major depressive disorder, such as cognitive behavioral therapy (CBT) or interpersonal therapy (IPT). None of the four subjects had failed to respond to an evidence-based treatment or FDA-approved treatment for depression during the current depressive episode. During the course of the trial, none of the participants started an antidepressant treatment.

Two of the four treatment-completers (50%) achieved remission (albeit not sustained) with HAM-D_{17}s of 4 and 3 at weeks 6 and 7, respectively. The mean HAM-D_{17} total score ($n = 3$) decreased from 17.7 ± 1.53 (SD) at baseline to 10.3 ± 0.57 (SD) at week 8 ($t = 8.315$; $df = 2$; $P = 0.014$). On the LOCF analysis, accounting for one missing value at week 8, the mean HAM-D_{17} total score ($n = 4$) decreased from 19.75 ± 4.35 (SD) to 13 ± 5.35 (SD) ($t = 7.905$; $df = 3$; $P = 0.004$). Figure 2 illustrates the mean HAM-D_{17} total scores over the course of the study for the four subjects. The NIR treatment was well tolerated with no adverse events; only one subject, already diagnosed with irritable bowel syndrome, reported transient, mild diarrhea, which was deemed unrelated to study treatment.

4. Discussion

We report findings on the safety and efficacy of multiple NIR sessions in patients with MDD. We observed, in four MDD subjects, that posttreatment depression ratings were significantly reduced from baseline, and the treatment was well tolerated.

Time to remission was 6-7 weeks, consistent with other antidepressant treatments. Since all four subjects who completed the 7-week treatment phase received NIR in their first 3 weeks (Figure 2), a carry-over effect from NIR is likely. In two prior reports, significant clinical and psychological effects were reported as early as week 2, after only a single NIR treatment [13, 17]. A possible explanation for this time to response discrepancy is that NIR in our study was delivered at higher irradiance (700 mW/cm^2) and fluence (84 J/cm^2) (Table 1). Alternatively, twice-weekly NIR sessions at four sites for 3 weeks might be suboptimal. A paradoxical dose-response, where higher power and energy densities might be less effective, has been postulated for NIR. Based on animal data, Xuan and colleagues [11] have postulated that

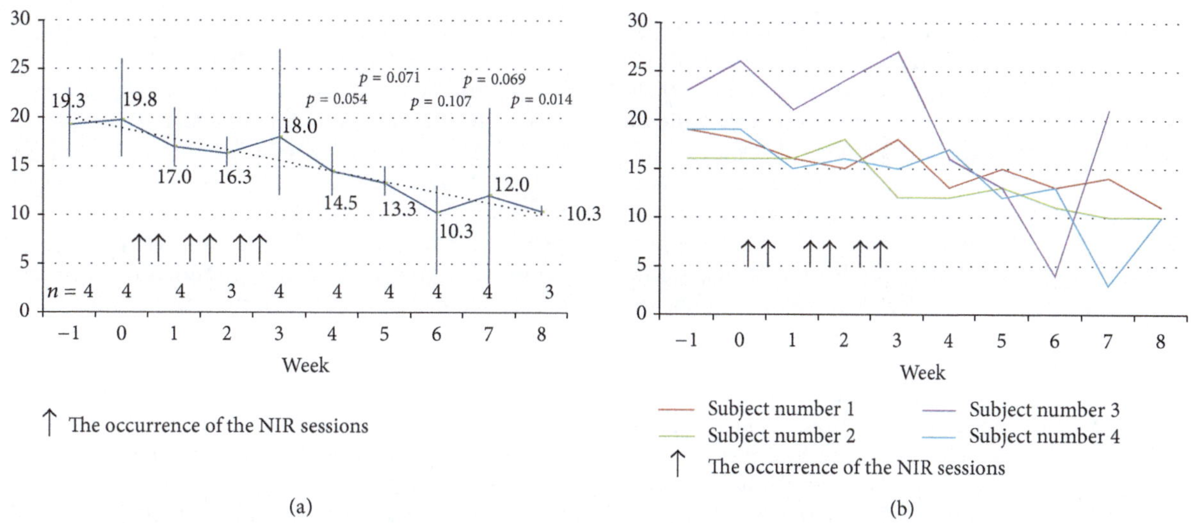

Figure 2: Mean and individual HAM-D_{17} total score ((a) and (b), resp.) for the 4 MDD subjects who sequentially received transcranial NIR and sham. All 4 treatment-completers had received NIR from week 0 to week 3.

an excessive exposure to NIR might be in fact counterproductive. This is somewhat in contrast with other reports in TBI patients, where daily NIR sessions appeared to be beneficial for cognition, although at a much lower NIR fluence (13–20 J/cm^2) [14, 15]. See Table 1 for the report of eleven cases from Naeser and colleagues [15].

Our 50% treatment remission rate (albeit not sustained) in this small sample size is consistent with the 60% remission rate reported in subjects with resistant MDD treated with NIR by Schiffer and colleagues [17]. Similar to Schiffer and colleagues [17], we used an augmentation design in which NIR was added to stable (at least 6 weeks) treatment. However, because none of our 4 subjects was taking antidepressant medications, we cannot ascribe the high remission rates to synergism. In contrast to Schiffer and colleagues [17], who used incoherent NIR (810 nm), our pilot was conducted with a laser device, coherent NIR. While coherent light (lasers) is likely to achieve deeper penetration into brain tissue [23], we did not observe any apparent advantage by comparing response rates in both studies.

The most important result of this pilot study on repeated NIR treatment is its tolerability and safety in patients with MDD. Our report is the first systematic assessment of tolerability and safety of repeated administration of transcranial NIR with a 5 W laser with high irradiance (700 mW/cm^2) in depressed subjects. Our finding is consistent with prior case-reports and case series suggesting that multiple transcranial NIR administrations could be safe in TBI subjects [14–16]. We encountered only one potential adverse event characterized by transient and mild diarrhea in a subject with irritable bowel syndrome. This event was attributed to the subject's preexisting medical illness and considered unrelated to the NIR treatment; it resolved within a week and did not require study discontinuation or other interventions. Consistent with our results, several large NIR stroke studies have shown no significant difference in rates of adverse events or serious adverse events between NIR and sham [18, 24].

5. Conclusions

Our findings are limited by our small sample size and by a probable carry-over effect. However, they support the hypothesis that TLT could be an effective treatment for MDD. If subsequent studies confirm that a brief course of TLT is effective for treating MDD, this intervention could have advantages over monotherapy with standard antidepressant medications because TLT is noninvasive, has few side effects, and might not require long-term administration. TLT and other treatments targeting brain mitochondria represent an innovative class of therapeutics (compared to standard antidepressant treatment) for patients with MDD.

Disclosure

This study was presented on October 25, 2013, at the 2013 New York Annual Symposium of the Brain and Behavior Research Foundation. This was an investigator initiated study; PhotoThera Inc. did not design the study per se (Dr. Maurizio Fava suggested the study design), but it contributed to the definition of imaging outcome variables that are not presented in this paper. The Brain and Behavior Research Foundation and the Dupont-Warren Committee at the Harvard Psychiatry Department did not contribute in any way to the design of the study. None of the funders had any input in the collection, analysis, and interpretation of the data. Dr. Luis De Taboada (ex-PhotoThera) joined as an author when the paper was nearly completed and reviewed the specifications of the instrument described in the paper.

Conflict of Interests

Dr. Paolo Cassano's salary was supported by the Harvard Psychiatry Department (Dupont-Warren Fellowship and Livingston Award), by the Brain and Behavior Research Foundation (NARSAD Young Investigator Award), and by the PhotoThera Inc. unrestricted grant. Drug donation was from TEVA. Travel reimbursement was from Pharmacia-Upjohn. Dr. Cristina Cusin's salary is supported by NIMH (R21 MH 095826-01), grant from the American Suicide Prevention Foundation and Department of Defense (V-SUBMGH-11-40, W81XWH-11-1-0073). Disclosures regarding financial relationships with commercial entities are as follows: Dr. David Mischoulon has received research support from the Bowman Family Foundation, Bristol-Myers Squibb Co., Cederroth, FisherWallace, Ganeden, Lichtwer Pharma, Nordic Naturals, Laxdale (Amarin), and SwissMedica. He has received honoraria for consulting, speaking, and writing from Pamlab, Bristol-Myers Squibb Co., Nordic Naturals, Virbac, Pfizer, and Reed Medical Education. He has received royalties from Back Bay Scientific for PMS Escape and from Lippincott Williams & Wilkins for published book *Natural Medications for Psychiatric Disorders: Considering the Alternatives*. No payment has exceeded $10,000. Dr. Michael R. Hamblin participated in only one session (12/17/13) of the DSMB for the ELATED study, which occurred after completion of the data collection for the same study. Research grants and consulting fees are from PhotoThera Inc. Scientific Advisory Board of Transdermal Cap Inc. (LLLT for hair regrowth). Michael R. Hamblin was supported by US NIH Grant R01AI050875. Disclosures regarding financial relationships with commercial entities are as follows: Mr. Luis De Taboada designed and developed the NeuroThera systems used for the study and received salary from PhotoThera Inc. as VP of Research and Development during a portion of this study. Mr. Luis De Taboada receives salary from LiteCure LLC (Newark, DE) as VP of research and development. Disclosures regarding patents are as follows: Mr. Luis De Taboada is a named inventor in multiple patents for the treatment of neurological disorders and injuries, including MDD. Ms. Angela Pisoni, Dr. Trina Chang, Dr. Albert Yeung, Dr. Dawn F. Ionescu, and Mr. Samuel R. Petrie have no conflict of interests to report regarding the publication of this paper. Dr. Andrew A. Nierenberg is a consultant for the Abbott Laboratories, American Psychiatric Association, Appliance Computing Inc. (Mindsite), Basliea, Brain Cells, Inc., Brandeis University, Bristol Myers Squibb, Clintara, Corcept, Dey Pharmaceuticals, Dainippon Sumitomo (now Sunovion), Eli Lilly and Company, EpiQ, L.P./Mylan Inc., Forest, Genaissance, Genentech, GlaxoSmithKline, Hoffman LaRoche, Infomedic, Lundbeck, Janssen Pharmaceutica, Jazz Pharmaceuticals, Medavante, Merck, Methylation Sciences, Naurex, Novartis, PamLabs, Parexel, Pfizer, PGx Health, Ridge Diagnostics Shire, Schering-Plough, Somerset, Sunovion, Takeda Pharmaceuticals, Targacept, and Teva, consulted through the MGH Clinical Trials Network and Institute (CTNI) for Astra Zeneca, Brain Cells, Inc., Dainippon Sumitomo/Sepracor, Johnson and Johnson, Labopharm, Merck, Methylation Science, Novartis, PGx Health, Shire, Schering-Plough, Targacept, and Takeda/Lundbeck Pharmaceuticals. He receives grant/research support from American Foundation for Suicide Prevention, AHRQ, Brain and Behavior Research Foundation, Bristol-Myers Squibb, Cederroth, Cephalon, Cyberonics, Elan, Eli Lilly, Forest, GlaxoSmithKline, Janssen Pharmaceutica, Lichtwer Pharma, Marriott Foundation, Mylan, NIMH, PamLabs, PCORI, Pfizer Pharmaceuticals, Shire, Stanley Foundation, Takeda, and Wyeth-Ayerst. Honoraria include Belvoir Publishing, University of Texas Southwestern Dallas, Brandeis University, Bristol-Myers Squibb, Hillside Hospital, American Drug Utilization Review, American Society for Clinical Psychopharmacology, Baystate Medical Center, Columbia University, CRICO, Dartmouth Medical School, Health New England, Harold Grinspoon Charitable Foundation, IMEDEX, Israel Society for Biological Psychiatry, Johns Hopkins University, MJ Consulting, New York State, Medscape, MBL Publishing, MGH Psychiatry Academy, National Association of Continuing Education, Physicians Postgraduate Press, SUNY Buffalo, University of Wisconsin, University of Pisa, University of Michigan, University of Miami, University of Wisconsin at Madison, APSARD, ISBD, SciMed, Slack Publishing and Wolters Klower Publishing ASCP, NCDEU, Rush Medical College, Yale University School of Medicine, NNDC, Nova Southeastern University, NAMI, Institute of Medicine, CME Institute, and ISCTM. He was currently or formerly on the advisory boards of Appliance Computing, Inc., Brain Cells, Inc., Eli Lilly and Company, Genentech, Johnson and Johnson, Takeda/Lundbeck, Targacept, and InfoMedic. He owns stock options in Appliance Computing, Inc., Brain Cells, Inc., and Medavante and has copyrights to the Clinical Positive Affect Scale and the MGH Structured Clinical Interview for the Montgomery Asberg Depression Scale exclusively licensed to the MGH Clinical Trials Network and Institute (CTNI). Dr. Fava received research support from the following for-profit and nonprofit private entities: Abbot Laboratories; Alkermes, Inc.; American Cyanamid; Aspect Medical Systems; AstraZeneca; BioResearch; BrainCells Inc.; Bristol-Myers Squibb; CeNeRx BioPharma; Cephalon; Clintara, LLC; Covance; Covidien; Eli Lilly and Company; EnVivo Pharmaceuticals, Inc.; Euthymics Bioscience, Inc.; Forest Pharmaceuticals, Inc.; Ganeden Biotech, Inc.; GlaxoSmithKline; Harvard Clinical Research Institute; Hoffman-LaRoche; Icon Clinical Research; i3 Innovus/Ingenix; Janssen R&D, LLC; Jed Foundation; Johnson & Johnson Pharmaceutical Research & Development; Lichtwer Pharma GmbH; Lorex Pharmaceuticals; MedAvante; National Alliance for Research on Schizophrenia & Depression (NARSAD); National Center for Complementary and Alternative Medicine (NCCAM); National Institute of Drug Abuse (NIDA); National Institute of Mental Health (NIMH); Neuralstem, Inc.; Novartis AG; Organon Pharmaceuticals; PamLab, LLC; Pfizer Inc.; Pharmacia-Upjohn; Pharmaceutical Research Associates, Inc.; Pharmavite LLC; PharmoRx Therapeutics; PhotoThera; Roche Pharmaceuticals; RCT Logic, LLC (formerly Clinical Trials Solutions, LLC); Sanofi-Aventis US LLC; Shire; Solvay Pharmaceuticals, Inc.; Synthelabo; Wyeth-Ayerst Laboratories; advisory/consulting: Abbott Laboratories; Affectis Pharmaceuticals AG; Alkermes, Inc.; Amarin Pharma Inc.; Aspect Medical Systems; AstraZeneca; Auspex Pharmaceuticals; Bayer AG; Best Practice Project Management, Inc.; BioMarin Pharmaceuticals, Inc.; Biovail Corporation; BrainCells Inc.; Bristol-Myers Squibb; CeNeRx BioPharma; Cephalon, Inc.; Cerecor; CNS Response, Inc.; Compellis Pharmaceuticals; Cypress Pharmaceutical, Inc.; DiagnoSearch Life Sciences

(P) Ltd.; Dinippon Sumitomo Pharma Co. Inc.; Dov Pharmaceuticals, Inc.; Edgemont Pharmaceuticals, Inc.; Eisai Inc.; Eli Lilly and Company; EnVivo Pharmaceuticals, Inc.; ePharmaSolutions; EPIX Pharmaceuticals, Inc.; Euthymics Bioscience, Inc.; Fabre-Kramer Pharmaceuticals, Inc.; Forest Pharmaceuticals, Inc.; GenOmind, LLC; GlaxoSmithKline; Grunenthal GmbH; i3 Innovus/Ingenis; Janssen Pharmaceutica; Jazz Pharmaceuticals, Inc.; Johnson & Johnson Pharmaceutical Research & Development, LLC; Knoll Pharmaceuticals Corp.; Labopharm Inc.; Lorex Pharmaceuticals; Lundbeck Inc.; MedAvante, Inc.; Merck & Co., Inc.; MSI Methylation Sciences, Inc.; Naurex, Inc.; Neuralstem, Inc.; Neuronetics, Inc.; NextWave Pharmaceuticals; Novartis AG; Nutrition 21; Orexigen Therapeutics, Inc.; Organon Pharmaceuticals; Otsuka Pharmaceuticals; Pamlab, LLC; Pfizer Inc.; PharmaStar; Pharmavite LLC; PharmoRx Therapeutics; Precision Human Biolaboratory; Prexa Pharmaceuticals, Inc.; Puretech Ventures; PsychoGenics; Psylin Neurosciences, Inc.; RCT Logic, LLC (formerly Clinical Trials Solutions, LLC); Rexahn Pharmaceuticals, Inc.; Ridge Diagnostics, Inc.; Roche; Sanofi-Aventis US LLC; Sepracor Inc.; Servier Laboratories; Schering-Plough Corporation; Solvay Pharmaceuticals, Inc.; Somaxon Pharmaceuticals, Inc.; Somerset Pharmaceuticals, Inc.; Sunovion Pharmaceuticals; Supernus Pharmaceuticals, Inc.; Synthelabo; Takeda Pharmaceutical Company Limited; Tal Medical, Inc.; Tetragenex Pharmaceuticals, Inc.; TransForm Pharmaceuticals, Inc.; Transcept Pharmaceuticals, Inc.; Vanda Pharmaceuticals, Inc.; additional conflict of interests might arise for Dr. Fava from compensations related to speaking and publishing; he received compensations from the following entities: Adamed, Co.; Advanced Meeting Partners; American Psychiatric Association; American Society of Clinical Psychopharmacology; AstraZeneca; Belvoir Media Group; Boehringer Ingelheim GmbH; Bristol-Myers Squibb; Cephalon, Inc.; CME Institute/Physicians Postgraduate Press, Inc.; Eli Lilly and Company; Forest Pharmaceuticals, Inc.; GlaxoSmithKline; Imedex, LLC; MGH Psychiatry Academy/Primedia; MGH Psychiatry Academy/Reed Elsevier; Novartis AG; Organon Pharmaceuticals; Pfizer Inc.; PharmaStar; United BioSource, Corp.; Wyeth-Ayerst Laboratories; Dr. Fava holds patents and equities related to Compellis; PsyBrain, Inc. Royalty/patent, another income: Patent for Sequential Parallel Comparison Design (SPCD), which are licensed by MGH to RCT Logic, LLC; and patent application for a combination of ketamine plus scopolamine in Major Depressive Disorder (MDD). Dr. Fava owns copyrights in connection to the following publications: the MGH Cognitive and Physical Functioning Questionnaire (CPFQ), Sexual Functioning Inventory (SFI), Antidepressant Treatment Response Questionnaire (ATRQ), Discontinuation-Emergent Signs and Symptoms (DESS), and SAFER; Lippincott, Williams & Wilkins; Wolkers Kluwer; World Scientific Publishing Co. Pte. Ltd. In the last three years Dan V. Iosifescu has been a consultant for CNS Response, Otsuka, Servier, and Sunovion and has received research support through Mount Sinai from Astra Zeneca, Brainsway, Euthymics, Neosync, Roche, and Shire. Dr. Iosifescu's lifetime conflict of interests is detailed hereafter: he has received research support from Aspect Medical Systems, Forest Laboratories, and Janssen Pharmaceutica, he has been a consultant for Forest Laboratories, Gerson Lehrman Group, and Pfizer, Inc., and he has received speaking honoraria from Eli Lilly & Co., Forest Laboratories, Pfizer, Inc., and Reed-Elsevier.

Authors' Contribution

Paolo Cassano conceived the study, conducted the study, evaluated study subjects, delivered treatment, and wrote first draft of paper for depression. Cristina Cusin evaluated study subjects, delivered treatment, and reviewed paper for depression. David Mischoulon evaluated study subjects, delivered treatment, and reviewed paper for depression. Michael R. Hamblin reviewed paper for transcranial light therapy. Luis De Taboada reviewed paper for instrument specifications. Angela Pisoni assisted with subjects management during the study and preparation of tables, figures, references, and editing of paper. Trina Chang evaluated study subjects, delivered treatment, and reviewed paper for depression. Albert Yeung evaluated study subjects, delivered treatment, and reviewed paper for depression. Dawn F. Ionescu reviewed paper for depression. Samuel R. Petrie assisted with preparation of tables, figures, references, and editing of paper. Andrew A. Nierenberg reviewed paper with specific focus on presenting data in abbreviated format. Maurizio Fava contributed to the conception of the study. Dan V. Iosifescu contributed to the conception of the study and to the writing of the first draft. All authors have approved the final version of the paper.

Acknowledgments

The authors thank Dr. Marc J. Kaufman and Dr. Fei Du from the McLean Imaging Center, McLean Hospital, who kindly supervised Dr. Paolo Cassano and performed the MRS scans on the study subjects, respectively, and Dr. Clark E. Tedford from LumiThera Inc. who provided them with the training for the use of the PhotoThera devices. The Harvard Psychiatry Department (Dupont-Warren Fellowship and Livingston Award), the Brain and Behavior Research Foundation (NARSAD Young Investigator Award), and PhotoThera Inc. sponsored this investigation.

References

[1] W. Yu, J. O. Naim, M. McGowan, K. Ippolito, and R. J. Lanzafame, "Photomodulation of oxidative metabolism and electron chain enzymes in rat liver mitochondria," *Photochemistry and Photobiology*, vol. 66, no. 6, pp. 866–871, 1997.

[2] N. Mochizuki-Oda, Y. Kataoka, Y. Cui, H. Yamada, M. Heya, and K. Awazu, "Effects of near-infra-red laser irradiation on adenosine triphosphate and adenosine diphosphate contents of rat brain tissue," *Neuroscience Letters*, vol. 323, no. 3, pp. 207–210, 2002.

[3] U. Oron, S. Ilic, L. De Taboada, and J. Streeter, "Ga-As (808 nm) laser irradiation enhances ATP production in human neuronal cells in culture," *Photomedicine and Laser Surgery*, vol. 25, no. 3, pp. 180–182, 2007.

[4] M. T. T. Wong-Riley, H. L. Liang, J. T. Eells et al., "Photobiomodulation directly benefits primary neurons functionally inactivated by toxins: role of cytochrome c oxidase," *Journal of Biological Chemistry*, vol. 280, no. 6, pp. 4761–4771, 2005.

[5] A. Giuliani, L. Lorenzini, M. Gallamini, A. Massella, L. Giardino, and L. Calzà, "Low infra red laser light irradiation on cultured neural cells: effects on mitochondria and cell viability after oxidative stress," *BMC Complementary and Alternative Medicine*, vol. 9, article 8, 2009.

[6] J. C. Rojas, J. Lee, J. M. John, and F. Gonzalez-Lima, "Neuroprotective effects of near-infrared light in an in vivo model of mitochondrial optic neuropathy," *Journal of Neuroscience*, vol. 28, no. 50, pp. 13511–13521, 2008.

[7] J. T. Eells, M. M. Henry, P. Summerfelt et al., "Therapeutic photobiomodulation for methanol-induced retinal toxicity," *Proceedings of the National Academy of Sciences of the United States of America*, vol. 100, no. 6, pp. 3439–3444, 2003.

[8] T. Ando, W. Xuan, T. Xu et al., "Comparison of therapeutic effects between pulsed and continuous wave 810-nm wavelength laser irradiation for traumatic brain injury in mice," *PLoS ONE*, vol. 6, no. 10, Article ID e26212, 2011.

[9] Q. Wu, W. Xuan, T. Ando et al., "Low-level laser therapy for closed-head traumatic brain injury in mice: effect of different wavelengths," *Lasers in Surgery and Medicine*, vol. 44, no. 3, pp. 218–226, 2012.

[10] A. Oron, U. Oron, J. Streeter et al., "Low-level laser therapy applied transcranially to mice following traumatic brain injury significantly reduces long-term neurological deficits," *Journal of Neurotrauma*, vol. 24, no. 4, pp. 651–656, 2007.

[11] W. Xuan, F. Vatansever, L. Huang et al., "Transcranial low-level laser therapy improves neurological performance in traumatic brain injury in mice: effect of treatment repetition regimen," *PLoS ONE*, vol. 8, no. 1, Article ID e53454, 2013.

[12] S. Michalikova, A. Ennaceur, R. van Rensburg, and P. L. Chazot, "Emotional responses and memory performance of middle-aged CD1 mice in a 3D maze: effects of low infrared light," *Neurobiology of Learning and Memory*, vol. 89, no. 4, pp. 480–488, 2008.

[13] D. W. Barrett and F. Gonzalez-Lima, "Transcranial infrared laser stimulation produces beneficial cognitive and emotional effects in humans," *Neuroscience*, vol. 230, pp. 13–23, 2013.

[14] M. A. Naeser, A. Saltmarche, M. H. Krengel, M. R. Hamblin, and J. A. Knight, "Improved cognitive function after transcranial, light-emitting diode treatments in chronic, traumatic brain injury: two case reports," *Photomedicine and Laser Surgery*, vol. 29, no. 5, pp. 351–358, 2011.

[15] M. A. Naeser, R. Zafonte, M. H. Krengel et al., "Significant improvements in cognitive performance post-transcranial, red/near-infrared light-emitting diode treatments in chronic, mild traumatic brain Injury: open-protocol study," *Journal of Neurotrauma*, vol. 31, no. 11, pp. 1008–1017, 2014.

[16] L. D. Morries, P. Cassano, and T. A. Henderson, "Treatments for traumatic brain injury with emphasis on transcranial near-infrared laser phototherapy," In press.

[17] F. Schiffer, A. L. Johnston, C. Ravichandran et al., "Psychological benefits 2 and 4 weeks after a single treatment with near infrared light to the forehead: a pilot study of 10 patients with major depression and anxiety," *Behavioral and Brain Functions*, vol. 5, no. 1, article 46, 2009.

[18] J. A. Zivin, R. Sehra, A. Shoshoo et al., "NeuroThera Efficacy and Safety Trial-3 (NEST-3): a double-blind, randomized, sham-controlled, parallel group, multicenter, pivotal study to assess the safety and efficacy of transcranial laser therapy with the NeuroThera Laser System for the treatment of acute ischemic stroke within 24 h of stroke onset," *International Journal of Stroke*, vol. 9, no. 7, pp. 950–955, 2014.

[19] W. Hacke, P. D. Schellinger, G. W. Albers et al., "Transcranial laser therapy in acute stroke treatment: results of neurothera effectiveness and safety trial 3, a phase III clinical end point device trial," *Stroke*, vol. 45, no. 11, pp. 3187–3193, 2014.

[20] Y. Lampl, J. A. Zivin, M. Fisher et al., "Infrared laser therapy for ischemic stroke: a new treatment strategy. Results of the NeuroThera Effectiveness and Safety Trial-1 (NEST-1)," *Stroke*, vol. 38, no. 6, pp. 1843–1849, 2007.

[21] B. N. Huisa, A. B. Stemer, M. G. Walker, K. Rapp, B. C. Meyer, and J. A. Zivin, "Transcranial laser therapy for acute ischemic stroke: a pooled analysis of NEST-1 and NEST-2," *International Journal of Stroke*, vol. 8, no. 5, pp. 315–320, 2013.

[22] W. Guy, W. H. Wilson, B. Brooking, G. Manov, and O. Fjetland, "Reliability and validity of SAFTEE: preliminary analyses," *Psychopharmacology Bulletin*, vol. 22, no. 2, pp. 397–401, 1986.

[23] J. Tuner and P. Jenkins, "Complications in comparing lasers and LED. Comment on Esper MA, Nicolau RA, Arisawa EA (2011) The effect of two phototherapy protocols on pain control in orthodontic procedure—a preliminary clinical study. Lasers Med Sci 26:657-663," *Lasers in Medical Science*, vol. 27, no. 6, pp. 1257–1258, 2012.

[24] J. A. Zivin, G. W. Albers, N. Bornstein et al., "Effectiveness and safety of transcranial laser therapy for acute ischemic stroke," *Stroke*, vol. 40, no. 4, pp. 1359–1364, 2009.

3

Prevalence of Depressive Symptoms and Related Factors in Japanese Employees: A Comparative Study between Surveys from 2007 and 2010

Masahito Fushimi[1,2]

[1]*Akita Prefectural Mental Health and Welfare Center, 2-1-51 Nakadori, Akita City, Akita Prefecture 010-0001, Japan*
[2]*Akita Occupational Health Promotion Center, 6-6 Senshukubota-machi, Akita City, Akita Prefecture 010-0874, Japan*

Correspondence should be addressed to Masahito Fushimi; fushimi@sings.jp

Academic Editor: Nicola Magnavita

Aims. The aim of this study was to examine the prevalence of depressive symptoms and their related factors in Japan. The results were analyzed to identify the relationship between high scores on the CES-D, sociodemographic status, and employment-related variables. *Methods.* Employees in Akita prefecture completed the Center for Epidemiologic Studies Depression Scale (CES-D) during a survey period between November and December 2010. The cutoff point for the CES-D scores was 16 or above (high scorers). *Results.* Data from 1,476 employees indicated that 44.2% had high scores on the CES-D. Sociodemographic and occupation-related factors associated with a high risk of depression were being female, young age, fewer hours of sleep on weekdays, and working over 8 hours per day, whereas drinking alcohol one to two days per week, albeit only in men, was significantly associated with a low risk of depression. The present results were consistent with the results of a previous survey completed in 2007; however, the present results regarding job categories and smoking behavior were not significantly associated with depression and thus were inconsistent with the 2007 survey data. *Conclusions.* These results can be useful as benchmark values for the CES-D and might help predict depressive disorders.

1. Introduction

The suicide rate in Japan steadily increased during the 1990s and sharply escalated in 1998. The main factor contributing to this surge was the sudden increase in suicide rates among middle-aged men (i.e., working age), often considered to be related to the drastic social changes occurring around that time, such as the national economic crisis (Japan's recession) and the termination of lifetime employment practices by many major companies. Currently, Japan has one of the highest suicide rates among developed countries, making suicide an important national problem. Health problems are regarded as the cause of the majority of the reported suicides in Japan [1]. It is important that occupational safety and health programs adopt an approach that is built on proactive prevention, screening, and early intervention, as well as the notion that mental health problems among employees are associated with a decline in employee productivity—thus, effective interventions alleviate mental health symptoms, thereby increasing employee productivity [2–4]. Depressive disorder is one of the most common mental disorders and is a major public health problem in Japan [1]. Previous surveys on the prevalence of depression and depressive symptoms in Japan have yielded widely different results [5, 6]. Occupational safety and health programs typically invite employees to complete a voluntary health assessment questionnaire at their workplace, involving brief self-report health scales (i.e., nondiagnostic methods), to determine the prevalence and severity of depressive symptoms. The Center for Epidemiologic Studies Depression Scale (CES-D), a self-report depression scale, has been widely used in population surveys across the world and has satisfactory levels of reliability and validity in numerous cultures [7, 8]. The CES-D has been translated into Japanese, and its reliability and validity have been confirmed in the Japanese general population [9, 10]. In the present study, a universal cutoff point of 16 was employed, since it most effectively detects and covers "probable" depression symptoms [5].

In this study, the prevalence of depressive symptoms using the CES-D among a probability sample of Japanese employees in Akita prefecture was examined. In addition, the predictors of these symptoms were analyzed. We had previously conducted an occupational mental health study in 2007 [11]. The present study, conducted in 2010, is a follow-up study that adopted similar methods to the 2007 study. In this report, the results of these two studies are compared, and these results can be used as benchmarks for comparisons of future employee health-risk assessment surveys using the CES-D. The data presented in this paper will help identify employees at high risk of depressive disorders and detect the contributing sociodemographic and work-related factors.

2. Materials and Methods

2.1. Participants. The information presented in this report was collected as part of the Northern-Japan Occupational Health Promotion Centers Collaboration Study for Mental Health (NOCS-MH), conducted by the occupational health promotion centers located in the seven prefectures of northern Japan (Hokkaido, Aomori, Iwate, Miyagi, Akita, Yamagata, and Fukushima). The NOCS-MH investigates stress situations and stress management skills and assesses depressive symptoms in employees [11]. The information from the Akita region was taken from the NOCS-MH. Participants were recruited first by randomly selecting their employers (random systematic sampling) and then by encouraging the employers to ask their employees to answer the survey. The companies ("employers") requested in the 2007 survey—which were selected by random systematic sampling—were asked to participate in this survey as well. Thus, requests in the 2010 survey were made to the same employers; however, since participation was voluntary, participant companies were not quite identical between the two surveys. The survey period was from November to December 2010. Twenty employers from Akita's public and private sectors agreed to participate in the study. Participation in the paper-based survey was voluntary and confidential. Of the 1,813 employees who were administered the questionnaire, 1,670 responded (a response rate of 92.1%). The Japan Labour Health and Welfare Organization, which has occupational health promotion centers established in each administrative division, approved the study protocol.

2.2. Instruments and Analysis. To determine the prevalence and severity of depressive symptoms, the CES-D was used. Each of the 20 items on the CES-D is rated on a four-point scale ranging from "rarely or none of the time" (0) to "most or all of the time" (3) and refers to how often the respondent felt what the item described in the previous week. The sum of the response scores can range from 0 to 60. Calibration studies of the CES-D indicate that scores of 16 or above represent "probable" depression symptoms; therefore, a cutoff score of 16 indicates significant current depressive symptomatology [5]. Sociodemographic information, including sex, age, which was divided into groups of 29 years and below, 30 to 39 years, 40 to 49 years, and 50 years and above, and highest level of education obtained (compulsory and senior high school, tertiary education, and graduate degree or higher), was also collected. Additionally, the questionnaire collected information about the employees' occupational characteristics (full-time work, managerial class, and job category). The employees had to choose one of the following job categories: clerical or administrative support (e.g., administrative assistant, office supervisor), professional (e.g., engineer, doctor, and nurse), sales- or service-related occupation (e.g., sales representative, retail sales staff), technical support (e.g., laboratory technician, computer programmer), and others (e.g., on-site worker, driver). The survey included items on the average number of working hours per day (≤8 and >8 h). In the present study, participants were also asked about their sleep duration per day, which was then sorted by hours of sleep per day during the weekdays (<6, 6, 7, and >7 h) and hours per day on holidays (<6, 6, 7, 8, and >8 h). In our previous 2007 study, questions regarding sleep were not categorized this way [11]. The survey also included items on the smoking behavior (nonsmoker, ceased smoker, and current smoker). In the present study, alcohol consumption was measured by days of consumption per week (none/rare, 1-2 days/week, 3–5 days/week, and 6-7 days/week); these items were more detailed than those used in the 2007 study (i.e., none/rare, sometimes, and daily consumption) [11].

Statistical analyses took the form of cross tabulations of the prevalence of depressive symptoms versus sociodemographic and employment variables, performed using SPSS version 11.0J for Windows (SPSS, Tokyo, Japan). Statistical differences were measured using three binomial multivariate logistic regressions with CES-D score (<16 or ≥16) as the dependent variable. Sex was included as an independent variable in one regression. The remaining two had separate data sets for men and women.

3. Results

The number of effective respondents, excluding those with insufficient data, was 1,476 (81.4%), including 883 men and 593 women. Table 1 presents the numbers, means, and standard deviations of the CES-D by sex and age. The mean score for the CES-D for all respondents was 16.12 (SD = 9.23; mean = 15.29 and SD = 8.66 for men; mean = 17.37 and SD = 9.90 for women), with lower mean scores among men than among women in all age groups. Table 2 distinguishes employees with a CES-D score of 16 or above (high scorers) from the others (low scorers). It also presents the sociodemographic status and employment-related variables and shows the percentages of high scorers on the CES-D by the demographics of each category. The overall prevalence of high scorers on the CES-D was 44.2% (41.1% for men, 48.7% for women), with a lower prevalence of high scorers among men than among women in all age groups. Further, a lower prevalence of high scorers was observed in the older age groups.

Table 3 shows the adjusted odds ratios (OR) from the binomial multivariate logistic regression for high scorers on the CES-D (16 or above) by sociodemographic status and employment-related variables. It indicates that the independent effect of sex on the prevalence of high scorers was

TABLE 1: Numbers, mean scores, and standard deviations of the CES-D scores according to sex and age in the 2010 survey.

Age	Total			Men			Women		
	Number	Mean	SD	Number	Mean	SD	Number	Mean	SD
≤29	291	19.02	10.46	174	17.16	8.77	117	21.80	12.07
30–39	396	15.82	8.44	255	15.47	8.38	141	16.45	8.54
40–49	394	15.89	9.29	229	15.23	9.29	165	16.80	9.25
≥50	395	14.51	8.49	225	13.68	7.93	170	15.62	9.08
Total	1476	16.12	9.23	883	15.29	8.66	593	17.37	9.90

significant. Namely, being female was significantly associated with a greater likelihood of being a high scorer. Among women, the prevalence of high scorers varied significantly by age ("50 years or above" had the lowest OR) and sleep duration on weekdays ("6 h" was associated with a decreased OR). However, these associations were not observed for men. In contrast, for men, the prevalence of high scorers on the CES-D varied significantly by sleep duration on weekdays ("7 h" was associated with a decreased OR) and alcohol consumption ("1-2 days/week" was associated with a decreased OR). On average, among men and women, participants aged "50 years or above" had the lowest likelihood of being high scorers; working more than eight hours per day was significantly associated with an increased likelihood; and those who selected six and seven hours of sleep on weekdays had significantly lower likelihoods of being high scorers.

4. Discussion

In the present study, the mean CES-D score was 16.12, and 44.2% of employees exhibited high CES-D scores (16 or above). These results were similar to our previous findings in 2007 (16.09 and 45.0%, resp.). Several studies using the CES-D, in Japan and abroad, showed mean CES-D scores of approximately 5–10, with prevalence rates of high CES-D scorers (also using the cutoff point of 16) ranging from 10% to 20% [9, 11–13]. The mean CES-D score and the prevalence rate of high scorers in this study are higher than the findings of previous studies. Our results clearly show that employers and managers cannot assume that their employees are free from mental health problems and suggest that screening and early intervention for problems such as depression might be an appropriate course of action. To prevent the negative consequences of mental health problems in the workplace, including high absenteeism, low productivity, and employee attrition, employers need to invest in mental health resources. Previous studies suggest that case management programs for employees with mental health problems lead to superior clinical outcomes, decreased unemployment, and increased employee productivity. Therefore, such programs have the potential to provide the employer with positive returns on their investment [2–4, 14]. It is unclear why so many respondents in the present study scored high on the CES-D. This might be partly explained by drastic social changes in job opportunities or the work environment and by a culturally different response styles to certain questions (e.g., Japanese are reluctant to express their positive affect) [1, 5, 9, 10, 15, 16]. Further studies are required to clarify this point.

In this study, the adjusted OR from the binomial multivariate logistic regression for high scorers on the CES-D also showed that the prevalence of high scorers on the CES-D varied significantly by sex, age, working hours, sleep duration on weekdays, and alcohol consumption, whereas it did not vary significantly by job category, sleep duration on holidays, and smoking behavior. In contrast, our previous results showed that the prevalence of high scorers on the CES-D varied significantly by job category and smoking behavior [11]. Therefore, sex, age, daily working hours, sleep durations, and alcohol consumption may be highly reproducible variables that predict CES-D score, whereas job category and smoking behavior may be insufficiently reproducible. Furthermore, it can be said that dividing sleep durations by weekdays and holidays is meaningful.

Previous studies using the CES-D scale have reported that gender, young age, and low educational level are independent risk factors for depressive symptoms [5, 7, 17–20], and the results of our study supported these findings to some extent. However, educational level was not significantly associated with high scores on the CES-D. Previous reports are inconsistent in terms of the relationship between depressive symptoms and educational levels [15, 16]. It has been widely accepted that as educational level decreases, the prevalence of mental health problems increases [5]. However, according to another report, significantly high levels of psychological distress were noted among employees with a postgraduate degree [21].

In this study, job category was not significantly associated with the prevalence rates of high scorers on the CES-D. However, in our previous study [11], job category was significantly associated with the prevalence rates (i.e., women in professional roles were highly likely to be high scorers on the CES-D). Therefore, it is believed that these results may not be reproducible. In several previous studies, lower rates of depressive symptoms were found among those who were highly educated and employed in professional/managerial positions. People in these groups seem to have less difficulty adjusting to changes in the social environment and controlling work-related distress [5]. In brief, there is no consistent evidence of the relationship between job category and psychological distress in the previous literature, no doubt due to the complexity of the relationship [16, 22].

Another indicator of psychological distress was hours spent working. Generally, high work demand is associated with a decline in mental well-being [23, 24] as is the pressure to work overtime. Increased working hours might also produce a negative work-to-family spillover, which is

Table 2: Demographics of sample and the comparison between nonhigh scorers on the CES-D (<16) and high scorers on the CES-D (≥16) in the 2010 survey.

	Nonhigh scorers on the CES-D (<16)						High scorers on the CES-D (≥16)						% of high scorers on the CES-D		
	Number			% of each category			Number			% of each category					
	Total	Men	Women	Total	Men	Women	Total	Men	Women	Total	Men	Women	Total	Men	Women
Sex	824	520	304	100	63.1	36.9	652	363	289	100	55.7	44.3	44.2	41.1	48.7
Age															
≤29	130	87	43	15.8	16.7	14.1	161	87	74	24.7	24.0	25.6	55.3	50.0	63.2
30–39	220	147	73	26.7	28.3	24.0	176	108	68	27.0	29.8	23.5	44.4	42.4	48.2
40–49	222	136	86	26.9	26.2	28.3	172	93	79	26.4	25.6	27.3	43.7	40.6	47.9
≥50	252	150	102	30.6	28.8	33.6	143	75	68	21.9	20.7	23.5	36.2	33.3	40.0
Education															
Compulsory/senior high school	491	331	160	59.6	63.7	52.6	375	237	138	57.5	65.3	47.8	43.3	41.7	46.3
Some tertiary education	194	82	112	23.5	15.8	36.8	177	64	113	27.1	17.6	39.1	47.7	43.8	50.2
Graduate degree or higher	137	106	31	16.6	20.4	10.2	98	60	38	15.0	16.5	13.1	41.7	36.1	55.1
Employment status															
Full-time work	667	451	216	80.9	86.7	71.1	555	331	224	85.1	91.2	77.5	45.4	42.3	50.9
No full-time work	94	31	63	11.4	6.0	20.7	58	16	42	8.9	4.4	14.5	38.2	34.0	40.0
Employee type															
Nonmanagerial class	570	326	244	69.2	62.7	80.3	472	255	217	72.4	70.2	75.1	45.3	43.9	47.1
Managerial class	160	126	34	19.4	24.2	11.2	106	65	41	16.3	17.9	14.2	39.8	34.0	54.7
Job category															
Clerical/administrative	195	110	85	23.7	21.2	28.0	136	67	69	20.9	18.5	23.9	41.1	37.9	44.8
Professional	191	79	112	23.2	15.2	36.8	167	46	121	25.6	12.7	41.9	46.6	36.8	51.9
Sales/service	64	50	14	7.8	9.6	4.6	43	32	11	6.6	8.8	3.8	40.2	39.0	44.0
Technical	176	146	30	21.4	28.1	9.9	149	116	33	22.9	32.0	11.4	45.8	44.3	52.4
Others (on-site workers)	184	126	58	22.3	24.2	19.1	143	92	51	21.9	25.3	17.6	43.7	42.2	46.8
Working hours per day															
≤8 h	467	266	201	56.7	51.2	66.1	323	167	156	49.5	46.0	54.0	40.9	38.6	43.7
>8 h	350	250	100	42.5	48.1	32.9	327	195	132	50.2	53.7	45.7	48.3	43.8	56.9
Sleep duration (weekdays)															
<6 h	105	56	49	12.7	10.8	16.1	172	84	88	26.4	23.1	30.4	62.1	60.0	64.2
6 h	332	190	142	40.3	36.5	46.7	241	146	95	37.0	40.2	32.9	42.1	43.5	40.1
7 h	257	182	75	31.2	35.0	24.7	154	83	71	23.6	22.9	24.6	37.5	31.3	48.6
>7 h	114	83	31	13.8	16.0	10.2	71	48	23	10.9	13.2	8.0	38.4	36.6	42.6
Sleep duration (holidays)															
<6 h	30	19	11	3.6	3.7	3.6	55	31	24	8.4	8.5	8.3	64.7	62.0	68.6
6 h	148	97	51	18.0	18.7	16.8	118	61	57	18.1	16.8	19.7	44.4	38.6	52.8
7 h	183	114	69	22.2	21.9	22.7	126	76	50	19.3	20.9	17.3	40.8	40.0	42.0
8 h	194	132	62	23.5	25.4	20.4	129	78	51	19.8	21.5	17.6	39.9	37.1	45.1
>8 h	35	24	11	4.2	4.6	3.6	48	25	23	7.4	6.9	8.0	57.8	51.0	67.6
Smoking behavior															
Nonsmoker	331	112	219	40.2	21.5	72.0	268	81	187	41.1	22.3	64.7	44.7	42.0	46.1
Ceased smoker	188	149	39	22.8	28.7	12.8	123	85	38	18.9	23.4	13.1	39.5	36.3	49.4
Current smoker	302	259	43	36.7	49.8	14.1	260	197	63	39.9	54.3	21.8	46.3	43.2	59.4
Alcohol consumption															
None/rare	287	118	169	34.8	22.7	55.6	259	108	151	39.7	29.8	52.2	47.4	47.8	47.2
1-2/week	164	103	61	19.9	19.8	20.1	133	61	72	20.4	16.8	24.9	44.8	37.2	54.1
3–5/week	102	71	31	12.4	13.7	10.2	75	48	27	11.5	13.2	9.3	42.4	40.3	46.6
6-7/week	269	227	42	32.6	43.7	13.8	185	146	39	28.4	40.2	13.5	40.7	39.1	48.1

TABLE 3: Effects of sociodemographic and employment-related factors on the prevalence of high scorers on the CES-D (≥16) in the 2010 survey.

	Total			Male			Female		
	OR	95% CI	*p* value	OR	95% CI	*p* value	OR	95% CI	*p* value
Sex									
Men		Ref.							
Women	1.49	1.03–2.15	<0.05						
Age									
≤29		Ref.			Ref.			Ref.	
30–39	0.67	0.44–1.01	0.06	0.90	0.54–1.52	0.69	0.39	0.18–0.81	<0.05
40–49	0.72	0.46–1.11	0.14	1.07	0.60–1.90	0.81	0.39	0.19–0.83	<0.05
≥50	0.52	0.33–0.83	<0.01	0.70	0.37–1.34	0.29	0.30	0.14–0.67	<0.005
Education									
Compulsory/senior high school		Ref.			Ref.			Ref.	
Some tertiary education	0.98	0.66–1.46	0.93	1.02	0.60–1.73	0.94	0.78	0.40–1.50	0.45
Graduate degree or higher	0.77	0.50–1.20	0.25	0.77	0.45–1.31	0.33	0.69	0.29–1.64	0.40
Employment status									
Full-time work		Ref.			Ref.			Ref.	
No full-time work	0.80	0.50–1.30	0.38	1.04	0.47–2.31	0.92	0.88	0.44–1.74	0.70
Employee type									
Nonmanagerial class		Ref.			Ref.			Ref.	
Managerial class	0.91	0.60–1.38	0.65	0.64	0.38–1.07	0.09	1.82	0.76–4.34	0.18
Job category									
Clerical/administrative		Ref.			Ref.			Ref.	
Professional	0.73	0.47–1.12	0.15	0.62	0.34–1.15	0.13	0.81	0.41–1.60	0.54
Sales/service	1.08	0.57–2.07	0.81	0.92	0.42–2.05	0.85	1.36	0.36–5.09	0.65
Technical	0.76	0.48–1.20	0.23	0.68	0.39–1.19	0.18	0.83	0.33–2.12	0.70
Others (on-site workers)	0.92	0.57–1.47	0.72	0.83	0.46–1.49	0.52	0.82	0.34–1.98	0.66
Working hours per day									
≤8 h		Ref.			Ref.			Ref.	
>8 h	1.42	1.04–1.94	<0.05	1.34	0.90–1.99	0.15	1.63	0.94–2.81	0.08
Sleep duration (weekdays)									
<6 h		Ref.			Ref.			Ref.	
6 h	0.56	0.37–0.86	<0.01	0.57	0.32–1.02	0.06	0.51	0.26–0.97	<0.05
7 h	0.46	0.28–0.76	<0.005	0.34	0.17–0.67	<0.005	0.67	0.31–1.46	0.32
>7 h	0.85	0.45–1.61	0.61	0.61	0.27–1.39	0.24	1.92	0.55–6.73	0.31
Sleep duration (holidays)									
<6 h		Ref.							
6 h	0.72	0.37–1.40	0.33	0.62	0.26–1.50	0.29	1.11	0.37–3.31	0.85
7 h	0.61	0.31–1.20	0.15	0.72	0.29–1.75	0.46	0.59	0.20–1.71	0.33
8 h	0.55	0.27–1.09	0.09	0.58	0.23–1.45	0.24	0.57	0.18–1.75	0.33
>8 h	1.09	0.49–2.46	0.83	1.04	0.36–2.98	0.95	1.60	0.41–6.26	0.50
Smoking behavior									
Nonsmoker		Ref.			Ref.			Ref.	
Ceased smoker	0.99	0.64–1.51	0.95	0.95	0.55–1.66	0.87	1.00	0.46–2.19	1.00
Current smoker	0.99	0.68–1.43	0.94	1.03	0.64–1.66	0.90	1.01	0.51–1.99	0.98
Alcohol consumption									
None/rare		Ref.			Ref.			Ref.	
1-2/week	0.75	0.50–1.12	0.16	0.52	0.30–0.91	<0.05	1.08	0.58–2.01	0.82
3–5/week	0.78	0.48–1.27	0.32	0.71	0.37–1.36	0.30	0.92	0.43–1.98	0.84
6-7/week	0.90	0.61–1.34	0.61	0.81	0.49–1.33	0.41	1.05	0.49–2.24	0.90

OR: odds ratio; CI: confidence interval; Ref.: reference group to which all other categorical variables are compared (binomial multivariate logistic regression).

associated with an increased risk of depression. A proportion of employees with high psychological distress possibly work longer hours to keep up with an excessive workload [21]. Further, several studies pointed out an association between insomnia and depression [25, 26]. Moreover, some studies from Japan examined the relationship between depressive symptoms, as assessed using the CES-D, and sleep state [27, 28]. Another study investigated the relationship between lifestyle, as defined by common health habits like sleeping habits, and symptoms of depression [29].

Many previous studies suggest sleep disturbances as a risk factor for depression. The results of both our 2007 and 2010 studies have shown that short sleep duration was associated with a high risk of depression. Moreover, when sleep duration (per day) was divided by weekdays and holidays, it was found that sleep duration on weekdays might be a useful indicator of depression.

Regarding alcohol consumption, men who consumed alcohol "1-2 days/week" had a relatively low risk to be high scorers on the CES-D compared with those who drank nothing or rarely. In our previous 2007 study [11], "sometimes" consuming alcohol was associated with a higher risk of depression compared with daily consumption. The reason for this trend is unclear; however, it is possible that participants that reported "none/rare" consumption already have a declining health status (i.e., they cannot consume due to their ill health). Further studies are required to clarify this point.

The limitation of this study lies in its cross-sectional design, which makes it difficult to determine whether these correlations between sociodemographic characteristics and depressive symptoms indicate antecedents or consequences of depressive disorders. In order to make inferences with regard to causality, a longitudinal follow-up study will be needed. The present study applied measures for different periods (i.e., the 2010 survey was a follow-up to the 2007 survey) and adopted a similar method to our previous study. From this, it is thought that the distinction between the result which is with the plasticity and the result which is not so is enabled. However, it is necessary to survey participants more than twice to show this thoroughly. While our use of 16 as the cutoff point for depressive disorders was justified by previous studies, this does not specifically indicate a clinical diagnosis of depression [5, 9]. Thus, it is difficult to compare the results of this study with that of other surveys, which used diagnostic approaches. As such, another type of epidemiological survey that applies a standardized diagnostic instrument in addition to a nondiagnostic one will be needed.

Conflict of Interests

The author declares that there is no conflict of interests regarding the publication of this paper.

Acknowledgments

The author would like to thank all of the occupational physicians from the seven administrative occupational health promotion centers located in the prefectures of northern Japan (Hokkaido, Aomori, Iwate, Miyagi, Akita, Yamagata, and Fukushima prefectures) and their assistants for their help during the course of the investigation and also all the operators who contributed to the study.

References

[1] M. Fushimi, J. Sugawara, and T. Shimizu, "Suicide patterns and characteristics in Akita, Japan," *Psychiatry and Clinical Neurosciences*, vol. 59, no. 3, pp. 296–302, 2005.

[2] A. Tsutsumi, M. Nagami, T. Yoshikawa, K. Kogi, and N. Kawakami, "Participatory intervention for workplace improvements on mental health and job performance among blue-collar workers: a cluster randomized controlled trial," *Journal of Occupational & Environmental Medicine*, vol. 51, no. 5, pp. 554–563, 2009.

[3] R. Umanodan, Y. Kobayashi, M. Nakamura, K. Kitaoka-Higashiguchi, N. Kawakami, and A. Shimazu, "Effects of a worksite stress management training program with six short-hour sessions: a controlled trial among Japanese employees," *Journal of Occupational Health*, vol. 51, no. 4, pp. 294–302, 2009.

[4] P. S. Wang, G. E. Simon, J. Avorn et al., "Telephone screening, outreach, and care management for depressed workers and impact on clinical and work productivity outcomes: a randomized controlled trial," *Journal of the American Medical Association*, vol. 298, no. 12, pp. 1401–1411, 2007.

[5] M. J. Cho, J. J. Nam, and G. H. Suh, "Prevalence of symptoms of depression in a nationwide sample of Korean adults," *Psychiatry Research*, vol. 81, no. 3, pp. 341–352, 1998.

[6] L. Stallones, M. B. Marx, and T. F. Garrity, "Prevalence and correlates of depressive symptoms among older U.S. adults," *The American Journal of Preventive Medicine*, vol. 6, no. 5, pp. 295–303, 1990.

[7] L. S. Radloff, "The CES-D scale: a self-report depression scale for research in the general population," *Applied Psychological Measurement*, vol. 1, no. 3, pp. 385–401, 1977.

[8] R. E. Roberts and S. W. Vernon, "The center for epidemiologic studies depression scale: its use in a community sample," *American Journal of Psychiatry*, vol. 140, no. 1, pp. 41–46, 1983.

[9] N. Iwata, Y. Okuyama, Y. Kawakami, and K. Saito, "Prevalence of depressive symptoms in a Japanese occupational setting: a preliminary study," *The American Journal of Public Health*, vol. 79, no. 11, pp. 1486–1489, 1989.

[10] N. Iwata, M. Umesue, K. Egashira et al., "Can positive affect items be used to assess depressive disorders in the Japanese population?" *Psychological Medicine*, vol. 28, no. 1, pp. 153–158, 1998.

[11] M. Fushimi, S. Saito, and T. Shimizu, "Prevalence of depressive symptoms and related factors in Japanese employees as measured by the center for epidemiologic studies depression scale (CES-D)," *Community Mental Health Journal*, vol. 49, no. 2, pp. 236–242, 2013.

[12] G. E. Barnes, R. F. Currie, and A. Segall, "Symptoms of depression in a Canadian urban sample," *Canadian Journal of Psychiatry*, vol. 33, no. 5, pp. 386–393, 1988.

[13] Y.-W. Ying, "Depressive symptomatology among Chinese-Americans as measured by the CES-D," *Journal of Clinical Psychology*, vol. 44, no. 5, pp. 739–746, 1988.

[14] J. W. Williams Jr., M. Gerrity, T. Holsinger, S. Dobscha, B. Gaynes, and A. Dietrich, "Systematic review of multifaceted interventions to improve depression care," *General Hospital Psychiatry*, vol. 29, no. 2, pp. 91–116, 2007.

[15] M. Fushimi, "The relationship between individual personality traits (internality-externality) and psychological distress in employees in Japan," *Depression Research and Treatment*, vol. 2011, Article ID 731307, 6 pages, 2011.

[16] M. Fushimi, S. Saito, T. Shimizu, Y. Kudo, M. Seki, and K. Murata, "Prevalence of psychological distress, as measured by the kessler 6 (K6), and related factors in Japanese employees," *Community Mental Health Journal*, vol. 48, no. 3, pp. 328–335, 2012.

[17] G. W. Comstock and K. J. Helsing, "Symptoms of depression in two communities," *Psychological Medicine*, vol. 6, no. 4, pp. 551–563, 1976.

[18] B. A. Husaini, J. A. Neff, J. B. Harrington, M. D. Houghs, and R. H. Stone, "Depression in rural communities: validating the CES-D scale," *Journal of Community Psychology*, vol. 8, no. 1, pp. 20–27, 1980.

[19] M. G. Madianos, V. Tomaras, A. Kapsali, N. Vaidakis, J. Vlachonicolis, and C. N. Stefanis, "Psychiatric case identification in two Athenian communities: estimation of the probable prevalence," *Acta Psychiatrica Scandinavica*, vol. 78, no. 1, pp. 24–31, 1988.

[20] W. E. Narrow, D. S. Rae, E. K. Moscicki, B. Z. Locke, and D. A. Regier, "Depression among Cuban Americans: the Hispanic Health and Nutrition Examination Survey," *Social Psychiatry and Psychiatric Epidemiology*, vol. 25, no. 5, pp. 260–268, 1990.

[21] M. F. Hilton, H. A. Whiteford, J. S. Sheridan et al., "The prevalence of psychological distress in employees and associated occupational risk factors," *Journal of Occupational and Environmental Medicine*, vol. 50, no. 7, pp. 746–757, 2008.

[22] M. Fushimi, T. Shimizu, S. Saito, Y. Kudo, M. Seki, and K. Murata, "Prevalence of and risk factors for psychological distress among employees in Japan," *Public Health*, vol. 124, no. 12, pp. 713–715, 2010.

[23] R. M. D'Souza, L. Strazdins, D. H. Broom, B. Rodgers, and H. L. Berry, "Work demands, job insecurity and sickness absence from work. How productive is the new, flexible labour force?" *Australian and New Zealand Journal of Public Health*, vol. 30, no. 3, pp. 205–212, 2006.

[24] S. A. Stansfeld, R. Fuhrer, M. J. Shipley, and M. G. Marmot, "Work characteristics predict psychiatric disorder: prospective results from the Whitehall II study," *Occupational and Environmental Medicine*, vol. 56, no. 5, pp. 302–307, 1999.

[25] P. P. Chang, D. E. Ford, L. A. Mead, L. Cooper-Patrick, and M. J. Klag, "Insomnia in young men and subsequent depression. The Johns Hopkins Precursors Study," *The American Journal of Epidemiology*, vol. 146, no. 2, pp. 105–114, 1997.

[26] D. Riemann and U. Voderholzer, "Primary insomnia: a risk factor to develop depression?" *Journal of Affective Disorders*, vol. 76, no. 1–3, pp. 255–259, 2003.

[27] Y. Kaneita, T. Ohida, M. Uchiyama et al., "The relationship between depression and sleep disturbances: a Japanese nationwide general population survey," *Journal of Clinical Psychiatry*, vol. 67, no. 2, pp. 196–203, 2006.

[28] A. Nakata, T. Haratani, M. Takahashi et al., "Association of sickness absence with poor sleep and depressive symptoms in shift workers," *Chronobiology International*, vol. 21, no. 6, pp. 899–912, 2004.

[29] T. Frederick, R. R. Frerichs, and V. A. Clark, "Personal health habits and symptoms of depression at the community level," *Preventive Medicine*, vol. 17, no. 2, pp. 173–182, 1988.

4

Do Panic Symptoms Affect the Quality of Life and Add to the Disability in Patients with Bronchial Asthma?

A. D. Faye,[1] S. Gawande,[1] R. Tadke,[1] V. C. Kirpekar,[1] S. H. Bhave,[1] A. P. Pakhare,[2] and B. Tayade[3]

[1]*Department of Psychiatry, NKP Salve Institute of Medical Sciences and Lata Mangeshkar Hospital, Digdoh Hills, Hingna Road, Nagpur, Maharashtra 440019, India*
[2]*Department of Community and Family Medicine, All India Institute of Medical Sciences, Bhopal 462020, India*
[3]*Department of Chest Medicine, NKP Salve Institute of Medical Sciences and Lata Mangeshkar Hospital, Digdoh Hills, Hingna Road, Nagpur, Maharashtra 440019, India*

Correspondence should be addressed to A. D. Faye; abhijeetfaye12@gmail.com

Academic Editor: Yvonne Forsell

Background. Anxiety and panic are known to be associated with bronchial asthma with variety of impact on clinical presentation, treatment outcome, comorbidities, quality of life, and functional disability in patients with asthma. This study aims to explore the pattern of panic symptoms, prevalence and severity of panic disorder (PD), quality of life, and disability in them. *Methods.* Sixty consecutive patients of bronchial asthma were interviewed using semistructured proforma, Panic and Agoraphobia scale, WHO Quality of life (QOL) BREF scale, and WHO disability schedule II (WHODAS II). *Results.* Though 60% of the participants had panic symptoms, only 46.7% had diagnosable panic attacks according to DSM IV TR diagnostic criteria and 33.3% had PD. Most common symptoms were "sensations of shortness of breath or smothering," "feeling of choking," and "fear of dying" found in 83.3% of the participants. 73.3% of the participants had poor quality of life which was most impaired in physical and environmental domains. 55% of the participants had disability score more than a mean (18.1). *Conclusion.* One-third of the participants had panic disorder with significant effect on physical and environmental domains of quality of life. Patients with more severe PD and bronchial asthma had more disability.

1. Introduction

Asthma is a major public health problem and its prevalence is increasing in both developed and developing countries in recent years [1, 2]. As it is a chronic illness, it has psychological consequences also. Though studies have suggested an association between asthma (especially of severe grade) and mental disorders, there are very few Indian studies that demonstrate the association of asthma and panic disorder (PD). Few studies have found higher rates of anxiety disorders (particularly panic disorder) and major depression among adults with asthma [3–6]. Though there is an increased rate of psychological comorbidity in patients with asthma [7–9], anxiety can be a normal reaction to extreme breathing difficulty [10] and may even be functional in moderation [11, 12]. High levels of panic fear can lead to poor management. Panic and anxiety can directly exacerbate asthma symptoms through hyperventilation, patients' overuse of as-needed asthma medications, more frequent hospital admissions, and longer hospital stays and with more frequent steroid treatment. All of these are independent of degree of objective pulmonary impairment [13, 14].

It has been reported that the prevalence rate of PD is two to six times more among asthma patients compared to general population [15]. The reason for this observation is yet not clear. There is also a symptom overlap and many symptoms of acute asthma can be misunderstood for panic and vice versa. There is limited data on the impact of anxiety comorbidity on functional status and asthma quality of life [9]. Effects of asthma symptoms and physical limitations along with phobic avoidance of a feared situation or trigger factors all can lead to poor quality of life. Similarly there is a sociooccupational impairment in panic disorder. It is also shown that asthma patients with PD had greater perceived impairment from asthma and health care utilization [16]. The study of panic disorder among asthmatics can contribute to improved medical outcome for this subgroup, while also improving our understanding of the biological and psychological etiology of panic. This study was conducted to review this relationship by examining the pattern of panic symptoms, prevalence of panic disorder, how panic disorder and panic symptoms affect the course of asthma and quality of life (QOL) in these patients, and the consequent research implications of this relationship.

2. Material and Methods

A hospital based cross-sectional study was conducted in Psychiatry and Chest Medicine Outpatient Department of tertiary care hospital between January 2012 and June 2013. Considering logistic feasibility, we decided to enroll 60 consecutive asthma patients so that this study would act as pilot for further research. Patients were selected from outpatient department of chest medicine. Bronchial asthma was diagnosed and categorized according to the severity by a qualified chest physician in tertiary care hospital (where the study was carried out), on the basis of clinical history, pulmonary function test, and GINA (Global Initiative for Asthma) pocket guide updated in 2011. A chest physician identified asthma patients between 18 to 60 years of age who were maintained (stable) on treatment. Enrolment was consecutive. Then, these patients were informed about the study and referred to psychiatry outpatient department where a qualified psychiatrist ascertained eligibility criterion. Patients who had already been diagnosed with other axis I psychiatric disorders and those with active symptoms or having acute exacerbation of asthma and unable to give informed consent were excluded from the study.

The whole interview process was semistructured which included clinical assessment, clinical psychiatric assessment, semistructured pro forma questionnaire, and DSM IV TR (Diagnostic and Statistical Manual for diagnosing mental disorders, 4th edition revised version) criteria for diagnosis of panic attack and panic disorder. The panic attack symptoms were selected from the list of the symptoms for DSM IV TR criteria for panic attack. Then, those satisfying the DSM IV TR criteria for panic disorder were considered for the diagnosis of panic disorder. Panic disorder was assessed by clinical interview with patients and close family members by authors who are qualified psychiatrists and diagnosis is done with structured diagnostic criteria of DSM IV TR.

All patients were given detailed information of the study in local language and written informed consent was obtained before administering questionnaires.

Then following questionnaires were administered in order as described below. All the questionnaires used were in local language, that is, Marathi or Hindi. On an average, one interview lasted for 45 minutes. They were as follows:

(1) *Semistructured pro forma* includes sociodemographic data and details regarding asthma (duration, treatment, severity, comorbid medical illnesses, past and family history, history of substance use, and psychiatric history).

(2) *Diagnostic and Statistical Manual for diagnosing mental disorders, 4th edition revised version (DSM IV TR)* for assessment of panic symptoms and panic disorder [17]: panic attack is diagnosed if 4 or more of the symptoms, out of total 13 symptoms mentioned, are developed abruptly and reached a peak within 10 minutes, while panic disorder is diagnosed if there are recurrent unexpected panic attacks followed by one-month or more period of persistent concern about additional attacks or worry about the implications of the attack or significant change in behaviour related to the attack along with other criteria.

(3) *Panic and Agoraphobia scale (PAS)* [18] to assess the severity of panic disorder: it is a special instrument used to determine the severity of PD. The scale contains 13 questions (items) each with 5 possible answers (0–4). Five components have been taken into account: panic attacks, agoraphobic avoidance, anticipatory anxiety, disability, and worries about health. Severity is assessed as 0–8: lack of symptoms; 9–18: mild symptoms; 19–39: severe symptoms; 40 or more: very severe symptoms.

(4) *WHO Quality of Life BREF scale* [19] for assessment of quality of life: from the overall quality of life and General Health facet: domain scores are scaled in a positive direction (i.e., higher scores denote higher quality of life). The mean score of items within each domain is used to calculate the domain score. Mean scores are then multiplied by 4 in order to make domain scores comparable with the scores used in the WHOQOL-100. It is an abbreviated version of WHO-QOL 100 scale, containing 26 items each rated on a 5-point Likert scale. It measures quality of life in 4 domains: physical, psychological, social, and environmental along with two items. The raw scores are converted into transformed scores to obtain the domain scores in the range of 0–100. The scale has high internal consistency (Cronbach alpha = 0.94).

(5) *World Health Organization Disability Assessment Schedule II (WHODAS II)*: this is a multidimensional questionnaire for measuring the level of disability across various conditions and interventions. It explores different areas of functioning in daily life (e.g., hygiene, work, concentration, and relationships). The short version of the scale is a 12-item scale covering the following six domains:

(1) Understanding and communicating with the world (cognition).

(2) Moving and getting around (mobility).

(3) Self-care (attending to one's hygiene, dressing, eating, and staying alone).

(4) Getting along with people (interpersonal interactions).

(5) Life activities (domestic responsibilities, leisure, and work).

(6) Participation in society (joining in community activities).

Scoring is based on averaging responses and then transforming scores into a standard scale. Two types of scoring

Table 1: Demographic profile of the participants.

Demographic factors		
Age in years	[Mean (SD)]	37 ± 7.4
Gender	Females	40% (24)
	Males	60% (36)
Marital status	Married	86.7% (52)
	Unmarried	13.3% (8)
Education status	Nil	10% (6)
	Up to primary	20% (12)
	Up to matriculation	43.3% (26)
	More than matriculation	26.7% (16)
Occupation status	Housewives	33.3% (20)
	Semiskilled	13.3% (8)
	Skilled	6.7% (4)
	Unskilled	46.7% (28)

(ways to compute the summary scores), namely, simple and complex scoring, are available. In simple scoring, the scores assigned to each of the items (none, 1; mild, 2; moderate, 3; severe, 4; and extreme, 5) are summed up without recoding or collapsing response categories. In complex scoring, also known as item response theory-based scoring, multiple levels of difficulty for each WHODAS 2.0 item are allowed for. Each item response (none, mild, moderate, severe, and extreme) is treated separately and the summary score is generated with a computer by differentially weighting the items and the levels of severity. Overall test-retest reliability of the scale is 0.94; reliability of each of the six domains ranges from 0.86 to 0.92.

3. Data Analysis

Data were entered in MS-Excel and analyzed in IBM SPSS version 21 (IBM Inc.) software. Categorical variables were summarized as counts and proportions, while numerical variables were summarized as mean and standard deviation. Prevalence was reported as proportion with its 95% confidence interval. Sociodemographic details, clinical data and scores of various scales were compared between asthmatics with and without panic disorder using Chi-square and unpaired t-test appropriately. Scores across the various domains of scales where weightage for each domain was equal were compared by related measure ANOVA which is popularly known as repeated measure ANOVA. A p value less than 0.05 was considered statistically significant.

4. Results

A total of 73 patients of asthma were screened for eligibility and administered consent to achieve desired sample size of 60 willing participants. Table 1 demonstrates the demographic profile of the study participants (Table 1).

Table 2 shows the profile of asthma with respect to duration, treatment taken, family history, and any substance abuse. Mean duration of bronchial asthma in this study group was 7.8 years. 66.7% (40 out of 60) of the participants were on treatment with both inhaler and oral drugs whereas 33.3% (20) were on inhaler only. 26.7% (16) of the patients were on (oral) steroid treatment. The majority (66.7%, i.e., 40) of the participants had history of multiple hospitalizations for asthma. Family history of bronchial asthma was found in only (12) 20% of the subjects and only 4 participants (6.7%) had history of psychiatric illness in the family. History of smoking was found in 53.3% (32) of the subjects while only 8 subjects (13.3%) had history of alcohol consumption. Other comorbid medical conditions like hypertension and chronic obstructive pulmonary disease were present in only 6.7% (4) of the subjects. Sixty percent (36) of the participants were suffering from moderate grade asthma whereas 33.3% (20) had mild asthma and only 4 (6.7%) had severe asthma (Table 2).

Table 2: Profile of asthma patients.

Variable	Number	Percent
Duration of asthma [mean (SD), years]	7.8	(4.0)
Treatment received		
Oral drugs and inhaler	40	(66.7)
Only inhaler	20	(33.3)
On steroid treatment	16	(26.7)
≤3 years	4	(25.0)
4–6 years	3	(18.8)
7–9 years	5	(31.3)
10–12 years	4	(25.0)
Hospitalizations		
Nil	4	(6.7)
1 to 5	16	(26.7)
Multiple (>5)	40	(66.7)
Family H/O asthma	12	(20.0)
Family H/O psychiatric disorder	4	(6.7)
H/O of exposure to smoking	32	(53.3)
H/O of alcohol consumption	8	(13.3)
Presence of medical comorbidity	4	(6.7)
Severity of asthma		
Mild	20	(33.3)
Moderate	36	(60.0)
Severe	4	(6.7)

This study (Table 3) that 33.3% (20) (95% CI 22.7 to 45.9) of the participants had panic disorder (PD), 16.7% (10) (95% CI 9.3 to 28.0) had adjustment disorder, and 13.3% (8) (95% CI 6.9 to 24.1) suffered panic attacks only (not fulfilling the criteria for panic disorder). Around 20% (12) (95% CI 11.8 to 31.8) did not have any diagnosable psychiatric disorder. Others had mild depression and mixed anxiety depression (Table 3).

60% (36) of the patients had 4 or more panic symptoms (not satisfying the criteria for panic attack). Out of this group, the most common symptoms were "sensations of shortness of breath or smothering," "feeling of choking," and "fear of dying" found in 83.3%. As these symptoms are similar to those of acute attack of asthma, these patients thought they have an acute episode of asthma while experiencing the above symptoms but they simultaneously explained some other symptoms which made us diagnose them as panic symptoms. Other symptoms were chest discomfort (72.2%), palpitations

TABLE 3: Profile of psychiatric problems and panic symptoms.

Variable	Number	Percent
Psychiatric problems ($n = 60$)		
Nil	12	(20.0)
Adjustment disorder	10	(16.7)
Mixed anxiety depression	4	(6.7)
Mild depression	6	(10.0)
Panic attacks (only)	8	(13.3)
Panic disorder	20	(33.3)
H/O of psychiatric treatment ($n = 48$)		
Benzodiazepines (BZDs), psychotherapy	20	(41.7)
Selective Serotonin Reuptake Inhibitors, BZDs	28	(58.3)
Presence of any panic symptom ($n = 60$)	36	(60.0)
Number of panic symptoms ($n = 36$)		
4	2	5.6
5	5	13.9
6	9	25.0
7	11	30.6
8	7	19.4
9	2	5.6
Number of panic attacks ($n = 28$)		
2	4	14.3
4	8	28.6
5 or more	16	57.1
Severity of panic disorder ($n = 20$)		
Mild	5	25.0
Severe	14	70.0
Very severe	1	5.0

TABLE 4: WHO QOL BREF scale and WHODAS II mean scores.

QOL domains	Mean	SD
QOL total score	195.5	(20.4)
QOL physical	47.6	(5.3)
QOL psychological	50.5	(7.9)
QOL social	51.1	(6.5)
QOL environmental	46.2	(4.7)
QOL-total		
<200—73.3% (44)		
>200—26.75% (16)		
WHODAS II	18.1	(9.2)
≤18.1—45% (27)		
>18.1—55% (33)		

TABLE 5: Association between panic disorder and WHO Quality of Life BREF scale domains.

QOL dimensions	Mean	95% confidence interval	
		Lower	Upper
No panic disorder			
Physical	49.3	47.8	50.8
Psychological	51.8	49.3	54.2
Social	50.7	48.6	52.7
Environmental	47.6	46.3	49.0
Presence of panic disorder			
Physical	**44.3**	42.1	46.4
Psychological	47.9	44.4	51.4
Social	52.1	49.2	55.0
Environmental	**43.5**	41.5	45.4

(58.33%), sweating (50%), tingling sensations in the extremities (47.2%), trembling of body (41.67%), feeling dizzy and unsteady (36.11%), and feeling of losing control (30.55%).

58.3% (28) of the patients with psychiatric diagnosis required treatment with psychotropic medications (Selective Serotonin Reuptake Inhibitors (SSRIs) and short course of Benzodiazepines (BZDs)) whereas 41.7% (20) were started on psychotherapy and BZDs on "as and when needed" basis. Though symptoms pattern was variable, 28 (46.7%) patients (out of total 60 patients) had diagnosable panic attack (only panic attacks (13.3%) + panic disorder (33.3%)) according to DSM IV TR. Out of this group, 57.1% (16 out of 28) had more than 4 panic attacks during the course of asthma. When patients of panic disorder were assessed for severity with Panic and Agoraphobia scale (PAS), 70% (14 out of 20) were found having "severe PD" whereas 25% (5 out of 20) had "mild PD."

In this study, 4 participants had panic symptoms (not diagnosable with panic attacks or panic disorder) before they developed asthma, out of which 3 had aggravation of panic symptoms during/after every attack of acute asthma. Subsequently, one turned up into panic disorder and the other two were diagnosed as having panic attacks. Out of 4, one continued to show panic symptoms only (not diagnosable with panic attacks or panic disorder). Further, it could not be differentiated whether panic symptoms newly developed in asthma patients were due to reaction to the severity of asthma or induced by asthma medication.

5. Quality of Life

In this study, 44 (73.3%) of the participants had poor quality of life with the total score of less than 200 on WHOQOL BREF scale (mean: 195.5 and standard deviation: 20.4). The mean score of disability on WHODAS II was 18.1 (standard deviation: 9.2). 55% (33) of the subjects had disability score of more than 18.1 (Table 4).

We also compared the scores of each domain of QOL among the participants with and without panic disorder. This was done by related measure ANOVA popularly known as repeated measure ANOVA. QOL scores among those without panic disorders were similar across all the domains. However, QOL scores were statistically significantly lower in physical and environmental dimensions among those with panic disorder (Table 5).

Though statistically nonsignificant, the majority of patients with moderate and severe asthma had quality of life score of less than 200. All the subjects with severe panic disorder as per the PAS scores were having poor quality of life with score of less than 200 which was statistically significant.

Table 6: Association between severity of asthma and PD with QOL.

	QOL				
	<200		>200		p value
	Number	Percent	Number	Percent	
Severity of asthma					
Mild	12	27.3%	8	50.0%	
Moderate	28	63.6%	8	50.0%	
Severe	4	9.1%	0	0.0%	0.162
Presence of PD					
No	28	63.6%	12	75.0%	
Yes	16	36.4%	4	25.0%	0.409
PAS					
Mild	1	2.3%	4	25.0%	
NA	28	63.6%	12	75.0%	
Severe	14	31.8%	0	0.0%	**0.005**
Very severe	1	2.3%	0	0.0%	

Table 7: Comparison between WHODAS II and QOL.

	QOL					
	<200		>200		Total	
	Mean	SD	Mean	SD	Mean	SD
WHODAS	20.91	8.32	10.31	6.98	18.08	9.23

This study also showed that the mere presence of asthma and absence of panic disorder can also lead to poor quality of life as indicated by 63.6% of the participants without panic disorder having QOL score less than 200 (Table 6).

On comparing the quality of life with disability (though statistically not significant), it was found that the more the disability score, the poorer the quality of life (score < 200) (Table 7).

Statistically significant difference was found between WHODAS score and severity of panic disorder and asthma. The more severe the panic disorder or asthma, the higher the disability ($p < 0.01$).

6. Discussion

Asthma is a major health problem, with increasing prevalence, morbidity, and mortality in the last few decades. It is also among the 4 most common chronic disorders in adult population, with a prevalence of approximately 5% [20]. Along with the environmental factors like indoor allergens, psychological factors are increasingly recognized to influence the onset and course of asthma. Literature shows that the prevalence of panic disorder is much more in patients with asthma compared to general population. This study is among the very few Indian studies to focus on this association with study of symptom profile and the prevalence of panic disorder in asthma and its effects on quality of life and functional disability.

The mean age of participants in this study was 37 ± 7.4. In a study [21] titled Demographic and Environmental Factors in Patients of Bronchial Asthma, including 398 subjects, mean age of the subjects was found as 35.5 years ± 12.19 years with the range between 18 and 60 years. Most of the participants were married and this was explainable by the mean age of the study population. 46.7% of the subjects were doing unskilled work which may be due to the rural and suburban population in the catering area of the institute. Family history of bronchial asthma was found in only 12% of study population. This finding was contradictory to the findings of other studies. Some studies documented that at least one of the first-degree family members may have asthma, while in few other studies family history of bronchial asthma was observed in 82.1% of patients [22]. We found low prevalence of family history of psychiatric illness in this study. In this study sample, the data related to family history was collected based on the information given by the patients, wherein likelihood of underreporting or not knowing on the part of the participants resulting in lesser prevalence of family history of psychiatric illness is possible.

Mean duration of bronchial asthma in this study was 7.8 ± 4 which suggests the chronic nature of the illness. The majority of the participants were on combination of inhaler and oral medications as 60% of the subjects had moderate grade asthma which is difficult to be managed by inhaler only. Also most of the subjects had history of multiple hospitalizations.

More than half of the subjects had a history of smoking exposure (active or passive). In this study, we found that one-third of the participants had diagnosable panic disorder; another common psychiatric diagnosis was adjustment disorder. Previous data from the studies in clinical and community settings suggest that asthma and mental disorders cooccur more often than expected by chance [23–29]. Several studies have found increased prevalence of anxiety disorder, including panic attacks and symptoms of generalized anxiety disorder (GAD), among clinical samples of patients with asthma [28, 30].

The prevalence of panic disorder in adults is 1% to 3% in community population [31] and 4% to 8% in primary care populations [32]. Many cross-sectional studies in adult population have suggested that the prevalence of panic disorder among patients with asthma ranges from 6.5% to 24% [9, 29].

Most of the adult and child studies of patients with asthma have shown an increased rate of comorbid anxiety disorders [28]. Studies have also shown a relatively specific association between the prevalence of bronchial asthma and panic [33, 34]. The association is specific even after adjusting the differences in demographics and psychiatric comorbidity. Severe asthma is associated with even greater likelihood of panic attacks [33]. Asthma medications can also have anxiogenic properties [35], and anxiety may further enhance the use of asthma medication.

We also found that, among the subjects with panic disorder, around 70% had severe PD which implicates the need to assess and treat the panic disorder, if associated with bronchial asthma.

A large community sample of 4181 adults from Germany, which included physician confirmation of asthma using a physician interview, found that current severe asthma (in the last 4 weeks) was associated with a significantly increased likelihood of having any anxiety disorder including panic disorder. Lifetime severe asthma was also associated with an increased risk of having any anxiety disorder, panic disorder, social phobia, generalized anxiety disorder, and bipolar disorder [13]. Anxiety and depressive disorders are even more common in patients who present with severe life-threatening episodes of asthma as well as those hospitalized with acute asthma exacerbations [36].

In this study, mixed anxiety depression and mild depression were found in around 16.7% of the participants.

Sixty percent of the subjects had some or other panic symptoms which suggests that asthma and panic have strong correlation. Literature shows that this relation can be direct (as the asthmatic attack may mimic panic attack, medications used to treat asthma may cause panic symptoms, and chronicity of the illness also contributes to it) or indirect as panic can be a psychological reaction to the asthma episode and fear about future asthmatic attack.

In this study, we found that the quality of life was impaired (poor) in the majority of the subjects specifically in physical and environmental dimensions. It was also found that presence of panic disorder was associated with significantly lower quality of life in physical and environmental domains. Though the correlation between QOL total score and presence of PD was not significant, the severity of panic disorder was significantly correlated with poor (overall) quality of life. The (feared situation) avoidant behaviour along with the physical limitation due to asthma symptoms may be severely disabling and isolating. This may lead to the functional restriction much greater than objectively measured physiologic level of impairment [37]. It may be speculated that anxiety, panic, and fear avoidance can further manifest with depressive symptoms leading to further deterioration in quality of life. Depressive symptoms are known to affect treatment adherence and lead to a vicious cycle of poorer asthma control and quality of life [38]. This in turn may be manifested in increased utilization of health resources, as suggested by a study including 1406 adult asthma patients in whom the asthma quality of life significantly predicted subsequent Emergency Department utilization [39]. Thus, poor asthma quality of life has an impact on treatment and asthma control along with many aspects of the individual's personal and social life. In turn, it can also be said that better treatment of asthma may also be worth achieving, if it is the asthma that drives the panic.

The mean score on disability scale was 18.1 and more than half of the participants had scored more than 18.1. Panic disorder severity was also associated with more disability. The disability score was still higher in those with impaired quality of life (score $\leq$ 200). Quality of life in turn was impaired more with moderate to severe asthma and associated severe panic disorder. These correlation findings can be explained, as asthma and panic disorder and its severity can cause physical disability and limitations in social and routine activities (because of the symptom profile and effect of capacity of a person) and overall functioning which in turn affects the quality of life. Literature shows that the negative impact of asthma is usually estimated on the basis of mortality, number of asthma attacks, and number of hospitalizations. However, the effects of the asthma can impair other important aspects, such as the quality of life and physical well-being of patients and can affect performance at school or work [40, 41].

7. Conclusion

Most common panic symptoms found in this study population were "sensations of shortness of breath or smothering," "feeling of choking," and "fear of dying" (found in 83.3% of those with panic symptoms). 46.7% of the participants had diagnosable panic attack according to DSM IV TR and more than half of them had more than 4 panic attacks during the course of asthma.

Panic disorder was found in about 1/3rd of the participants out of which the majority had severe panic disorder. Quality of life was poor in the majority of the subjects with statistically significant impairment in physical and environmental domains found in those with severe PD. Patients with more severe panic disorder and bronchial asthma had more disability. Poor quality of life was found to have positive correlation with disability.

This is an important study to document the extent of comorbidity and whether comorbid anxiety, especially panic disorder, is associated with higher symptom load, impaired functioning, and poor quality of life.

As the comorbid rate was high, future studies need to be planned to enhance the understanding of biological and cognitive mechanisms that might explain this association. Large-scale studies are needed for patients with asthma and panic disorder to help validate the cooccurrence of these 2 conditions by measuring the effect of comorbidity on symptom burden, functioning, adherence to asthma self-care regimens, quality of life, and medical costs for controlling asthma.

Limitations

Though this study is among the very few Indian studies to focus on symptom profile and prevalence of panic disorder in asthma, there are few limitations of the study that cannot be overlooked. The sample size of this study was small for the aim of finding the prevalence of panic disorder in patients with asthma. Secondly as the study was carried out in only one centre with a nonrandom selection of sample, it is hard to determine what a true point prevalence of panic disorder is. As this was a cross-sectional single interview study, the answers to the questionnaire might have been affected by the state of mind at the time of interview and no follow-up assessment was done. Psychiatric comorbidities that may be present along with the panic disorder were not analyzed statistically. Lastly, though it was expected that patients attending a tertiary referral centre are likely to be on medium to higher grade of treatments, details about the asthma medications, exact doses, and compliance could not be analyzed statistically for the correlation.

Conflict of Interests

The authors declare that there is no conflict of interests regarding the publication of this paper.

References

[1] N. Pearce, J. Douwes, and R. Beasley, "The rise and rise of asthma: a new paradigm for the new millennium?" *Journal of Epidemiology and Biostatistics*, vol. 5, no. 1, pp. 5–16, 2000.

[2] S. Holt and N. Pearce, "Asthma in New Zealand: myths and realities," *New Zealand Medical Journal*, vol. 113, no. 1103, pp. 39–41, 2000.

[3] E. Brown, D. Khan, and S. Mahadi, "Psychiatric diagnosis in inner city outpatients with moderate to severe asthma," *The International Journal of Psychiatry in Medicine*, vol. 30, pp. 295–297, 2000.

[4] R. D. Goodwin, M. Olfson, S. Shea et al., "Asthma and mental disorders in primary care," *General Hospital Psychiatry*, vol. 25, no. 6, pp. 479–483, 2003.

[5] N. Afari, K. B. Schmaling, S. Barnhart, and D. Buchwald, "Psychiatric comorbidity and functional status in adult patients with asthma," *Journal of Clinical Psychology in Medical Settings*, vol. 8, no. 4, pp. 245–252, 2001.

[6] I. Nascimento, A. E. Nardi, A. M. Valença et al., "Psychiatric disorders in asthmatic outpatients," *Psychiatry Research*, vol. 110, no. 1, pp. 73–80, 2002.

[7] V. M. Deshmukh, B. G. Toelle, T. Usherwood, B. O'Grady, and C. R. Jenkins, "Anxiety, panic and adult asthma: a cognitive-behavioral perspective," *Respiratory Medicine*, vol. 101, no. 2, pp. 194–202, 2007.

[8] C. T. Thoren and F. Petermann, "Reviewing asthma and anxiety," *Respiratory Medicine*, vol. 94, no. 5, pp. 409–415, 2000.

[9] W. J. Katon, L. Richardson, P. Lozano, and E. McCauley, "The relationship of asthma and anxiety disorders," *Psychosomatic Medicine*, vol. 66, no. 3, pp. 349–355, 2004.

[10] A. G. Gift, "Psychologic and physiologic aspects of acute dyspnea in asthmatics," *Nursing Research*, vol. 40, no. 4, pp. 196–199, 1991.

[11] P. Spinhoven, A. S. Van Peski-Oosterbaan, A. J. W. Van der Does, L. N. A. Willems, and P. J. Sterk, "Association of anxiety with perception of histamine induced bronchoconstriction in patients with asthma," *Thorax*, vol. 52, no. 2, pp. 149–152, 1997.

[12] R. E. Carr, "Panic disorder and asthma," *Journal of Asthma*, vol. 36, no. 2, pp. 143–152, 1999.

[13] R. D. Goodwin, F. Jacobi, and W. Thefeld, "Mental disorders and asthma in the community," *Archives of General Psychiatry*, vol. 60, no. 11, pp. 1125–1130, 2003.

[14] G. Hasler, P. J. Gergen, D. G. Kleinbaum et al., "Asthma and panic in young adults. A 20-year prospective community study," *The American Journal of Respiratory and Critical Care Medicine*, vol. 171, no. 11, pp. 1224–1230, 2005.

[15] K. L. Lavoie, S. L. Bacon, S. Barone, A. Cartier, B. Ditto, and M. Labrecque, "What is worse for asthma control and quality of life: depressive disorders, anxiety disorders, or both?" *Chest*, vol. 130, no. 4, pp. 1039–1047, 2006.

[16] J. M. Feldman, P. M. Lehrer, S. Borson, T. S. Hallstrand, and M. I. Siddique, "Health care use and quality of life among patients with asthma and panic disorder," *Journal of Asthma*, vol. 42, no. 3, pp. 179–184, 2005.

[17] American Psychiatric Association, *Diagnostic and Statistical Manual of Mental Disorders*, American Psychiatric Association, Washington, DC, USA, 4th edition, 1994.

[18] A. Potoczek, "The panic disorder prevalence and it's influence on the severity of aspirin-induced asthma," *Archives of Psychiatry and Psychotherapy*, vol. 13, no. 1, pp. 17–20, 2011.

[19] K. Yamada, "Quality of life in patients treated with Kampo medicine: a complementary alternative to modern medicine," *Journal of Alternative and Complementary Medicine*, vol. 12, no. 8, pp. 799–803, 2006.

[20] T. G. Rundall, S. M. Shortell, M. C. Wang et al., "As good as it gets? Chronic care management in nine leading US physician organisations," *The British Medical Journal*, vol. 325, no. 7370, pp. 958–961, 2002.

[21] S. Kaur, D. Behera, D. Gupta, and S. K. Verma, "Demographic and Environmental factors in patients of bronchial asthma," *Indian Journal of Allergy, Asthma and Immunology*, vol. 22, no. 2, pp. 85–89, 2008.

[22] F. Forastiere, J. Balmes, M. Scarinci, and I. B. Tager, "Occupation, asthma, and chronic respiratory symptoms in a community sample of older women," *The American Journal of Respiratory and Critical Care Medicine*, vol. 157, no. 6, pp. 1864–1870, 1998.

[23] J. W. Goethe, R. Maljanian, S. H. Wolf, P. Hernandez, and Y. Cabrera, "The impact of depressive symptoms on the functional status of inner-city patients with asthma," *Annals of Allergy, Asthma and Immunology*, vol. 87, no. 3, pp. 205–210, 2001.

[24] I. Nascimento, A. E. Nardi, A. M. Valença et al., "Psychiatric disorders in asthmatic outpatients," *Psychiatry Research*, vol. 110, no. 1, pp. 73–80, 2002.

[25] H. Swadi, "Psychiatric morbidity in a community sample of Arab children with asthma," *Journal of Tropical Pediatrics*, vol. 47, no. 2, pp. 106–107, 2001.

[26] G. Vila, C. Nollet-Clemençon, J. de Blic, M.-C. Mouren-Simeoni, and P. Scheinmann, "Prevalence of DSM-IV anxiety and affective disorders in a pediatric population of asthmatic children and adolescents," *Journal of Affective Disorders*, vol. 58, no. 3, pp. 223–231, 2000.

[27] A. N. Ortega, S. E. Huertas, G. Canino, R. Ramirez, and M. Rubio-Stipec, "Childhood asthma, chronic illness, and psychiatric disorders," *Journal of Nervous and Mental Disease*, vol. 190, no. 5, pp. 275–281, 2002.

[28] R. D. Goodwin, D. S. Pine, and C. W. Hoven, "Asthma and panic attacks among youth in the community," *Journal of Asthma*, vol. 40, no. 2, pp. 139–145, 2003.

[29] R. D. Goodwin and D. S. Pine, "Respiratory disease and panic attacks among adults in the United States," *Chest*, vol. 122, no. 2, pp. 645–650, 2002.

[30] J. Von Behren, R. Kreutzer, and A. Hernandez, "Self-reported asthma prevalence in adults in California," *Journal of Asthma*, vol. 39, no. 5, pp. 429–440, 2002.

[31] R. C. Kessler, K. A. McGonagle, S. Zhao et al., "Lifetime and 12-month prevalence of DSM-III-R psychiatric disorders in the United States. Results from the National Comorbidity Survey," *Archives of General Psychiatry*, vol. 51, pp. 8–19, 1994.

[32] T. S. Zaubler and W. Katon, "Panic disorder and medical comorbidity: a review of the medical and psychiatric literature," *Bulletin of the Menninger Clinic*, vol. 60, no. 2, supplement A, pp. A12–A38, 1996.

[33] R. D. Goodwin and W. W. Eaton, "Asthma and the risk of panic attacks among adults in the community," *Psychological Medicine*, vol. 33, no. 5, pp. 879–885, 2003.

[34] A. Ten Brinke, M. E. Ouwerkerk, E. H. Bel, and P. Spinhoven, "Similar psychological characteristics in mild and severe asthma," *Journal of Psychosomatic Research*, vol. 50, no. 1, pp. 7–10, 2001.

[35] N. W. Dahlem, R. A. Kinsman, and D. J. Horton, "Panic-fear in asthma: requests for as-needed medications in relation to pulmonary function measurements," *The Journal of Allergy and Clinical Immunology*, vol. 60, no. 5, pp. 295–300, 1977.

[36] J. Kolbe, W. Fergusson, M. Vamos, and J. Garrett, "Case-control study of severe life threatening asthma (SLTA) in adults: psychological factors," *Thorax*, vol. 57, no. 4, pp. 317–322, 2002.

[37] P. M. Yellowlees and R. S. Kalucy, "Psychobiological aspects of asthma and the consequent research implications," *Chest*, vol. 97, no. 3, pp. 628–634, 1990.

[38] R. D. Goldney, R. Ruffin, L. J. Fisher, and D. H. Wilson, "Asthma symptoms associated with depression and lower quality of life: a population survey," *Medical Journal of Australia*, vol. 178, no. 9, pp. 437–441, 2003.

[39] D. J. Magid, D. Houry, J. Ellis, E. Lyons, and J. S. Rumsfeld, "Health-related quality of life predicts emergency department utilization for patients with asthma," *Annals of Emergency Medicine*, vol. 43, no. 5, pp. 551–557, 2004.

[40] T. M. L. Eagan, A. Gulsvik, G. E. Eide, and P. S. Bakke, "The effect of educational level on the incidence of asthma and respiratory symptoms," *Respiratory Medicine*, vol. 98, no. 8, pp. 730–736, 2004.

[41] L. Ellison-Loschmann, J. Sunyer, E. Plana et al., "Socioeconomic status, asthma and chronic bronchitis in a large community-based study," *European Respiratory Journal*, vol. 29, no. 5, pp. 897–905, 2007.

5

Prevalence and Factors Associated with Perceived Stigma among Patients with Epilepsy in Ethiopia

Tolesa Fanta,[1] Telake Azale,[2] Dawit Assefa,[1] and Mekbit Getachew[1]

[1] *Amanuel Mental Specialized Hospital, Addis Ababa, Ethiopia*
[2] *Department of Psychiatry, Faculty of Medicine and Health Science, University of Gondar, Gondar, Ethiopia*

Correspondence should be addressed to Tolesa Fanta; ftolesa@yahoo.com

Academic Editor: Veit Roessner

Background. Epilepsy stigma is considered to be one of the most important factors that have a negative influence on people with epilepsy. Among all types of stigma perceived stigma further exerts stress and restricts normal participation in society. *Methods.* Hospital based cross-sectional study was conducted from May 1, 2013, to May 30, 2013. All patients with epilepsy in Ethiopia were source population. The sample size was determined using single population proportion formula and 347 subjects were selected by using systematic random sampling method. Data was analyzed by using SPSS version 20. *Results.* A total of 346 participants with mean age of 29.3 ± 8.5 SD participated with a response rate of 99.7%. The prevalence of perceived stigma was 31.2%. Age range between 18 and 24 [AOR = 2.84, 95%CI: 1.02, 7.92], difficulty to attend follow-up because of stigma [AOR = 3.15, 95%CI: 1.19, 8.34], seizure related injury [AOR = 1.88, 95%CI: 1.12, 3.15], and contagion belief [AOR = 1.88, 95%CI: 1.10, 5.08] were significantly associated with perceived stigma. *Conclusions.* Perceived stigma was found to be a common problem among patients suffering from epilepsy. The results reinforce the need for creating awareness among patients with epilepsy and addressing misconceptions attached to epilepsy.

1. Introduction

Epilepsy is a chronic brain disorder characterized by recurrent derangement of the nervous system due to sudden excessive discharge of the cerebral neurons [1]. It is a neurological condition that knows no geographic, social, or racial boundaries, occurring in men and women and affecting people of all ages [2]. It affects approximately 50 million people worldwide [3].

The population prevalence of epilepsy varies across countries from 0.5 to 5%. The higher levels tend to be seen in developing countries where fewer than 50% of cases are on medication [4]. In a large community-based epidemiological study, the prevalence of epilepsy in Ethiopia was reported as 5.2/1000 population [5, 6]. The incidence was 64/100,000 population as reported in a community-based study conducted in Mescal and Marko districts of rural central Ethiopia [7].

Stigma is social process or related personal experience characterized by exclusion, rejection, blame, and devaluation and is a phenomenon associated with many chronic health conditions. Stigma and its psychosocial consequences cause indescribable suffering to those who are stigmatized. In addition, stigma has indirect but strongly negative implications for public health efforts to combat the diseases concerned. Epilepsy has a considerable psychological and emotional impact on PWE. Uncontrolled seizures can be very unsettling. People may fear even going outside their homes unaccompanied. They may fear what people might think of them if they were to have a seizure in public [8].

Across the world and throughout history, epilepsy has been a culturally devalued condition and awareness about epilepsy is usually very low. Such devaluing and lack of awareness often make people with epilepsy be stigmatized, discriminated, and excluded from society to problems at work and economic difficulties, bearing a psychosocial burden as well as inappropriate treatment [9–21]. From the patient's view, the diagnosis of epilepsy triggers a change in perception, bringing on fears of being different and anxiety about the future in the community, with apprehension about getting a job or starting a family [22–31]. Understanding and reducing epilepsy-associated stigma are one of the stated aims of the World Health Organization's Global Campaign against Epilepsy "Out of the Shadows" initiative [32].

According to study conducted among more than 5,000 patients living in 15 countries in Europe 51% reported feeling stigmatized with 18% reporting feeling highly stigmatized and people with epilepsy who experienced injury during seizure attack reported high feeling of stigma [30]. Another study conducted in Via Christi Comprehensive Epilepsy Center, Wichita, KS, USA, on PWE indicates that about 34% of the respondents who were on AEDs indicated they had belief that the general public had negative feelings and reactions towards individuals with epilepsy [33].

The case-control study conducted in Cambodia reveals that about 46% cases reported highest stigma score [34]. Another institutional based cross-sectional study conducted at Brooklyn Hospital Academic Medical Center on patients with epilepsy reveals that 69% of respondents fulfill the criteria of perceived stigma [35]. According to community-based cross-sectional study conducted in Campinas, Brazil, on 1850 PWE, the median of the general stigma score was 42 and low educational level, female sex, and religion were sociodemographic factors that made great association with perceived stigma [36]. According to the institutional based cross-sectional study conducted in Iran, the Gulf, and Near East on 3,889 people with epilepsy attending epilepsy clinic, about one-third (~33%) of the patients felt stigmatized by their epilepsy [37]. A community-based cross-sectional study conducted in Benin reveals that the proportion of PWE who felt stigmatized by their condition was 68.7%, and 38.8% of them reported high feelings of stigma [38]. According to case-control study conducted in Zambia, Lusaka, on 169 adults who were on follow-up at epilepsy clinic the median stigma score was 2.5 and higher stigma scores were associated with community disclosure, forced disclosure either through a public seizure or through someone else revealing their condition to the community. People who believed epilepsy to be contagious also had higher felt stigma [39]. A descriptive cross-sectional survey conducted in Kilifi, Kenya, on 673 respondents reported that 33% felt stigmatized as measured by the KSSE; and younger age was significantly associated with perceived stigma [40]. According to the institutional based cross-sectional study which was conducted in Butajira, Ethiopia, on 831 respondents the prevalence estimate of perceived stigma was 81%. Male sex and age group of 45 years and above were sociodemographic factors which were significantly associated with PS.

Those who had more frequent seizures also reported experiencing more stigma compared to those who had less frequent seizures [41].

2. Objective

The aim of the study is to assess the prevalence of perceived stigma and factors associated with it among patients with epilepsy in Ethiopia.

3. Method

Institutional based quantitative cross-sectional study was conducted from May 1, 2013, to May 30, 2013, at Amanuel Mental Specialized Hospital which is the only mental hospital in the country. The minimum number of samples required for this study was determined by using single population proportion formula and found to be 347. The adults aged 18 years and above were included in the study and subjects who had major cognitive impairments or intellectual disability were not included in the study. A systematic random sampling technique was used to select participants. People with epilepsy who were already diagnosed by neuropsychiatrist as having epilepsy and were on regular follow-up at Amanuel Hospital Epilepsy Department were interviewed using the Kilifi Stigma Scale of Epilepsy which was developed and validated in Kilifi, Kenya, with high internal consistency, Cronbach's α of 0.91, and excellent test-retest reliability with r of 0.92. It is a simple three-point Likert scoring system scored as "not at all" (score of 0), "sometimes" (score of 1), and "always" (score of 2). It has fifteen items and a total score was calculated by addition of all item scores. The score above the value on 66th percentile of the data indicated presence of perceived/felt stigma [40, 42]. Questions used to assess sociodemographic data and other relevant information were designed by the investigator.

There were also some questions to assess clinical factors, patients' belief about a nature of their illness, and disclosure status of the patient. Data was collected by four trained psychiatry nurses and data collectors were supervised by two B.S. nurses. The questionnaire was translated to local language (Amharic) to be understood by all participants and translated back to English. The translation and back translation were done by neuropsychiatrists and neurologists working in Amanuel Hospital. Data was entered, cleaned, and stored by using EPI info version 3.5.1 and then exported into Statistical Package for the Social Sciences (SPSS) version 20 for analysis. Frequency and percentage were used to describe the data. Crude and adjusted OR was analyzed using logistic regression and the level of significance of association was determined at p value < 0.05. Ethical clearance was obtained from the Institutional Review Board of College of Medicine and Health Sciences, University of Gondar, and from Amanuel Mental Specialized Hospital. Written informed consent for participation in the study was obtained from participants just after start of the interview.

4. Results

A total of 347 patients with epilepsy were recruited in the study. Out of 347 patients with epilepsy 346 responded to the questionnaire with overall response rate of 99.7%.

4.1. Sociodemographic Characteristics. All of the respondents were in the age group of 18–57 years with the mean age of 29.3 ± 8.5 SD. Among all participants, 216 (62.4%) were male. The participants from urban area were (268) (77.5%) and the rest were from rural area. Among the total study subjects

Table 1: Distribution of study subjects by sociodemographic factors.

Variables	(*n*/346)	(%)
Age		
18–24	112	32.4
25–34	136	39.3
35–44	57	16.5
≥45	41	11.8
Sex		
Male	216	62.4
Female	130	37.6
Residence		
Rural	78	22.5
Urban	268	77.5
Ethnicity		
Amhara	122	35.5
Oromo	110	31.8
Tigre	26	7.5
Gurage	78	22.5
Others	10	2.9
Marital status		
Married	125	36.1
Single	177	51.2
Divorced	23	6.6
Widowed	21	6.1
Religion		
Orthodox	232	67.1
Protestant	52	15
Muslim	57	16.5
Educational status		
No formal education	45	13
1–8	145	41.9
9–12	123	35.5
12+	33	9.5
Occupational status		
Employed	134	38.7
Farmer	50	14.5
Student	49	14.2
Daily laborer	97	28
Others	16	4.6

232 (67.1%) were Orthodox religion followers and 177 (51.2%) were single (Table 1).

4.2. Description of Respondents by Clinical Factors. Majority of the study subjects (150 (43.4%)) were living with epilepsy for more than 11 years and 114 (33%) were on AEDs for more than 11 years. Among the study subjects who had seizure in past three months (81 (23.4%)) majority of them (58 (71.6%)) reported that they experienced seizure less than six times in past three months (Table 2).

4.3. Description of Respondents by Disclosure Status, Patient's Contagion Belief, and Causal Belief of Epilepsy. Majority of the respondents (241 (69.7%)) reported that their condition is disclosed to the society, and among these 196 (81.3%) reported that their condition is disclosed involuntarily (attack occurred at public place and/or other persons disclosed their condition). Forty-two percent of the participants believe that the cause of their epilepsy is evil spirit (Table 3).

Table 2: Distribution of study subjects by clinical factors.

Variables	(*n*/346)	(%)
Duration of the illness		
≤1 yr	21	6.1
2–5 yr	90	26
6–10 yr	85	24.6
≥11 yr	150	43.4
Duration on AEDs		
≤1 yr	56	16.2
2–5 yr	106	30.6
6–10 yr	70	20.2
≥11 yr	114	32.9
Seizure in last 3 m		
No	265	76.6
Yes	81	23.4
Frequency of seizure in three months		
≤6x/3 m	58	71.6
>6x/3 m	23	28.4
Difficulty in attending follow-up because of fear of stigma		
No	312	90.2
Yes	34	9.8
Difficulty in taking AEDs daily because of fear of stigma		
Yes	28	8.1
No	318	91.9
Injury during seizure		
No	212	61.3
Yes	134	38.7

4.4. Perceived Stigma Scores of Participants. Most of the participants reported that they feel disappointed in their self which is followed by feeing embarrassed (Table 4). The lowest score of the data was 0 and the highest score was 30. The lower, median, and upper quartile values were 1, 4, and 9, respectively. The 66th percentile of the data was 7, so that scores above 7 were considered to show the PWE who felt stigmatized (Figure 1). Accordingly, out of the 346 study subjects recruited in the study, 31.2% fulfilled the criteria for perceived stigma as measured by the KSSE.

4.5. Multivariate Analysis of Perceived Stigma and Explanatory Variables. The multivariate logistic regression which controls the effect of confounding variables was used by taking all covariates into account simultaneously for perceived stigma. Analysis was done after adjusting for age, residence, educational status, difficulty in attending follow-up, difficulty in

Table 3: Distribution of study subjects by disclosure status, patient's contagion belief, and causal belief of epilepsy.

Variables	(n/346)	(%)
Cause of epilepsy		
Supernatural force	90	26
Evil spirit	147	42.5
Other	15	4.3
I do not know	94	27.2
Contagion belief		
No	306	88.4
Yes	40	11.6
Disclosure status		
Not disclosed	105	30.3
Disclosed	241	69.7
Way of disclosure		
Voluntary disclosure	45	18.7
Forced disclosure	196	81.3

Table 4: Proportion of responses to KSSE by study participants.

	Items	n/346	%
1	Do you feel different from other people?	119	34.4
2	Do you feel lonely?	125	36.1
3	Do you feel embarrassed?	166	48
4	Do you feel disappointed in yourself?	181	52.3
5	Do you feel that you cannot have a rewarding life?	135	39
6	Do you feel that you cannot contribute anything in society?	86	24.8
7	Do you feel that you cannot join others in public places?	106	30.6
8	Do you feel that other people are uncomfortable with you?	105	30.4
9	Do you feel that other people do not want to go to occasions with you?	80	23.1
10	Do you feel that other people treat you like an inferior person?	110	31.8
11	Do you feel that other people would prefer to avoid you?	106	30.6
12	Do you feel that other people avoid exchanging greetings with you?	62	17.9
13	Do you feel that you are mistreated by other people?	60	17.3
14	Do you feel that other people discriminate against you?	83	24
15	Do you feel that other people treat you like an outcast?	51	14.7

taking medication daily, seizure related injury, and contagion belief of epilepsy. Accordingly age group between 18 and 24 years were about 2.8 times more likely to have perceived stigma as compared to age group ≥ 45 years (AOR = 2.84, 95% CI: 1.02, 7.92). Those who reported difficulty in attending follow-up because of stigma were 3 times more likely to have

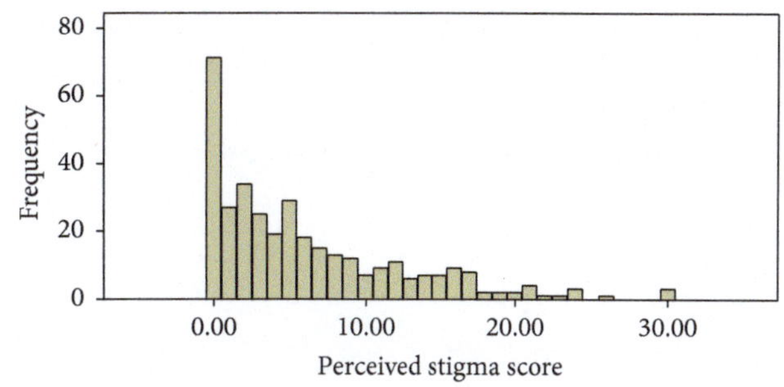

Figure 1: Scores for the Kilifi Stigma Scale for Epilepsy.

perceived stigma compared to those who have no difficulty in attending follow-up because of stigma (AOR = 3.15, 95% CI: 1.19, 8.34). The patients with epilepsy who had seizure related injury were about 1.8 times more likely to have perceived stigma when compared to those who have no seizure related injury (AOR = 1.88, 95% CI: 1.12, 3.15). The participants who believe that epilepsy is contagious were 2.4 times more likely to have perceived stigma as compared to those who believe that epilepsy is not contagious (AOR = 2.37, 95% CI: 1.10, 5.08) (Table 5).

5. Discussion

The study found that the prevalence of perceived stigma among patients with epilepsy in Ethiopia in year 2013 was 31.2%. The prevalence of PS in current study is lower when compared with other studies conducted in Butajira, Ethiopia, which was 81% [41]. The discrepancy might be due to difference in study setting and difference in instrument used. The prevalence of PS in our study is in line with that of Kenya which was 33% [40].

The prevalence of perceived stigma in our study is lower when compared to that of Benin which was 68.7% [38]. The variation might be due to difference in instrument they used which was Jacoby Stigma Scale and difference in study setting. The study conducted in Brazil and Zambia reported that the median stigma score of patients with epilepsy was 42 and 2.5, respectively [36, 39]. The median score of current study which is 4 is lower when compared with median stigma score in Brazil and is higher when compared to that of Zambia. This could be due to instrument difference which was Stigma Scale of Epilepsy in case of Brazil and Jacoby Stigma Scale in case of Zambia. The other reason might be population difference.

The prevalence of perceived stigma reported by our study is lower when compared with the studies conducted in European countries, Cambodia, Kansas, and Brooklyn which was 51%, 46%, 34%, and 69%, respectively [30, 33–35]. This is explained by population difference, instrument difference which was Jacoby Stigma Scale in all, large sample size they used, and difference in study setting. In other ways the prevalence of perceived stigma found in our study is in line with that of Iran, the Gulf, and Near East, which was 33% [37].

Age group between 18 and 24 were more likely to have perceived stigma (AOR = 2.84, 95% CI: 1.02, 7.92) when

TABLE 5: Factors associated with perceived stigma of people with epilepsy (bivariate and multivariate analysis).

Explanatory variables	Perceived stigma		Bivariate and multivariate analysis	
	Yes	No	COR (95% CI)	AOR (95% CI)
Age				
18–24	38	74	2.49 (1.01, 6.15)	**2.84 (1.02, 7.92)****
25–34	40	96	2.02 (0.83, 4.94)	2.23 (0.82, 6.06)
35–44	23	34	3.29 (1.25, 8.67)	3.04 (0.34, 9.13)
≥45	7	34	1.00	1.00
Educational status				
No formal education	22	23	2.99 (1.11, 8.03)	2.52 (0.84, 7.58)
1–8	49	96	1.59 (0.67, 3.79)	1.24 (0.47, 3.28)
9–12	29	94	0.96 (0.39, 2.37)	0.72 (0.27, 1.96)
12+	8	25	1.00	1.00
Residence				
Rural	33	45	1.89 (1.12, 3.18)	0.65 (0.34, 1.22)
Urban	75	193	1.00	1.00
Difficulty in attending follow-up				
Yes	23	11	5.58 (2.61, 11.95)	**3.15 (1.19, 8.34)***
No	85	227	1.00	1.00
Difficulty in taking medication daily				
Yes	18	10	4.56 (2.03, 10.26)	2.02 (0.70, 5.81)
No	90	228	1.00	1.00
Injury during seizure attack				
Yes	53	81	1.87 (1.18, 2.93)	**1.88 (1.12, 3.15)***
No	55	157	1.00	1.00
Contagion belief				
Yes	20	20	2.48 (1.27, 4.83)	**2.37 (1.10, 5.08)***
No	88	218	1.00	1.00

*Statistically significant at p value <0.05. **Statistically significant at p value <0.001.

compared to those who were 44 years and above. This result is in line with that of Kenya [40]. This is explained by older people who were less likely to report feeling stigmatized because discriminatory attitudes towards epilepsy may have less importance to them than younger people. The younger people want to fit in with peers.

Participants who reported that they had difficulty in attending follow-up because of fear of stigma were more likely to have perceived stigma (AOR = 3.15, 95% CI: 1.19, 8.34) when compared to those who had no difficulty in attending follow-up because of fear of stigma. This could be due to fear of enacted stigma if the society knows that they were on follow-up for epilepsy case.

Participants who experienced injury during seizure attack were more likely to feel stigmatized (AOR = 1.88, 95% CI: 1.12, 3.15) compared to those who did not experience injury during seizure attack. This finding is in line with that of European countries [30]. This may be explained by the physical deformity and scars due to the fact that injury may easily disclose their condition. The scar and the deformity may also cause another stigma or potentiate the existing stigma.

The participants who believe that epilepsy is contagious were more likely to have perceived stigma compared to those who believe that epilepsy is not contagious (AOR = 2.37, 95% CI: 1.10, 5.08). This result is in line with that of Zambia [39]. The possible explanation is because they thought that the society also believes that epilepsy is contagious, so they felt that they were stigmatized by society.

Among the variables entered into multivariate analysis, residence, educational status, difficulty in taking AEDs daily because of fear of stigma, and disclosure status were not associated with perceived stigma.

6. Conclusion

The prevalence of perceived stigma, even if it seems low, is not negligible and is showing a significant public health issue among patients with epilepsy that requires great emphasis. Age, difficulty in attending follow-up, seizure related injury, and contagion belief were significantly associated with perceived stigma among patients with epilepsy.

Abbreviations

AEDs: Antiepileptic drugs
AMSH: Amanuel Mental Specialized Hospital
KSSE: Kilifi Stigma Scale of Epilepsy
PS: Perceived stigma
PWE: People with epilepsy.

Conflict of Interests

The authors declare that they have no competing interests.

Authors' Contribution

Tolesa Fanta is involved in the design of the study and Telake Azale, Dawit Assefa, and Mekbit Getachew were involved in revising the paper critically for important intellectual content and analysis of data. All authors read and approved the final paper.

Acknowledgments

The study was funded by Amanuel Mental Specialized Hospital. The authors are grateful to Ephraim Mabrate and Ibsa Dagne for providing important materials when they were conducting this research. Their gratitude also goes to all study participants, data collectors, and supervisors.

References

[1] M. Kabir, Z. Iliyasu, I. S. Abubakar, Z. S. Kabir, and A. U. Farinyaro, "Knowledge, attitude and beliefs about epilepsy among adults in a northern Nigerian urban community," *Annals of African Medicine*, vol. 4, no. 3, pp. 107–112, 2005.

[2] J. W. Sander, "The epidemiology of epilepsy revisited," *Current Opinion in Neurology*, vol. 16, no. 2, pp. 165–70, 2003.

[3] A. Jacoby and G. Baker, *Quality of Life in Epilepsy: Beyond Seizure Counts in Assessment and Treatment*, Psychology Press, 2001.

[4] World Health Organization (WHO), *Initiative of Support to People with Epilepsy*, Division of Mental Health, Geneva, Switzerland, 1990.

[5] R. Tekle-Haimanot, M. Abebe, L. Forsgren et al., "Attitudes of rural people in central Ethiopia toward epilepsy," *Social Science and Medicine*, vol. 32, no. 2, pp. 203–209, 1991.

[6] R. Tekle-Haimanot, M. Abebe, A. Gebre-Mariam et al., "Community-based study of neurological disorders in rural central Ethiopia," *Neuroepidemiology*, vol. 9, no. 5, pp. 263–277, 1990.

[7] R. Tekle-Haimanot, L. Forsgren, and J. Ekstedt, "Incidence of epilepsy in rural central Ethiopia," *Epilepsia*, vol. 38, no. 5, pp. 541–546, 1997.

[8] H. Wim and M. D. van Brakel, "Measuring health-related stigma," vs2.doc.2005:3.

[9] P. T. Fernandes and E. A. P. De Souza, "Identification of family variables in parents' groups of children with epilepsy," *Arquivos de Neuro-Psiquiatria*, vol. 59, no. 4, pp. 854–858, 2001.

[10] N. Buchanan, *Understanding Epilepsy: What It Is and How It Can Affect Your Life*, Simon & Schuster, Sydney, Australia, 2002.

[11] M. Bishop and B. Hermann, "Impact of epilepsy on quality of life: a review," in *Quality of Life in Epilepsy: Beyond Seizure Counts in Assessment and Treatment*, G. A. Baker and A. Jacoby, Eds., pp. 103–120, Harwood Academic, Amsterdam, The Nrtherlands, 2000.

[12] E. Goffman, *Stigma: Notes on the Management of Spoiled Identity*, Touchstone, New York, NY, USA, 1963.

[13] W. M. McLin and H. M. de Boer, "Public perceptions about epilepsy," *Epilepsia*, vol. 36, no. 10, pp. 957–959, 1995.

[14] J. A. Collings, "Psychosocial well-being and epilepsy: an empirical study," *Epilepsia*, vol. 31, no. 4, pp. 418–426, 1990.

[15] L. L. Min and J. W. A. S. Sander, "National demonstration project on epilepsy in Brazil," *Arquivos de Neuro-Psiquiatria*, vol. 61, no. 1, pp. 153–156, 2003.

[16] C. A. Guerreiro, M. M. Guerreiro, F. Cendes, and I. Lopes-Cendes, "Considerações gerais," in *Lemos Editorial*, pp. 1–10, Epilepsia, São Paulo, Brazil, 2000.

[17] J. Ablon, "The nature of stigma and medical conditions," *Epilepsy & Behavior*, vol. 3, no. 6, pp. 2–9, 2002.

[18] A. Jacoby, "Stigma, epilepsy, and quality of life," *Epilepsy & Behavior*, vol. 3, pp. 10–20, 2002.

[19] W. M. McLin and H. M. de Boer, "Public perceptions about epilepsy," *Epilepsia*, vol. 36, no. 10, pp. 957–959, 1995.

[20] P. T. Fernandes and L. M. Li, *Estigmanaepilepsia [Ph.D. thesis]*, Departamento de Neurologia—FCM/UNICAMP, 2005.

[21] P. T. Fernandes, P. C. B. Salgado, A. L. A. Noronha, F. D. Barbosa, E. A. P. Souza, and L. M. Li, "Stigma scale of epilepsy: conceptual issues," *Journal of Epilepsy and Clinical Neurophysiology*, vol. 10, no. 4, pp. 213–218, 2004.

[22] M. Rätsepp, A. Õun, S. Haldre, and A.-E. Kaasik, "Felt stigma and impact of epilepsy on employment status among Estonian people: exploratory study," *Seizure*, vol. 9, no. 6, pp. 394–401, 2000.

[23] H. M. de Boer, M. Mula, and J. W. Sander, "The global burden and stigma of epilepsy," *Epilepsy and Behavior*, vol. 12, no. 4, pp. 540–546, 2008.

[24] G. Scambler and A. Hopkins, "Generating a model of epileptic stigma: the role of qualitative analysis," *Social Science & Medicine*, vol. 30, no. 11, pp. 1187–1194, 1990.

[25] R. Ryan, K. Kempner, and A. C. Emlen, "The stigma of epilepsy as a self-concept," *Epilepsia*, vol. 21, no. 4, pp. 433–444, 1980.

[26] J. L. Dell, "Social dimensions of epilepsy, stigma and response," in *Psychopathology in Epilepsy: Social Dimensions*, S. Whitman and B. P. Hermann, Eds., Oxford University Press, New York, NY, USA, 1986.

[27] L. M. Li, P. T. Fernandes, A. L. Noronha et al., "Demonstration project on epilepsy in Brazil: situation assessment," *Arquivos de Neuro-Psiquiatria*, vol. 65, supplement 1, pp. 5–13, 2007.

[28] A. Kleinman, W.-Z. Wang, S.-C. Li et al., "The social course of epilepsy: chronic illness as social experience in interior China," *Social Science and Medicine*, vol. 40, no. 10, pp. 1319–1330, 1995.

[29] M. Ahmad, "Epilepsy: stigma and management," *Current Research in Neuroscience*, vol. 1, no. 1, pp. 1–14, 2011.

[30] G. A. Baker, J. Brooks, D. Buck, and A. Jacoby, "The stigma of epilepsy: a European perspective," *Epilepsia*, vol. 41, no. 1, pp. 98–104, 2000.

[31] W. van Brakeletal, *ILEP Guidelines to Reduce Stigma*, The International Federation of Anti-Leprosy Associations (ILEP), London, UK; The Netherlands Leprosy Relief (NLR), Amsterdam, The Netherlands, 2011.

[32] R. Reis and H. Meinardi, "ILAE/WHO 'out of the shadows campaign' stigma: does the flag identify the cargo?" *Epilepsy & Behavior*, vol. 3, no. 6, pp. 33–37, 2002.

[33] A. M. Paschal, S. R. Hawley, T. S. Romain et al., "Epilepsy patients' perceptions about stigma, education, and awareness: preliminary responses based on a community participatory approach," *Epilepsy & Behavior*, vol. 11, no. 3, pp. 329–337, 2007.

[34] D. Bhalla, K. Chea, C. Hun et al., "Population-based study of epilepsy in Cambodia associated factors, measures of impact, stigma, quality of life, knowledge-attitude-practice, and treatment gap," *PLoS ONE*, vol. 7, no. 10, Article ID e46296, 2012.

[35] N. Prus and A. C. Grant, "Patient beliefs about epilepsy and brain surgery in a multi-cultural urban population," *Epilepsy & Behavior*, vol. 17, no. 1, p. 46, 2010.

[36] P. T. Fernandes, P. C. B. Salgado, A. L. A. Noronha et al., "Epilepsy stigma perception in an urban area of a limited-resource country," *Epilepsy & Behavior*, vol. 11, no. 1, pp. 25–32, 2007.

[37] G. A. Baker, A. Jacoby, J. Gorry, J. Doughty, and V. Ellina, "Quality of life of people with epilepsy in Iran, the Gulf, and Near East," *Epilepsia*, vol. 46, no. 1, pp. 132–140, 2005.

[38] F. Rafael, D. Houinato, P. Nubukpo et al., "Sociocultural and psychological features of perceived stigma reported by people with epilepsy in Benin," *Epilepsia*, vol. 51, no. 6, pp. 1061–1068, 2010.

[39] M. Atadzhanov, A. Haworth, E. N. Chomba, E. K. Mbewe, and G. L. Birbeck, "Epilepsy-associated stigma in Zambia: what factors predict greater felt stigma in a highly stigmatized population?" *Epilepsy & Behavior*, vol. 19, no. 3, pp. 414–418, 2010.

[40] C. K. Mbuba, A. Abubakar, P. Odermatt, C. R. Newton, and J. A. Carter, "Development and validation of the Kilifi Stigma Scale for Epilepsy in Kenya," *Epilepsy and Behavior*, vol. 24, no. 1, pp. 81–85, 2012.

[41] T. Shibre, A. Alem, R. Tekle-Haimanot, and G. Medhin, "Perception of stigma in people with epilepsy and their relatives in Butajira, Ethiopia," *Ethiopian Journal of Health Development*, vol. 20, no. 3, 2006.

[42] C. KathomiMbuba, *Epilepsy treatment gap, associated risk factors and intervention strategies in Kilifi, Kenya*, University of Basel, Basel, Switzerland, 2011.

6

Psychiatric Patients Experiences with Mechanical Restraints

Klas Lanthén,[1] Mikael Rask,[2] and Charlotta Sunnqvist[3]

[1]*Skåne University Hospital, Södra Förstadsgatan 101, 214 28 Malmö, Sweden*
[2]*Department of Health and Caring Sciences, Linnaeus University, Lückligs Plats, 351 95 Växjö, Sweden*
[3]*Department of Care Science, Faculty for Health and Society, Malmö University, Jan Waldenströms Gata 25, 205 06 Malmö, Sweden*

Correspondence should be addressed to Charlotta Sunnqvist; charlotta.sunnqvist@mah.se

Academic Editor: Nicola Magnavita

Objective. To examine psychiatric patients' experience of mechanical restraints and to describe the care the patients received. *Background.* All around the world, threats and violence perpetrated by patients in psychiatric emergency inpatient units are quite common and are a prevalent factor concerning the application of mechanical restraints, although psychiatric patients' experiences of mechanical restraints are still moderately unknown. *Method.* A qualitative design with an inductive approach were used, based on interviews with patients who once been in restraints. *Results.* This study resulted in an overbridging theme: *Physical Presence, Instruction and Composed Behaviour Can Reduce Discontent and Trauma*, including five categories. These findings implicated the following: information must be given in a calm and sensitive way, staff must be physically present during the whole procedure, and debriefing after the incident must be conducted. *Conclusions.* When mechanical restraints were unavoidable, the presence of committed staff during mechanical restraint was important, demonstrating the significance of training acute psychiatric nurses correctly so that their presence is meaningful. Nurses in acute psychiatric settings should be required to be genuinely committed, aware of their actions, and fully present in coercive situations where patients are vulnerable.

1. Introduction

All around the world, threats and violence (termed aggressive incidents) perpetrated by patients in psychiatric emergency inpatient units are quite common and are prevalent factors concerning the application of mechanical restraints [1–3]. Aggressive incidents are attributed to numerous causes, such as frustration, pathology, or staff influence on the environment or even staff, patient relationships [4–7]. The majority of the patients subjected to mechanical restraints in Sweden are diagnosed with borderline personality disorder and suffer from self-injury behaviour patterns [8]. In Norway, two separate studies conducted in psychiatric inpatient units from different hospitals found that mechanical restraints were most commonly used on young, male patients [9, 10].

A Polish study found psychotic episodes to be the most common diagnosis for patients in mechanical restraints [11]. In addition, a Japanese study [12] found that restrained patients are significantly more likely than nonrestrained patients to be diagnosed with organic mental disorders or substance disorder and schizophrenia but are less likely to be diagnosed with a mood disorder or a neurotic disorder.

In 2011, mechanical restraints were used 3,400 times on 1,142 patients in Swedish psychiatric inpatient units in connection to violence or self-harm. In 2012, mechanical restraints were used 4,123 times on 1,327 individuals and hence 2156 times on women and 1967 times on men. The statistics showed that it was common that one patient was placed in mechanical restraints several times and it was more common among women. The use of mechanical restraints seems to have increased in Sweden between 2010 and 2013 [8].

In Scandinavian countries, systematic risk assessments to predict aggressive behaviour or special methods for handling aggressive patients have been implemented in several psychiatric inpatient wards [6, 13]. Assessment aims are to avoid outbursts of aggression, to minimize risk of injury, to reduce the need for restrictive coercive measures, and to help the patients control their behaviour.

Although coercive measures occur [14], research into patients' experiences is rare. There are some studies describing both negative and more neutral reactions. Chien et al. [15] found from interviews that patients felt afraid, humiliated, or being punished having been placed in mechanical restraints. Some patients felt more frustrated and found that mechanical interventions brought back frightening memories; many studies have stated that mechanical restraints elicit traumatic memories [16–21]. Less negative or neutral reactions sometimes occurred when the health professionals were able to provide psychological and informational support to patients throughout the mechanical restraints [15].

Nurses in psychiatric intensive care units are frequently confronted with patient aggression, and many nurses in such settings have experienced patient violence during the course of their careers [22]. Nurses in general do not experience the use of coercion as positive [23], but at times they still need to perform coercive measures. According to Olofsson et al. [23], nurses understand the necessity of performing coercive measures, but at the same time they ought to perform the coercive measure as a nonoffensive action. A Norwegian study about staff attitudes to coercion in psychiatric inpatient units [24] showed that male and unskilled staff were significantly more prone to use a highly restrictive intervention against violent patients than the rest of the staff.

Both patients and staff describe their relationship as an important issue [5, 25]. The interpersonal relationship and being a human are two important issues between the nurse and the patient when a coercive measure is performed [25]. Carlsson [5] found that this was explicated by seven themes of meaning: respecting the individual's fear and respecting the client, touch, dialogue, situated knowledge, stability, mutual regard, and pliability.

Quality and Safety Education for Nurses (QSEN) has described six core competencies for advanced nursing [26], and the overall goal is to prepare future nurses to continuously improve the quality and safety of the healthcare system. Person-centred care, one of the six core competencies, aims to provide compassionate and coordinated care based on respect for patients' preferences, values, and needs. The therapeutic relationship between the psychiatric nurse and the patient is at risk when applying mechanical restraints [27]. Consequently, it is also important to examine this interaction further. Many studies on coercive measures focus on the nurses' experience and official reports of violent incidents [28]; thus, psychiatric patients' experiences of mechanical restraints are still moderately unknown. Their experiences are the main factors that may improve care when coercive measure ought to be performed. Therefore, the aims of this study are to examine psychiatric patients' experience of mechanical restraints and to describe the care the patients received.

2. Methods

2.1. Design. The restrained individuals themselves can only answer what it actually means to be fixed in restraints. Consequently, a qualitative design with an inductive approach based on interviews was chosen.

2.2. Participants and Data Collection. Psychiatric outpatient units, as well as patient organizations, were contacted by mail or visited by the first author. Posters giving information about the study were placed at outpatient units and at the houses of patient organization. Patients from inpatient units were not included. The reason for this was to avoid informants with current acute mental illness. Inclusion criteria included proficiency in the Swedish language and having been mechanically restrained at least once, while the exclusion criteria included those less than 18 years of age and those who currently had been admitted to a psychiatric inpatient unit because of acute mental illness.

The participants responded in different ways: two participants responded by e-mail, two responded by telephone, two participants gave verbal consent through their contact person at the outpatient unit so that the first author could contact them, and two participants gave verbal consent at a patient organization to the first author. Three participants were contacted by the first author because two participants gave verbal consent to the first author through another informant, while one gave verbal consent through the third author. All participants provided written, informed consent before the interview, having received verbal information from the first author.

The participants constituted ten former psychiatric patients (five men and five women) who were currently, or had been previously (at some point in life), subjected to compulsory psychiatric care and who had experienced mechanical restraints. The ages ranged from 32 to 70, and the mean age was 47.3 ± 14.3 years. By their own admission, the participants had been treated for psychosis, self-harming, and bipolar disorders.

The informants themselves decided the time and location of the interviews. The one-on-one interviews began with demographic questions followed by two open-ended questions, such as *"Can you describe for me how the restraints procedure was performed and how you experienced the situation?"* followed by *"How did the staff act and how did you want them to act?"* The interviewees were encouraged to talk freely to enrich their story. However, the author also had an interview guide with supportive questions to use if the informants found it difficult to speak of their own accord. The interviews were conducted during Spring Term 2013 and were duly recorded. The median time for an interview was 24 minutes, ranging from 12 to 45 minutes, and was transcribed verbatim by the first author. One (of eleven interviews) was excluded due to a tape recording failure.

2.3. Analysis. The interviews were analysed using quantitative content analysis according to Miles and Huberman [29] and Berg [30]. The use of both manifest and latent analyses facilitated the apparent structure, as well as the deep structural meaning of the interviews. Both the first and the third authors read the transcribed material separately. The first author read the transcriptions several times and identified meanings units, which described how psychiatric patients' experienced the mechanical restraints. After the meanings units were identified, they were condensed into codes. The process continued with the organization of the subcategories into categories. Both the first and the third authors separately formulated subcategories into categories, and consensus was extended after comparison and discussions. Five categories were identified after comparisons, and finally a theme was formulated.

The first author has experienced being a nurse at an intensive psychiatric care unit and had acted as a team leader in many situations where mechanical restraints had been used. The author brought his preconception of the experience of patients who have been in restraints into the interviews. All authors have worked for several years as psychiatric and mental health nurses, and they also have deeper knowledge about the context.

2.4. Ethical Considerations. Ethical approval was granted from the Ethical Advisory Board at Malmö University, Department of Health and Society, Malmö, Sweden (Dnr: HS60-2012/1047:13). Participants were told that they could opt to discontinue the study at any time before, during, or after the interviews. All participants gave both verbal and written informed consents.

3. Results

The findings are presented within the structure of a category system based on an overall theme entitled *Physical Presence, Instruction and Composed Behaviour Can Reduce Discontent and Trauma*, which is based on the categories created from the subcategories (Table 1).

3.1. Physical Presence, Instruction and Composed Behaviour Can Reduce Discontent and Trauma. The importance of an appropriate attitude and care from staff when placing the patient in mechanical restraints was stressed repeatedly in the interviews; in many cases, it was the determining factor as to how the mechanical restraint situation was experienced. Different dimensions of attitude and actions arose from the narratives. The informants pointed out the significance of receiving clear information during the mechanical restraints situation. Having knowledge about what was happening and what was going to happen gave the participants a sense of control, calm, and security. It was suggested that this information should be given by one person only during the mechanical restraints situation. Clear information was described by some informants as being the most important aspect of quality care in a mechanical restraints situation. The interviews also revealed that the physical presence of staff was crucial for the patient's positive experience during his or her time in mechanical restraints. Feelings of safety and warmth in connection to the presence of a staff were reported.

If the nursing care during the mechanical restraints situation was carried out according to the above-mentioned criterion, there was a chance for a positive experience from the procedure for the patient. The mechanical restraints situation would, in such cases, perhaps not lead to discontent or traumatisation.

Table 1: Theme and categories.

Theme	Categories	Subcategories
Physical Presence, Instruction and Composed Behaviour Can Reduce Discontent and Trauma	Safety and understanding	Positive emotions Feeling of necessity
	Fear, powerlessness, and feelings of unreality	Negative emotions Uncertainty Feelings of unreality and splitting
	Composed and professional attitude	Impersonal and clinical approach The attitude is important Risk for trauma Calm and sober behaviour
	Physical presence and giving information	Communication is important Presence and body contact
	Debriefing and processing	Follow-up interventions

3.2. Safety and Understanding. Several informants reported feelings such as calm and safety from the mechanical restraints situation. Being restrained was described as security (safety) because it prevented the patient from self-harming behaviour. It was also described as an ultimate and resolute method of stopping a growing feeling of loss of control and degeneration. The calmness emerged from the feeling of safety. The informants perceived the calmness as a positive feeling in a situation that was otherwise unusual and unpleasant:

> *That part I remember quite a lot of was not who did it and so on, but just that they did it and that it made me feel safe. (Interview 3)*

Thoughts and feelings about the mechanical restraints as necessary and inevitable reappear. The mechanical restraints were sometimes described as unavoidable or essential. The informants had, in these cases, an understanding of the situation and that it perhaps was the only option left:

> *It was, it was like the only way there was, so to speak, since nothing else worked. I wasn't able to speak, so it was a little hard to, like, just take a few deep breaths. (Interview 1)*

Mechanical restraints were defined as an intervention that becomes necessary for calming a person who is extremely anxious and violent. Therefore, some informants regarded it as an intervention that fulfilled a purpose.

3.3. Fear, Powerlessness, and Feelings of Unreality. The fear that the mechanical restraints sometimes reappears in many of the interviews. In some descriptions, the fear was manifested as anger and as a feeling of violation. One of the informants described a feeling of pure fear in connection with the mechanical restraints. The fear was described as a strong negative feeling and was many times characterised as one of the worst fears they had ever experienced:

> *It's mostly fear really, a real horror show, it was terrible. (Interview 7)*

> *I have never been so afraid in my entire life. (Interview 4)*

The fear was often caused by a sense of ambiguity about what was going to happen next and how long the mechanical restraints would stay in place. The patients often lost the concept of time in the mechanical restraints room, and this led to anxiety.

Being in mechanical restraints also led to a feeling of powerlessness and being excluded or exposed. The feeling was partially connected to the feeling of insecurity, but it was also manifested as an experience of its own. Some informants described a total loss of control and how they experienced a position of dependence on the staff. The feeling was experienced as negative, and the idea of no longer having control over what was going to happen was perceived as frightening:

> *To be left to someone else's good will because you do not have, sort of, it's not possible for you to get up, you cannot talk yourself out of the situation, you cannot sort of.... (Interview 1)*

Feelings of unreality occurred for some informants when they were in mechanical restraints. They described what was going on as absurd and different, so much that they could not really take it in:

> *It felt a bit like a movie, sort of, eeeh it felt a bit like, sort of eeeh, it's just like this sort of, this is just fake almost kind of... this is just not real. (Interview 2)*

The difficulties in taking in what was happening were sometimes described as a sudden flight and a screen from reality. The feelings were described as a condition of splitting and sudden disintegration.

3.4. Composed and Professional Attitude. It appears that the informants experienced the staff in different ways during the mechanical restraints procedure. Both negative and more beneficial experiences of the staff's attitude and care were noted.

The informants described a composed, soft, and well-balanced attitude and care as well as actions, which often resulted in a dignified and respectful "care" during the mechanical restraints procedure. The care was described as nonhectic, and it helped the person to calm down or to stabilize an already escalated and troublesome situation:

> *When, with a shit load of people, fix what they are supposed to fix and then out again fast and then there were only the few left to carry on further contact with me, so it was very, it was like an isolation measure, sort of. Everyone in and step on the gas and then out again. So it became as calm as possible as fast as possible, so I think that it was quite professionally done actually. (Interview 1)*

Experience of an emotionally cold and clinical attitude, as well as behaviour, also emerged from the interviews. Impersonal and negligent behaviour concerning the feelings of the person in restraints was described: a procedure where barely a word was uttered and the staff acted out of routine. If something was said, it was said in a negative and accusatory tone. One informant even experienced that she had been taunted and verbally ridiculed by the staff under restraint. Many times, it emerged from the informants that staff had been talking *about* them rather than *with* them or *to* them:

> *Everything happens in total silence and eh it's sort of just, the only thing that happens is that you feel that they are talking over your head; you just hear, "Yes you take that one there and you take this and have you got that buckle?" And stuff like that. (Interview 9)*

In several interviews, the informants corroborated that the attitude and level of care of the staff were significant to how they experienced the situation. If the staff kept calm, acted in a stable manner, and managed to deal with their feelings, the mechanical restraints situation was experienced as quite neutral and, in retrospect, meaningful. It could, in some cases, have also been avoided. If the staff, on the other hand, acted unprofessionally, with a cold and harsh attitude, this affected the experience of the mechanical restraints situation negatively. Furthermore, this could affect the entire experience of the hospitalization period and lead to increased suspiciousness towards psychiatry in general:

> *I remember it was a total horror show, and then you get imprinted by that if you think about the psychiatry and so how you perceive the psychiatry and doctors and all that; you are a little cautious with doctors what you tell them and such, so they do not misinterpret you. (Interview 7)*

In addition, many informants described the mechanical restraints situation as traumatic. They believed that they had been so frightened and violated by the incident that it had marked them. Some described sleeping problems and that they thought about the mechanical restrain situation on a daily basis. They could feel poorly long after the incident when they thought about it, and it had created worry and feelings of fear within them. Thoughts about disproportionate measures in psychiatry emerged and the restraining procedure had not been performed the way it should have been according to directions:

> *This is probably, I believe, quite a major intervention and too many actually. Maybe then especially*

if you are, so to say, "clear in the head" when it happens and so and that you remember it, then it becomes kind of like a trauma. (Interview 4)

A point of view that permeated almost all the interviews was that the negative reactions to the mechanical restraints situation could have been prevented. It could have been avoided with the use of a professional, composed, and stable attitude and quality care from the staff.

3.5. Physical Presence and Giving Information. The importance of physical presence and contact just after the mechanical restraint was performed and emphasized in several interviews. The presence of the staff during the time in restraint was important for informants' feeling of safety. If the staff sat at a distance from the restrained person and did not engage sufficiently with the patient, this was experienced as negative. Contact with staff and being active were described as important. Physical contact, such as placing a hand on the shoulder or on the arm, could additionally contribute to the feeling of safety, decrease anxiety, and induce calm:

A psychiatric nurse was left, and he touched my arm and just asked if there was something he could do for me; and then I said yes you can keep holding your arm there, because it felt so safe. (Interview 2)

The experience of vagueness in connection with the mechanical restraint has shown itself to be troublesome for many of the informants. In many interviews, the wish to be informed about what was going to happen next emerged. Clear information from the staff about their intentions in connection with the mechanical restraint was requested. Information and communication with, preferably, one person during the procedure were the best according to many informants. Knowing what was going on, what the staff were doing with them, and how long they were going to be restrained provided a sense of safety. In the interviews, the fact that the informants had not always been told what was going to happen and that the staff had not communicated with them emerged. Many of the informants stated that it was important to get information during the procedure about how and why the mechanical restraint was being performed:

I think that it is enormously important that you get to know what is going on, that you, that someone tells you what is going on and what you are supposed to do. (Interview 8)

3.6. Debriefing and Processing. The informants expressed a desire to talk about their experience in the mechanical restraints situation. The possibility of debriefing with staff was seen as a way to process the experience. If an understanding of the situation that occurred could be reached through hearing the staff's version, the processing of the experience was supported. A successful adoption of the situation was crucial if the experience was to develop into trauma or not. The informants proposed debriefing as a good method. It included both a verbal follow-up and a written follow-up with the staff, with the written follow-up being in the form of a questionnaire. Several informants saw a later reduction of the drama of the mechanical restraints situation as essential, so that they could move on from the experience:

After experiencing a mechanical restraints situation like this, I think it's really good to have a debriefing session just like after an incident. (Interview 4)

4. Discussion

This study resulted in an overall theme: *Physical Presence, Instruction and Composed Behaviour Can Reduce Discontent and Trauma.* The results disclosed that the physical presence of staff was crucial for the patient's positive experience during his or her period in mechanical restraints. An appropriate attitude and level of care from the staff when placing the patient in mechanical restraints were the determining factors concerning how the situation was experienced. The informants pointed out the significance of receiving clear instruction during the mechanical restraints situation. Receiving knowledge about what was happening and what was going to happen provided the participants with a sense of control, calm, and safety. Similar results have been described previously; for example, [15, 31, 32] have shown how a calm and professional attitude towards patients in a mechanical restraints situation increases the chances of a positive experience for the patient. The importance of giving clear information to the patient has also been reported [15, 33]. The value of the presence of a staff member has partially been reported [32]. The essential issue in the present study was the importance of the physical presence of a supporting staff during the procedure and the debriefing procedure afterwards. Otherwise, as this study has shown, the mechanical restraints can be experienced as abusive and, in some cases, as creating trauma.

Consequently, it is important to identify risk patients so that coercive restraint can be prevented. In Sweden, a noncommercial violence prevention and management programme has been introduced. This model was originally developed in Haukeland University Hospital, Department of Forensic Psychiatry, Bergen, Norway [13]. Among other things, this model emphasises that the staff maintain neutral body language and a calm tone when communicating with a patient exhibiting aggressive behaviour. This approach demonstrates that the staff are not seeking confrontation with the patient. Similar guidelines are used in the Project BETA (Best practices in Evaluation and Treatment of Agitation), a noncoercive deescalation with the goal to calm an agitated patient and to gain his or her cooperation in the evaluation and treatment [34]. There is strong international focus on reducing and possibly eliminating restraint [35–37] which is important and necessary, but still mechanical restraints occur, and some are unavoidable considering the violence-controlling methods that exist today.

Several participants in the study explained that they thought that mechanical restraint was necessary in certain extreme situations, and they expressed an understanding for the use of this intervention. The patients described a perceived feeling of safety because staff were helping them to control their aggressive symptoms, that is, to be put in restraints to prevent behaviour dangerous to other patients or to staff [15, 38]. A competency clarified by QSEN [26] is safety, which means minimising risk of harm to patients and care providers through both system effectiveness and individual performance. Therefore, there must be skills present to establish effective use of strategies in order to maintain safety and understanding when mechanical restraint is necessary, for example, to communicate and inform the patient throughout the entire procedure with a calm voice, as well as being physically present.

The interviews in this study describe varying quality in staff attitude and care towards patients during the mechanical restraints procedure. Informants described both gentle and not-so-gentle approaches. If the staff kept their calm, acted in a stable manner, and managed to deal with emotions, the mechanical restraints situation felt satisfactory for the patients and, in retrospect, meaningful. If the staff, on the other hand, acted unprofessionally, being cold and harsh in their attitudes and care, this affected the experience of this situation negatively.

The diversity of the care described during mechanical restraint shows the importance of further discussions on the standardization of safety for patients when using mechanical restraints. Here, it also becomes important to apply the QSEN [26] competency: person-centred care in order to provide compassionate and coordinated care based on respect for patients' preferences, values, and needs.

In order to reduce negative feelings, it was important that staff were present during the mechanical restraints period. The physical presence of staff was described as significant and was seen as important for feelings of safety. To the best of the authors' knowledge, this has been only ambiguously reported previously. The expressed need of receiving information before and during the mechanical restraints procedure and the significance of the staff communicating with patients was another important component in this study. Another important factor was to be able to discuss the process and the experience of mechanical restraints with the staff after the event. The opportunity of debriefing with staff was seen as a way to adapt to the experience. This included both a verbal follow-up and a written follow-up with the staff. Similar findings are reported by [21, 39], who came to the conclusion that debriefing after mechanical restraints was essential for the patient and also for the staff, so they could jointly ascertain how mechanical restraints could be avoided in the future.

This study is important as it confirms earlier studies' findings of negative feelings, importance of communication, and debriefing in connection with mechanical restraints [13, 15, 16, 19, 22, 32, 39–41]. It also brings new knowledge with the narrated importance of physical presence of staff when mechanical restraints are deemed inevitable.

5. Limitations

There are several limitations to this study, for example, the small sample of ten informants and the fact that all informants came from outpatients units. Consequently, the informants gave their narratives retrospectively and might have reconstructed their experiences. It might have been different if the narratives came from inpatients with a fresh memory of the event. The difficulty with such a method was to obtain ethical permission for research on patients in compulsory institutional care. Five of the ten interviews were coded by the first and third authors, leaving five interviews coded solely by one researcher. Yet, we aimed to achieve reliability in agreement with the standard criteria for qualitative research [42].

6. Conclusions

When mechanical restraints are unavoidable, a nursing perspective must be taken into consideration. Information must be given in a calm and sensitive manner, the staff must be physically present during the entire procedure, and debriefing must be conducted thereafter. If this is accomplished, the overall goals of QSEN to improve the quality and safety of healthcare systems are on their way to be achieved [26]. The importance of the presence of committed staff during mechanical restraints that this study shows demonstrates the significance of training acute psychiatric nurses correctly so that their presence is meaningful. Nurses in acute psychiatric settings should be required to be genuinely committed, be aware of their actions, and be fully present in coercive situations where patients are vulnerable. This entails that managers of acute psychiatric settings ensure that staff get appropriate training in empathy and violence prevention. Furthermore, this could form the basis of consensus when creating nationwide routines for nursing care in mechanical restraints situations.

Disclaimer

The authors alone are responsible for the content and writing of the paper.

Conflict of Interests

The authors report no actual or potential conflict of interests.

Authors' Contribution

Klas Lanthén designed the project and conducted the interviews. Both Klas Lanthén and Charlotta Sunnqvist made the analyses. Klas Lanthén drafted the paper with the help from Charlotta Sunnqvist and Mikael Rask, and all the authors (Klas Lanthén, Mikael Rask, and Charlotta Sunnqvist) read and approved the final content of the paper.

Acknowledgments

The informants are gratefully acknowledged.

References

[1] W. A. Fisher, "Restraint and seclusion: a review of the literature," *The American Journal of Psychiatry*, vol. 151, no. 11, pp. 1584–1591, 1994.

[2] R. Kaltiala-Heino, C. Tuohimäki, J. Korkeila, and V. Lehtinen, "Reasons for using seclusion and restraint in psychiatric inpatient care," *International Journal of Law and Psychiatry*, vol. 26, no. 2, pp. 139–149, 2003.

[3] R. Whittington, E. Baskind, and B. Paterson, "Coercive measurement in the management of imminent violence: restraint, seclusion and enhanced observation. I," in *Violence in Mental Health Settings. Causes, Consequences, Management*, D. Richer and R. Whittington, Eds., pp. 145–172, Springer, New York, NY, USA, 2006.

[4] G. Carlsson, K. Dahlberg, and N. Drew, "Encountering violence and aggression in mental health nursing: a phenomenological study of tacit caring knowledge," *Issues in Mental Health Nursing*, vol. 21, no. 5, pp. 533–545, 2000.

[5] G. Carlsson, *The phenomenology of violent encounters—threats and violence in psychiatric care [Ph.D. thesis]*, Linnaeus University, Kalmar, Sweden, 2003, Acta Wexionensia no. 32/2003, (Swedish).

[6] I. Needham, C. Abderhalden, R. Meer et al., "The effectiveness of two interventions in the management of patient violence in acute mental inpatient settings: report on a pilot study," *Journal of Psychiatric and Mental Health Nursing*, vol. 11, no. 5, pp. 595–601, 2004.

[7] J. Duxbury and R. Whittington, "Causes and management of patient aggression and violence: staff and patient perspectives," *Journal of Advanced Nursing*, vol. 50, no. 5, pp. 469–478, 2005.

[8] The Swedish Board of Health and Welfare, Socialstyrelsen, patientregistret, 2013, http://www.socialstyrelsen.se/register/halsodataregister/patientregistret.

[9] M. Knutzen, N. H. Mjosund, G. Eidhammer et al., "Characteristics of psychiatric inpatients who experienced restraint and those who did not: a case-control study," *Psychiatric Services*, vol. 62, no. 5, pp. 492–497, 2011.

[10] R. Wynn, "Medicate, restrain or seclude? Strategies for dealing with violent and threatening behaviour in a Norwegian university psychiatric hospital," *Scandinavian Journal of Caring Sciences*, vol. 16, no. 3, pp. 287–291, 2002.

[11] M. Kostecka and M. Zardecka, "The use of physical restraints in polish psychiatric hospitals in 1989 and 1996," *Psychiatric Services*, vol. 50, no. 12, pp. 1637–1638, 1999.

[12] T. Odawara, H. Narita, Y. Yamada, J. Fujita, T. Yamada, and Y. Hirayasu, "Use of restraint in a general hospital psychiatric unit in Japan," *Psychiatry and Clinical Neurosciences*, vol. 59, no. 5, pp. 605–609, 2005.

[13] A. Björkdahl, G. Hansebo, and T. Palmstierna, "The influence of staff training on the violence prevention and management climate in psychiatric inpatient units," *Journal of Psychiatric and Mental Health Nursing*, vol. 20, no. 5, pp. 396–404, 2013.

[14] L. Kjellin, "Forskning om vuxenpsykiatrisk tvångsvård," in *Tvingad till hjälp, om tvång, etik och tillit i barn-och ungdomspsykiatrisk vård*, I. Engström, Ed., pp. 171–199, Studentlitteratur, Lund, Sweden, 2006.

[15] W.-T. Chien, C. W. H. Chan, L.-W. Lam, and C.-W. Kam, "Psychiatric inpatients' perceptions of positive and negative aspects of physical restraint," *Patient Education and Counseling*, vol. 59, no. 1, pp. 80–86, 2005.

[16] G. Bonner, T. Lowe, D. Rawcliffe, and N. Wellman, "Trauma for all: a pilot study of the subjective experience of physical restraint for mental health inpatients and staff in the UK," *Journal of Psychiatric and Mental Health Nursing*, vol. 9, no. 4, pp. 465–473, 2002.

[17] R. Fish and E. Culshaw, "The last resort? Staff and client perspectives on physical intervention," *Journal of Intellectual Disabilities*, vol. 9, no. 2, pp. 93–107, 2005.

[18] R. Gallop, E. McCay, M. Guha, and P. Khan, "The experience of hospitalization and restraint of women who have a history of childhood sexual abuse," *Health Care for Woman International*, vol. 20, no. 4, pp. 401–416, 1999.

[19] H. Sequeira and S. Halstead, "Control and restraint in the UK: service user perspectives," *The British Journal of Forensic Practice*, vol. 4, no. 1, pp. 9–18, 2002.

[20] S. B. Smith, "Restraints: retraumatization for rape victims?" *Journal of Psychosocial Nursing & Mental Health Services*, vol. 33, no. 7, pp. 23–28, 1995.

[21] R. Wynn, "Psychiatric inpatients' experience with restraints," *Journal of Forensic Psychiatry & Psychology*, vol. 15, no. 1, pp. 124–144, 2004.

[22] S. A. Quintal, "Violence against psychiatric nurses. An untreated epidemic?" *Journal of Psychosocial Nursing and Mental Health Services*, vol. 40, no. 1, pp. 46–53, 2002.

[23] B. Olofsson, F. Gilje, L. Jacobsson, and A. Norberg, "Nurses' narratives about using coercion in psychiatric care," *Journal of Advanced Nursing*, vol. 28, no. 1, pp. 45–53, 1998.

[24] R. Wynn, A.-M. Kvalvik, and T. Hynnekleiv, "Attitudes to coercion at two Norwegian psychiatric units," *Nordic Journal of Psychiatry*, vol. 65, no. 2, pp. 133–137, 2011.

[25] B. Olofsson and A. Norberg, "Experiences of coercion in psychiatric care as narrated by patients, nurses and physicians," *Journal of Advanced Nursing*, vol. 33, no. 1, pp. 89–97, 2001.

[26] L. Cronenwett, G. Sherwood, J. Pohl et al., "Quality and safety education for advanced nursing practice," *Nursing Outlook*, vol. 57, no. 6, pp. 338–348, 2009.

[27] M. Cleary, "The challenges of mental health care reform for contemporary mental health nursing practice: relationships, power and control," *International Journal of Mental Health Nursing*, vol. 12, no. 2, pp. 139–147, 2003.

[28] D. Stewart, L. Bowers, A. Simpson, C. Ryan, and M. Tziggili, "Manual restraint of adult psychiatric inpatients: a literature review," *Journal of Psychiatric and Mental Health Nursing*, vol. 16, no. 8, pp. 749–757, 2009.

[29] M. B. Miles and M. Huberman, *Qualitative Data Analysis: A Sourcebook of New Methods*, SAGE Publications, Beverly Hills, Calif, USA, 2nd edition, 1994.

[30] B. L. Berg, *Qualitative Research Metods for the Social Sciences*, Allyn & Bacon, Boston, Mass, USA, 4th edition, 2001.

[31] J. Bak, V. Zoffmann, D. M. Sestoft, R. Almvik, and P. M. Brandt-Christensen, "Mechanical restraint in psychiatry. Preventive factors in theory and practice. A Danish-Norwegian association study," *Perspectives in Psychiatric Care*, vol. 50, no. 3, pp. 155–166, 2013.

[32] R. Kontio, G. Joffe, H. Putkonen et al., "Seclusion and restraint in psychiatry: patients' experiences and practical suggestions on how to improve practices and use alternatives," *Perspectives in Psychiatric Care*, vol. 48, no. 1, pp. 16–24, 2012.

[33] R. Kontio, M. Anttila, T. Lantta, K. Kauppi, G. Joffe, and M. Välimäki, "Toward a safer working environment on psychiatric wards: service users' delayed perspectives of aggression and violence-related situations and development ideas," *Perspectives in Psychiatric Care*, vol. 50, no. 4, pp. 271–279, 2014.

[34] D. K. Knox and G. H. Holloman Jr., "Use and avoidance of seclusion and restraint: consensus statement of the American

Association for emergency psychiatry project BETA seclusion and restraint workgroup," *Western Journal of Emergency Medicine*, vol. 13, no. 1, pp. 35–40, 2012.

[35] F. L. Bower, C. S. McCullough, and M. E. Timmons, "A synthesis of what we know about the use of physical restraints and seclusion with patients in psychiatric and acute care settings: 2003 update," *The Online Journal of Knowledge Synthesis for Nursing*, vol. 10, article 1, 2003.

[36] D. M. Lewis, "Responding to a violent incident: physical restraint or anger management as therapeutic interventions," *Journal of Psychiatric and Mental Health Nursing*, vol. 9, no. 1, pp. 57–63, 2002.

[37] A. M. Sullivan, J. Bezmen, C. T. Barron, J. Rivera, L. Curley-Casey, and D. Marino, "Reducing restraints: alternatives to restraints on an inpatient psychiatric service—utilizing safe and effective methods to evaluate and treat the violent patient," *The Psychiatric Quarterly*, vol. 76, no. 1, pp. 51–65, 2005.

[38] C. Haw, J. Stubbs, A. Bickle, and I. Stewart, "Coercive treatments in forensic psychiatry: a study of patients' experiences and preferences," *Journal of Forensic Psychiatry and Psychology*, vol. 22, no. 4, pp. 564–585, 2011.

[39] C. Larue, A. Dumais, R. Boyer, M.-H. Goulet, J.-P. Bonin, and N. Baba, "The experience of seclusion and restraint in psychiatric settings: perspectives of patients," *Issues in Mental Health Nursing*, vol. 34, no. 5, pp. 317–324, 2013.

[40] J. Bergk, E. Flammer, and T. Steinert, "'Coercion Experience Scale' (CES)—validation of a questionnaire on coercive measures," *BMC Psychiatry*, vol. 10, article 5, 2010.

[41] S. A. Simpson, J. M. Joesch, I. I. West, and J. Pasic, "Risk for physical restraint or seclusion in the psychiatric emergency service," *General Hospital Psychiatry*, vol. 36, no. 1, pp. 113–118, 2014.

[42] U. H. Graneheim and B. Lundman, "Qualitative content analysis in nursing research: concepts, procedures and measures to achieve trustworthiness," *Nurse Education Today*, vol. 24, no. 2, pp. 105–112, 2004.

7

Overcoming Recruitment Barriers in Urban Older Adults Residing in Congregate Living Facilities

Adam Simning,[1] Edwin van Wijngaarden,[2] and Yeates Conwell[1]

[1] *Department of Psychiatry, University of Rochester, 300 Crittenden Boulevard, Rochester, NY 14642, USA*
[2] *Department of Public Health Sciences, University of Rochester, 265 Crittenden Boulevard, Rochester, NY 14642, USA*

Correspondence should be addressed to Adam Simning; adam.simning@gmail.com

Academic Editor: Veit Roessner

Background. Participation of minority older adults in mental health research has been limited by mistrust, transportation difficulties, lack of knowledge, and insufficient community partnership. We describe strategies utilized to overcome these recruitment barriers. *Methods.* Our target population included 553 public housing residents of older adult high-rise buildings in Rochester, NY. We had a two-stage cross-sectional study: Stage 1 was a health survey for all residents and Stage 2 was a psychiatric interview of English-speaking residents aged 60 years and older. Recruitment occurred through mailings, onsite activities, and resident referrals. *Results.* Stage 1 had 358 participants (64.7% response) and Stage 2 had 190 (61.6% target population response), with higher participation among African Americans. We found some strategies effective for overcoming recruitment barriers. First, we partnered with a community agency and organized onsite educational activities to improve residents' trust. Second, the study occurred entirely onsite, which facilitated participation of functionally impaired residents. Third, onsite activities allowed the residents to learn about the study and complete surveys in person. Fourth, we provided immediate incentives that resulted in many study referrals. *Conclusions.* Although recruitment of minority older adults presents unique challenges, a multifaceted community-tailored approach mitigated several recruitment barriers in this mental health study.

1. Introduction

There is a great need to obtain better representation of diverse populations of older adults in mental health studies, and difficulty recruiting minority groups into research is well documented [1–3]. In response to the many barriers to recruitment, a science is slowly developing on how to increase participation of minority older adults in research. There remain, however, few concrete examples of strategies that can successfully recruit individuals from diverse populations into mental health studies.

Mistrust of medical researchers can be substantial, and a problematic issue for research recruitment is that African Americans—the second largest minority group in the United States [4]—do not trust doctors or medical research as much as others do [5]. There is a powerful history of mistreatment that has eroded African American trust in medical research [6, 7]. Among African Americans the term "medical research" triggered associations such as being lied to, corruption, deception, using people, and guinea pigs, and many had reservations about research scientists' motivations, which they thought were primarily a drive for money and prestige [8]. Such misgivings can be prominent in older African Americans because some may have witnessed or experienced medical research abuses [9, 10]. Some minority older adults may thereby feel uneasy in traditional research settings. To overcome mistrust, connecting with the community is a critical component of successful recruitment of minority older adults [11, 12], as is creating a common understanding between researchers and study participants [13, 14]. In particular, a key to recruiting underserved and hard-to-reach individuals is to involve people who are known and trusted within the community [15, 16]. Mistrust may also partly explain why solicitation methods that work well recruiting white older adults into research studies (e.g., advertisements) can have limited success with minority older adults [3, 17].

A second recruitment barrier is transportation difficulties. For many older adults, especially for those in minority groups which often are socioeconomically disadvantaged and tend to have worse health than whites [18], traveling to research sites can be difficult due to cost, illness, functional impairment, perceived inaccessibility of the research site, and security risks [7, 19]. Consequently, conducting research within the minority older adults' communities is one method to increase accessibility [3].

A third barrier to recruitment is that poor health literacy, limited mental illness knowledge, and not understanding the potential benefits of research participation can limit older adults from participating in research [3, 19–21]. In response, researchers have used community education projects, community-centered health fairs, and other venues to provide participants with knowledge regarding health- and research-related issues and to engage them with research staff [15, 19].

A fourth recruitment barrier is that relationships between the community and research institutions are often fleeting. Lack of meaningful feedback and little apparent concrete benefit of research to the community can foster reservations about investigators' motivations [8]. To strengthen community-academic relations, researchers can provide tangible benefits to the communities and maintain connections that may improve future research efforts within a community [12]. Disseminating findings back to the community also should be a component of community-based research [22] because it can help build lasting reciprocal relationships between researchers and the communities they study. To empower and more effectively engage communities, there is growing support for conducting community-based participatory research that represents a cooperative process in which both the researchers and community contribute to and learn from the research process [23].

In summary—although not necessarily unique to minority older adults or mental health research as recruitment of any sample of older adults can be difficult [19]—issues of mistrust, transportation difficulties, knowledge gaps, and a community-academic divide are considerable barriers limiting diverse populations of older adults from participating in mental health studies. Prior to the initiation of our two-stage mental health study, we devised a multifaceted recruitment approach that targeted these four anticipated recruitment barriers with strategies based on recommendations derived from prior recruitment efforts. Our objective here was to describe resident response to our recruitment strategies as a means of characterizing their apparent effectiveness. Our analytic goals were to estimate the study's response and characterize the demographic differences between responders and nonresponders. We hypothesized that nonresponders were more likely to be older, male, of African American race, and of Hispanic ethnicity. There are few empirical examples of how to recruit a diverse population of older adults into mental health studies, and this study's findings aim to provide guidance for future research efforts seeking to do so.

2. Materials and Methods

2.1. Study Setting. From May 2009 to June 2010, our two-stage cross-sectional epidemiologic study occurred within four public housing high-rises reserved for residents aged 50 years and older in Rochester, NY. Residents had a median age of 64.4 years and 46.8% were male, 24.8% were Hispanic, and 61.0% were African American; non-Hispanic whites only comprised 11.8% of the residents. The high-rise buildings housed between 73 in the smallest building and 299 public housing residents in the largest building and had differing ethnic (5.5% to 40.1% Hispanic) and racial (46.0% to 82.7% African American) compositions. The study's primary goals were to use a psychiatric research interview to characterize anxiety, depression, and service utilization among English-speaking residents aged 60 years and older. These findings will serve as a basis for better matching mental health services with need for such services.

2.2. Study Design. The study had two stages that corresponded to a health survey, which occurred in Stage 1 of the study, and the subsequent psychiatric research interview that comprised Stage 2. Stage 1's sampling frame consisted of all public housing residents, whereas Stage 2 targeted English-speaking residents aged 60 years and older with capacity to provide informed consent. Our recruitment was limited in that the Rochester Housing Authority did not permit us to initiate contact through telephone or door-to-door solicitation because it did not want the study to intrude upon residents uninterested in participating. The primary investigator (P.I.), a non-Hispanic white M.D./Ph.D. student, was responsible for all aspects of data collection and had received psychiatric research interview training through the University of Rochester's Psychiatry Department. Due to the limited research staff, data collection proceeded in one high-rise building at a time; the same recruitment strategies, however, were employed at each high-rise. The University of Rochester Human Subjects Review Board approved this study.

2.2.1. Stage 1. During the first stage, we sent mailings to all residents. Every mailing was translated using a professional translating service with Hispanic residents receiving mailings in both English and Spanish. Prior to study recruitment, Hispanic ethnicity was determined by the public housing demographic information that was provided to the study team. In general, the mailed surveys were rarely returned to the study team and most recruitment occurred in person. The objectives of Stage 1 were to engage residents and facilitate recruitment into Stage 2 as well as to collect health data that would allow for comparisons across demographic groupings not represented in Stage 2 (e.g., residents younger than 60 years). The first two mailings introduced the study and provided educational material on healthy aging and cognitive health, topics we thought would be relevant and interesting to this older adult community. More specifically, the first mailing addressed some aging myths (e.g., "To be old is to be sick," "You can't teach an old dog new tricks") while the second mailing had 10 tips for supporting memory such as "Exercise your body" and "Keep in touch [socially]." The 3rd mailing contained several questions on demographic information and a brief four-question health survey [24]; we made this mailing as brief as possible to maximize resident response. After the first round of Stage 2 research interviews, Stage 1 nonresponders received another health questionnaire mailing. On the Stage 1 survey, residents indicated their willingness to participate in Stage 2 via a "Yes/No" response to a question asking them if they would be interested in answering more questions about their health and participating in a follow-up study; residents endorsing "Yes" provided their phone number so that we could call them and schedule an interview. Several half-day onsite educational activities and recruitment sessions (conducted in English) coincided with each of the educational and health survey mailings, respectively. The onsite educational activities mirrored the content of the mailings (e.g., after the first mailing, a table was set up in the high-rise lobby where study staff would interact with residents and discuss the mailings). After completion of the study in each building, residents received a thank you letter summarizing the health survey results. There were no exclusion criteria for Stage 1. Most participants immediately received $5 when they turned in the health survey to the P.I. in person, while a few returned the survey by mail or gave it to the onsite social worker.

2.2.2. Stage 2. The second stage included Stage 1 respondents who were 60 years or older and English-speaking (non-English speakers were excluded) and had capacity to provide informed consent. Determination of capacity to provide informed consent occurred in person prior to commencing the research interview; we evaluated capacity for consent with a series of questions that assessed the participants' understanding of the study and excluded residents unable to adequately answer these questions. Due to the sensitive nature of psychiatric interviews, we did not utilize proxy informants. Literacy, medical comorbidities, and psychiatric comorbidities were not exclusion criteria. Stage 2 comprised a 1.5-hour interview and assessed anxiety and depression with the Structured Clinical Interview for the DSM-IV [25]. The interviews were in person and primarily occurred in the residents' apartments or other private onsite high-rise locations. Participants promptly received $25.

2.3. Recruitment Barrier Strategies. In our recruitment approach many strategies addressed recruiting issues relating to mistrust, transportation, lack of knowledge, and the community-academic divide. Although some strategies targeted multiple barriers, we have paired each strategy with the barrier it primarily targeted to avoid redundancy. We adopted three strategies to address the mistrust barrier: (1) partnered with a community services agency familiar to residents; (2) sent informational mailings; and (3) organized onsite educational activities. Our strategy for overcoming the transportation barrier was to conduct the study entirely within the high-rises. To address the lack of knowledge barrier, we relied on three strategies: (1) a series of recruitment mailings, (2) onsite recruitment sessions, and (3) attendance at resident council meetings. Lastly, we had four strategies to overcome the community-academic divide barrier: (1) immediately reimbursed residents $5 for the health survey and $25 for the psychiatric interview; (2) attempted to limit the interview's burdensomeness/length; (3) mailed residents a summary of the health survey findings and thanked them for participating; and (4) presented the findings to the resident council meetings, aging services agency assisting the residents, and Rochester Housing Authority.

2.4. Statistical Analysis. Basic descriptive statistics described the residents' demographics. We reported medians and interquartile ranges for variables not normally distributed. Bivariate analyses characterized the sociodemographic differences between responders and nonresponders. The Pearson chi-square test examined differences of categorical variables, while the nonparametric Wilcoxon rank sum test for nonnormal data contrasted differences in continuous variables. A p value of 0.05 or less indicated statistical significance, and we conducted analyses with SAS statistical software version 9.2 (SAS Institute, Inc., Cary, NC).

3. Results

3.1. Stage 1 Response. Stage 1 target sample was all public housing high-rise residents ($n = 553$), and most residents ($n = 358$; 64.7%) completed the health survey (Table 1). Non-Hispanics, African Americans, and women were in the majority, comprising 80.4%, 64.8%, and 55.3% of Stage 1 responders. While there were no age or gender differences between responders and nonresponders, Stage 1 responders were more likely to be of African American race and non-Hispanic ethnicity. Among residents completing Stage 1 brief health survey, 329 (91.9%) expressed an interest in participating in Stage 2 psychiatric interview.

3.2. Stage 2 Response. Our Stage 2 target sample consisted of non-Hispanic residents aged 60 years and older who were English-speaking and cognitively able to provide informed consent ($n = 292$), of whom we interviewed 180 (61.6%) (Table 2). Among non-Hispanic residents, Stage 2 responders were younger than nonresponders, but the response did not vary by gender or race.

We excluded Hispanic residents from Stage 2's response rate denominator because an unknown majority of Hispanic residents were not fluent in English: of Stage 1 Hispanic responders, 41.4% reported being able to speak English (many of these were not fluent), and we were only able to interview 10 Hispanic Stage 1 responders for a total of 190 interviewees.

3.3. Building-Specific Response Rates. Stage 1 response rates (included Hispanic residents in the denominator) varied from a low of 60.9% at the largest and most diverse building ($n = 299$ residents; 40.1% Hispanic; 46.0% African American) to a high of 75.3% at high-rise number 4, which had many fewer residents and a more homogenous population ($n = 81$; 6.2% Hispanic; 82.7% African American). Stage 2 building-specific response rates (did not include Hispanic residents in the denominator) mirrored those in Stage 1 (Table 3).

3.4. Overcoming Mistrust. To address mistrust, we adopted three strategies. The first strategy was to partner with an aging services provider that for many years has employed

Table 1: Stage 1 responders and nonresponders by sociodemographic groupings.

Demographics	Nonresponders n	Nonresponders % or median (interquartile range)	Responders n	Responders % or median (interquartile range)	p value*
Age	195	66.0 (59.0 to 74.0)	358	64.0 (59.0 to 70.8)	0.077
Gender					0.171
Female	96	49.2	198	55.3	
Male	99	50.8	160	44.7	
Ethnicity					<0.001
Hispanic	67	34.4	70	19.6	
Non-Hispanic	128	65.6	288	80.4	
Race					0.012
African American	104	53.9	232	64.8	
Non-African American	89	46.1	126	35.2	

*p values determined by the nonparametric Wilcoxon two sample tests, Pearson chi-square tests, or Fisher's exact test.

Table 2: Stage 2 responders and nonresponders by sociodemographic groupings.

Demographics	Nonresponders n	Nonresponders % or median (interquartile range)	Responders n	Responders % or median (interquartile range)	p value*
Age	112	71.5 (65.0 to 79.0)	180	66.3 (63.1 to 72.8)	<0.001
Gender					0.214
Female	57	50.9	105	58.3	
Male	55	49.1	75	41.7	
Race					0.202
African American	88	78.6	152	84.4	
Non-African American	24	21.4	28	15.6	

*p values determined by the nonparametric Wilcoxon two sample tests, Pearson chi-square tests, or Fisher's exact test.

onsite social workers that provided assistance to residents. This partnership allowed us to send 4 to 5 mailings to all residents that were signed by us and the building-specific social worker. This linkage with the aging services agency enabled residents to discuss concerns they had regarding the study with the social workers and also allowed the social worker to introduce us to residents.

The second strategy for overcoming mistrust was to use a series of informational mailings on healthy aging and cognitive health (described previously in Section 2). These initial mailings provided a service to the residents and acquainted many of them with us.

The third strategy was to organize educational activities in the high-rise lobbies that coincided with each mailing. Placing the educational activities in the lobbies generated much more resident contact than did having the activities in community rooms, which were often removed from the buildings' daily traffic. The onsite educational activities spanned two days, took place in either the mornings or afternoons, and contained free nutritious snacks, which facilitated interaction with many residents and helped build rapport. Because of these onsite activities, residents became accustomed to seeing the P.I. in the high-rise and many grew to interact with him on a friendly and casual level. Such residents would often later participate and actively recruit other residents into the study. Many residents were initially hesitant or neutral regarding participation, and when trusted residents endorsed our study, recruitment surged as knowledge and acceptance of the study spread through the public housing social networks.

3.5. Overcoming Lack of Transportation. We had one strategy to overcome recruitment difficulties related to transportation, which was to situate the study entirely within the high-rises and require no traveling by study participants. Bringing the study to the community was necessary because the residents were socioeconomically distressed and many had functional impairments that limited their mobility. Some residents also expressed strong reservations about traveling in winter due to safety concerns related to icy conditions. Conducting the psychiatric research interview in a convenient place and time helped convince many ambivalent residents to participate (e.g., some residents would only participate in an interview after returning home from their work; others were only

TABLE 3: Stage 1 and Stage 2 building-specific response rates.

	High-rise number 1		High-rise number 2		High-rise number 3		High-rise number 4		Total	
	n	%	*n*	%	*n*	%	*n*	%	*n*	%
Stage 1 survey response	47	64.4	68	68.0	182	60.9	61	75.3	358	64.7
Stage 2 interview response*	30	60.0	46	61.3	65	57.0	39	73.6	180	61.6

*Total eligible for Stage 2 includes public housing residents who were non-Hispanic, English-speaking, 60 years or older, and cognitively able to provide informed consent; we excluded Hispanic residents from Stage 2's response rate denominator because an unknown majority of Hispanic residents were not fluent in English.

willing to participate if the interview did not overlap with their favorite TV shows).

3.6. Overcoming the Knowledge Gap. Based on our interactions with the residents and feedback from onsite social workers, limited education, illiteracy, and lack of knowledge regarding mental illness were highly prevalent among the high-rise residents. To address the lack of knowledge recruitment barrier, we relied on three strategies: (1) a series of recruitment mailings, (2) onsite recruitment sessions, and (3) attendance at resident council meetings.

The series of recruitment mailings received a mixed reaction from the residents. While some residents read the mailings, and a few talked with us or the onsite social worker about the mailings, a large proportion of residents also did not read them: we saw many unopened mailings thrown away or in resident apartments during Stage 2 interviews. Of note is that a few residents voiced suspicion about the mass mailings due to the numerous scams that had targeted them.

The onsite recruitment sessions allowed us to interact verbally with residents and assist them in completing the health survey, which was particularly important for the many residents unable to read. Residents often had many questions about the study and these recruitment sessions did much to alleviate concerns and to increase knowledge of the study.

Throughout the course of the study, the P.I. attended some building-specific resident council meetings to introduce himself, discuss the study, and answer resident questions. After attending these meetings, some residents became friendlier and made a greater effort to refer others to the study.

3.7. Overcoming the Community-Academic Divide. We addressed the last recruitment barrier—that of community-academic relationship building issues—in four ways. First, we immediately reimbursed residents for the health survey and psychiatric interview. These reimbursements helped ensure that the study was of tangible benefit to the participants, garnered support for our study, and resulted in referrals as many participants actively recruited others.

Second, to foster community support of our research and minimize its possible negative impact, we attempted to limit the burdensomeness of the interview. If the interview was too burdensome, it may have discouraged residents from participating in this study and possibly in future research efforts, whereas a less exhaustive interview could have the opposite effect. Consequently, the median interview duration was 94 minutes, with an interquartile range of 77 to 119 minutes. Although we tried to have the interview be relatively brief, and this interview duration was well below other psychiatric epidemiology studies that had interviews lasting beyond 2 hours [26, 27], some interviewees—relatively many of whom were male—would have preferred a shorter interview.

Third, after we completed the interviews in a high-rise, the residents received a mailing thanking them for their participation and summarizing the health survey findings for their building.

Fourth, we presented the findings to the resident council meetings, aging services agency assisting the residents, and Rochester Housing Authority. In support of this strategy is that throughout the study many residents expressed a desire to learn about the study findings.

4. Discussion

4.1. Study Response. Achieving a robust response among diverse urban older adults can be challenging as participation in epidemiologic studies has been declining [28] and many urban older adults are African Americans, a group for which recruitment into research has been difficult [7]. In consideration of this environment, our response rate of 61.6% for the non-Hispanic target population is satisfactory and compares favorably with other public housing studies [15, 29, 30]. Importantly, we were able to achieve a 60% response rate without directly soliciting residents by cold-calling or knocking. These direct solicitation recruitment methods were used in prior public housing studies [10, 15, 30, 31] and national psychiatric epidemiology studies, which achieved a 70% response following multiple contacts of nonresponders and high monetary incentives [32]. Rather we organized onsite educational activities and recruitment sessions at which residents primarily approached us.

There were differences between responders and nonresponders to Stage 1 health survey and Stage 2 interview that partly supported our hypotheses: Stage 1 respondents were more likely to be non-Hispanic and African American, whereas Stage 2 interviewees were more likely to be younger (consistent with prior studies having younger respondents [33]) and only 5.3% were Hispanic. Stage 1's ethnicity difference suggests that the Spanish-translated mailings were insufficient to overcome the language barrier, and it is possible that many of the Spanish-speaking residents were also illiterate (as were many of the non-Hispanic residents). Having a Spanish-speaking researcher at the recruitment activities to facilitate interaction and rapport-building with Hispanic and Latino residents would have been highly beneficial. Overall, our approach to accommodating the non-English speakers seemed to be only partially effective in Stage 1 and was absent in Stage 2 because of study resource limitations.

Response also varied across buildings. The largest building had the worst response rate, which was likely due to two factors. First, at times the demand to participate in Stages 1 and 2 was too much for us to accommodate. In the largest building it took many months to complete the interviews and it was difficult to maintain momentum as some Stage 1 respondents forgot about the study before they were contacted to schedule a Stage 2 interview. Second, 4 in 10 of the largest building residents were Hispanic, the majority of whom was not fluent in English. This made it difficult for the English-speaking P.I. to have meaningful in-person interactions with a large portion of the residents. In contrast, the building with the best recruitment (high-rise number 4) was relatively small and had far fewer non-English speakers. The varied responses across building sites suggest that researchers should be flexible in their recruitment approach to cater to the different community cultures present even within a single target population. While one research staff member was adequate in some situations, additional bilingual research staff would have been very useful in other settings.

4.2. Recruitment Barriers Summary. We anticipated that many residents would have considerable misgivings towards university researchers. Our efforts to partner with a community agency and provide an educational service to the residents seemed to be partially successful in building residents' trust as many residents—some of whom were initially hesitant and skeptical about our motivations—became quite friendly. A cautionary note must be raised, however: each high-rise had unique internal politics resulting in different resident cliques, and courting of one could harm recruitment from other cliques. Issues such as these may explain how differing recruitment approaches can influence the outcomes observed [34]. A practical approach to limit such biased outcomes would be to use multiple recruitment approaches that cast a wider net for engaging a variety of individuals (e.g., mailings, fliers, in-person recruitment, and referrals by community agencies). Our study would have likely had more participation if we formally involved the onsite social workers, building staff, resident council members, and study participants in recruitment.

Bringing the study to the residents was probably our most important recruitment strategy. Analogous strategies may be applied in communities for which residents reside in their own houses (e.g., recruitment from places where the residents congregate such as churches and senior nutrition centers).

In acknowledgement of the community-academic divide, we sought to balance the benefit to and demand upon the community by providing monetary incentives and limiting the interview burdensomeness. Most seemed happy to have participated and many were eager to participate in future research efforts. Nonetheless, there were a few who expressed annoyance with the interview length for whom we could have had available an abbreviated interview containing the key study constructs.

Table 4: Recruitment recommendation summary.

(1) Partner with known and trusted community agencies.
(2) Perform study at community sites accessible to and frequently visited by the study target population.
(3) Prior to recruitment, conduct a series of educational/outreach activities to acquaint the community with research staff.
(4) Provide immediate reimbursement to generate enthusiasm for and increase referrals into the study.
(5) To the extent feasible, limit the research burden upon participants.
(6) Use a wide variety of recruitment strategies to limit sampling bias and improve recruitment rates.
(7) Have research staff that is fluent in the study target population's language(s).*
(8) Share study findings with participants.

* Our study did not do this and we were unable to adequately recruit Hispanic residents.

4.3. Limitations and Strengths. Our findings have a number of limitations to consider. First, this study was based in a single geographic locale with recruitment strategies designed to take advantage of the congregate living setting, which may limit its generalizability. Second, the study utilized one recruitment approach for all residents, thereby preventing a direct comparison of effectiveness across recruitment strategies. Third, we did not systematically use feedback from building residents in our evaluation of recruitment strategies (e.g., no formal qualitative interviews); rather we used unsolicited resident feedback to inform our narrative. Fourth, we had limited information on study nonresponders, which weakened our ability to characterize them. Fifth, due to the limited resources, a non-Spanish-speaking white doctoral student conducted the educational activities, recruitment efforts, and psychiatric research interviews. Although matching recruitment staff on race and ethnicity is ideal if possible, white and African American researchers can have similar recruitment yields among minority populations if properly trained [35]. Due to language barriers, however, our study had limited accessibility to the 24.8% of the residents who were Hispanic.

The study recruitment approach has some notable strengths. In less than 1.5 years we were able to collect general health information from 358 and detailed mental health and service utilization data from 190 residents. This study's multifaceted recruitment approach achieved a 60% response rate in spite of being limited by the inability to use unsolicited telephone and at-home recruitment. Furthermore, study responders had a larger proportion of African Americans than study nonresponders, which is encouraging as older African Americans are usually underrepresented in research studies. The study also relied on relatively few resources (training grants funded the study) and may be easily adapted to other research studies. Table 4 summarizes our recommendations for studies seeking to recruit urban older adults, especially those living in congregate settings, and we recommend that future studies formally evaluate our impressions regarding these recruitment strategies.

5. Conclusions

Our study and others [15] suggest that socioeconomically disadvantaged older adults living in urban congregate settings are receptive to research that concurrently combines research efforts with educational outreach to assist the individuals. Among these urban older adults, many of whom are racial minorities, the willingness and need to participate in research exist, but the impetus is on researchers to leave their academic institutions and meet these individuals in the communities in which they reside.

Disclosure

Some of this paper's findings were presented at The Gerontological Society of America's 63rd Annual Scientific Meeting, New Orleans, November 19–23, 2010.

Disclaimer

The content of this paper is solely the responsibility of the authors and does not necessarily reflect the official views of the National Institute of General Medicine Sciences, AHRQ, NIMH, NCRR, or NIH.

Conflict of Interests

The authors declare that there is no conflict of interests regarding the publication of this paper.

Authors' Contribution

Adam Simning designed and conducted the study, performed the analyses, and wrote the paper. Yeates Conwell and Edwin van Wijngaarden supervised the study, provided input on the analyses, and assisted with writing the paper. The study sponsors had no role in study design, analyses, data interpretation, or publication of this study.

Acknowledgments

The authors thank the staff of the Rochester Housing Authority and Eldersource for making this work possible. During this study, Adam Simning was a trainee in the University of Rochester's Medical Scientist Training Program funded by the National Institutes of Health (NIH) (T32 GM07356), and this research was supported in part by grants from the Agency for Healthcare Research and Quality (AHRQ) (R36 HS018246); National Institute for Mental Health (NIMH) (R24 MH071604); and the National Center for Research Resources (NCRR) (TL1 RR024135), a component of the NIH, and NIH Roadmap for Medical Research.

References

[1] V. L. Shavers-Hornaday, C. F. Lynch, L. F. Burmeister, and J. C. Torner, "Why are African Americans under-represented in medical research studies? Impediments to participation," *Ethnicity and Health*, vol. 2, no. 1-2, pp. 31–45, 1997.

[2] H. Gavaghan, "Clinical trials face lack of minority group volunteers," *Nature*, vol. 373, no. 6511, p. 178, 1995.

[3] P. A. Areán and D. Gallagher-Thompson, "Issues and recommendations for the recruitment and retention of older ethnic minority adults into clinical research," *Journal of Consulting & Clinical Psychology*, vol. 64, no. 5, pp. 875–880, 1996.

[4] U.S. Census Bureau, *Profile of General Population and Housing Characteristics: 2010*, U.S. Census Bureau, 2014, http://quickfacts.census.gov/qfd/states/00000.html.

[5] G. Corbie-Smith, S. B. Thomas, and D. M. M. S. George, "Distrust, race, and research," *Archives of Internal Medicine*, vol. 162, no. 21, pp. 2458–2463, 2002.

[6] J. Wasserman, M. A. Flannery, and J. M. Clair, "Rasing the ivory tower: the production of knowledge and distrust of medicine among African Americans," *Journal of Medical Ethics*, vol. 33, no. 3, pp. 177–180, 2007.

[7] C. D. Qualls, "Recruitment of African American adults as research participants for a language in aging study: example of a principled, creative, and culture-based approach.," *Journal of Allied Health*, vol. 31, no. 4, pp. 241–246, 2002.

[8] G. Corbie-Smith, S. B. Thomas, M. V. Williams, and S. Moody-Ayers, "Attitudes and beliefs of African Americans toward participation in medical research," *Journal of General Internal Medicine*, vol. 14, no. 9, pp. 537–546, 1999.

[9] C. E. Earl and P. J. Penney, "The significance of trust in the research consent process with African Americans," *Western Journal of Nursing Research*, vol. 23, no. 7, pp. 753–762, 2001.

[10] B. P. Dennis and J. B. Neese, "Recruitment and retention of african american elders into community-based research: lessons learned," *Archives of Psychiatric Nursing*, vol. 14, no. 1, pp. 3–11, 2000.

[11] L. Curry and J. Jackson, "The science of including older ethnic and racial group participants in health-related research," *The Gerontologist*, vol. 43, no. 1, pp. 15–17, 2003.

[12] G. Moreno-John, A. Gachie, C. M. Fleming et al., "Ethnic minority older adults participating in clinical research: developing trust," *Journal of Aging & Health*, vol. 16, no. 5, pp. 93S–123S, 2004.

[13] T. J. McCallum and C. R. Arlien, "Enhancing the matching model of recruitment through focus groups," *Aging & Mental Health*, vol. 10, no. 3, pp. 312–318, 2006.

[14] S. Levkoff and H. Sanchez, "Lessons learned about minority recruitment and retention from the centers on minority aging and health promotion," *The Gerontologist*, vol. 43, no. 1, pp. 18–26, 2003.

[15] S. K. Jeffries, W. Choi, J. Butler, K. J. Harris, and J. S. Ahluwalia, "Strategies for recruiting African-American residents of public housing developments into a randomized controlled trial," *Ethnicity & Disease*, vol. 15, no. 4, pp. 773–778, 2005.

[16] J. N. Henderson, M. Gutierrez-Mayka, J. Garcia, and S. Boyd, "A model for Alzheimer's disease support group development in African-American and Hispanic populations," *The Gerontologist*, vol. 33, no. 3, pp. 409–414, 1993.

[17] S. L. Bistricky, R. S. MacKin, J. P. Chu, and P. A. Areán, "Recruitment of African Americans and Asian Americans with late-life depression and mild cognitive impairment," *The American Journal of Geriatric Psychiatry*, vol. 18, no. 8, pp. 734–742, 2010.

[18] D. R. Williams, "African-American health: the role of the social environment," *Journal of Urban Health*, vol. 75, no. 2, pp. 300–321, 1998.

[19] E. L. Ballard, F. Nash, K. Raiford, and L. E. Harrell, "Recruitment of black elderly for clinical research studies of dementia: the CERAD experience," *The Gerontologist*, vol. 33, no. 4, pp. 561–565, 1993.

[20] M. S. Wolf, J. A. Gazmararian, and D. W. Baker, "Health literacy and functional health status among older adults," *Archives of Internal Medicine*, vol. 165, no. 17, pp. 1946–1952, 2005.

[21] M. Kutner, E. Greenberg, Y. Jin, and C. Paulsen, *The Health Literacy of America's Adults: Results from the 2003 National Assessment of Adult Literacy*, US Department of Education, National Center for Education Statistics, Washington, DC, USA, 2003.

[22] S. M. Stahl and L. Vasquez, "Approaches to improving recruitment and retention of minority elders participating in research: examples from selected research groups including the National Institute on Aging's Resource Centers for Minority Aging Research," *Journal of Aging & Health*, vol. 16, no. 5, pp. 9S–17S, 2004.

[23] M. W. Leung, I. H. Yen, and M. Minkler, "Community-based participatory research: a promising approach for increasing epidemiology's relevance in the 21st century," *International Journal of Epidemiology*, vol. 33, no. 3, pp. 499–506, 2004.

[24] D. G. Moriarty, M. M. Zack, and R. Kobau, "The Centers for Disease Control and Prevention's Healthy Days Measures—population tracking of perceived physical and mental health over time," *Health and Quality of Life Outcomes*, vol. 1, article 37, 2003.

[25] M. B. First, R. L. Spitzer, M. Gibbon, and J. B. W. Williams, *Structured Clinical Interview for DSM-IV-TR Axis I Disorders*, New York State Psychiatric Institute, Biometrics Research, New York, NY, USA, 2002.

[26] J. S. Jackson, M. Torres, C. H. Caldwell et al., "The National Survey of American Life: a study of racial, ethnic and cultural influences on mental disorders and mental health," *International Journal of Methods in Psychiatric Research*, vol. 13, no. 4, pp. 196–207, 2004.

[27] R. C. Kessler, P. Berglund, W. T. Chiu et al., "The US National Comorbidity Survey Replication (NCS-R): design and field procedures," *International Journal of Methods in Psychiatric Research*, vol. 13, no. 2, pp. 69–92, 2004.

[28] S. Galea and M. Tracy, "Participation rates in epidemiologic studies," *Annals of Epidemiology*, vol. 17, no. 9, pp. 643–653, 2007.

[29] P. V. Rabins, B. S. Black, R. Roca et al., "Effectiveness of a nurse-based outreach program for identifying and treating psychiatric illness in the elderly," *The Journal of the American Medical Association*, vol. 283, no. 21, pp. 2802–2809, 2000.

[30] J. Robison, J. J. Schensul, E. Coman et al., "Mental health in senior housing: racial/ethnic patterns and correlates of major depressive disorder," *Aging and Mental Health*, vol. 13, no. 5, pp. 659–673, 2009.

[31] P. V. Rabins, B. Black, P. German et al., "The prevalence of psychiatric disorders in elderly residents of public housing," *The Journals of Gerontology, Series A: Biological Sciences and Medical Sciences*, vol. 51, no. 6, pp. M319–M324, 1996.

[32] S. G. Heeringa, J. Wagner, M. Torres, N. Duan, T. Adams, and P. Berglund, "Sample designs and sampling methods for the Collaborative Psychiatric Epidemiology Studies (CPES)," *International Journal of Methods in Psychiatric Research*, vol. 13, no. 4, pp. 221–240, 2004.

[33] M. Michelet, A. Lund, and U. Sveen, "Strategies to recruit and retain older adults in intervention studies: a quantitative comparative study," *Archives of Gerontology and Geriatrics*, vol. 59, no. 1, pp. 25–31, 2014.

[34] M. Izal, R. Nuevo, I. Montorio, and G. Pérez-Rojo, "Method of recruitment and the scores of self-report measures: the example of worry in the elderly," *Archives of Gerontology and Geriatrics*, vol. 48, no. 1, pp. 45–49, 2009.

[35] E. E. Thompson and H. W. Neighbors, "Recruitment and retention of African American patients for clinical research: an exploration of response rates in an urban psychiatric hospital," *Journal of Consulting & Clinical Psychology*, vol. 64, no. 5, pp. 861–867, 1996.

8

Depression among Ethiopian Adults: Cross-Sectional Study

Getasew Legas Molla,[1] Haregwoin Mulat Sebhat,[2] Zebiba Nasir Hussen,[3] Amsalu Belete Mekonen,[4] Wubalem Fekadu Mersha,[5] and Tesfa Mekonen Yimer[5]

[1]*Debre Tabor Hospital, Debre Tabor, Ethiopia*
[2]*Psychiatry Department, University of Gondar, P.O. Box 196, Gondar, Ethiopia*
[3]*Amanuel Mental Specialized Hospital, P.O. Box 1971, Addis Ababa, Ethiopia*
[4]*College of Health Sciences, Debre Tabor University, P.O. Box 272, Debre Tabor, Ethiopia*
[5]*College of Medicine and Health Sciences, Wolaita Sodo University, P.O. Box 138, Wolaita Sodo, Ethiopia*

Correspondence should be addressed to Wubalem Fekadu Mersha; wubfek@gmail.com

Academic Editor: Benno Roozendaal

Background. Depression is one of the most common mental disorders worldwide and is the second leading cause of disability and major contributor to suicide. *Methods.* Community based cross-sectional study was conducted among 779 adults residing in Northwest Ethiopia. Multistage cluster sampling technique was used to select study participants. Depression was measured by Patient Health Questionnaire (PHQ-9). Bivariate as well as multivariate logistic regressions were used to identify associated factors. p value of < 0.05 was considered statistically significant. *Result.* The prevalence of depression was 17.5%, where 10.7% of patients were with mild depression, 4.2% were with moderate depression, 1.9% were with moderately severe depression, and 0.6% had severe depression. Being female, age of 55 years and above, poor social support, having a comorbidity medical illness, current tobacco smoking, and living alone were significantly associated with depression. *Conclusion and Recommendation.* The prevalence of depression in Ethiopia is as common as the other lower and middle income countries. Female gender, being currently not married, poor social support, low wealth index, tobacco smoking, older age, having comorbid illness, and living alone were significantly associated with depression. So, depression is a significant public health problem that requires a great emphasis and some factors like smoking habit are modifiable.

1. Background

Depression is a common mental disorder characterized by depressed mood, loss of interest or pleasure, feeling of worthlessness or inappropriate guilt, disturbed sleep and appetite, feeling of tiredness, and poor concentration for a minimum of two weeks [1]. It affects 350 million people in the world and is the second leading cause of disability. The mortality rate due to suicide is 20 times greater among depressed individuals than the general population [2–4].

The magnitude of depression varies across different regions. WHO health survey conducted among 245,404 adults of 60 courtiers indicated that the overall one-year prevalence of depression was 3.2% [5]. Eighteen-country adult based study reported that the life time prevalence of Major Depressive Disorder (MDD) was 14.6% in 10 high income countries and 11.1% in 8 low and middle income countries [6]. Depression was also reported as 4.8% in Canada [7], 11.1% in Estonian [8], 15.1% in India, and 45.6% in Pakistan [9, 10] and it ranges from 4.9% to 29.3% in different African countries including Ethiopia [11–13].

According to CDC mortality and morbidity report in US, depression was more common in females (4.0%) than males (2.7%) and in unemployed persons (9.8%) than employed persons (2.0%) [14]. Depression was also common among substance users, disrupted marital status, older age, and lower educational level [15–19]. Other factors associated with depression in different studies were lack of social support, rural residence, having chronic illness, smoking, and alcohol use [20–23].

Assessing the prevalence of depression and the associated factors is very important in order to give good impression for the policy makers and to provide an input for evidence based intervention of depression. It is also helpful to indicate the modifiable factors that can affect depression for clinicians.

2. Methods

Community based cross- sectional study was conducted in 2015 at Ebinat town, Northwest Ethiopia. The town is located in south Gondar, Ethiopia, which is 680 km far from Addis Ababa, and the main livelihood is farming.

The sample was calculated using single population proportion formula by assuming the prevalence of depression of 9.1%, margin of error of 3%, 95% confidence level, design effect of 2, and 10% nonrespondent rate which gives a total sample of 779. Participants were recruited by using cluster sampling technique. All individuals whose age was greater or equal to 18 years were included in the study.

The dependent variable was depression and sociodemographic characteristics (age, sex, marital status, educational status, occupational status, wealth index, and residence), clinical factors (comorbid medical or surgical illness, past history of mental illness, and family history of mental illness), substance related factors, and social support were independent variables.

In this study participants were considered to have depression if their PHQ-9 score was greater or equal to 5 (5–9 mild depression, 10–14 moderate depression, 15–19 moderately severe depression, and 20–27 severe depression). Social support was described by sum score of Oslo 3 social support scale (OSS-3) as strong social support (12–14), intermediate social support (9–11), and poor social support (3–8).

The data were collected by pretested structured interviewer administered questionnaire which includes sociodemographic characteristics, substance use, clinical factors, social support (OSS-3), and PHQ-9. PHQ-9 screening tool has nine items and was validated in Ethiopia with sensitivity of 86% and specificity of 67% [24]. To maintain the quality of data training was given for data collectors and supervisors. The collected data were checked on daily basis for completeness and consistency. The data were entered in to Epi-Info version 7 and exported to SPSS-20 for analysis. Descriptive statistics was used to describe the study population in relation to relevant variables. Both bivariate and multivariate logistic regression models were used to identify associated factors. Odds ratio and their respective 95% confidence intervals were computed and variables with p value less than 0.05 were considered significantly associated.

Ethical clearance was approved by the Institutional Review Board (IRB) of University of Gondar and Amanuel Mental Specialized Hospital. After the purpose and related issues of the study were clearly informed, verbal consent was obtained from each study participant. Confidentiality was maintained by using anonymous questionnaire and by keeping the data in secure place. Participation was voluntary based and participants had the right to refuse the interview whenever they want. Participants who were found severely depressed were linked to the nearby health facility.

TABLE 1: Sociodemographic characteristics of respondents in Ebinat town, Northwest Ethiopia, 2015.

Variable	Category	Frequency (n)	Percentage (%)
Age	18–24	234	30
	25–34	298	38.3
	35–44	131	16.8
	45–54	54	6.9
	≥55	62	8
Sex	Male	416	53.4
	Female	363	46.6
Ethnicity	Amhara	775	99.5
	Tigre	4	0.5
Educational status	Unable to read and write	204	26.2
	Primary	151	19.4
	Secondary and above	424	54.4
Religion	Orthodox	682	87.5
	Muslim	95	12.2
	Protestant	2	0.3
Marital status	Widowed & divorced	106	13.6
	Single	300	38.5
	Married	373	47.6
Living circumstance	With family	561	72
	Alone	204	26.2
	Other	14	1.8
Wealth index	Lower income	141	18.1
	Medium income	382	49
	High income	256	32.9

3. Results

A total of 779 residents of the town were included in the study. Among the respondents 416 (53.4%) were male. Majority of participants were in the age group of 25–34 years with median age of 28 years and interquartile range of 14. About 373 (47.9%) were married and 424 (54.1%) had educational status of secondary school and above (Table 1).

From the total study participants, 62.3% of them drink alcohol, 9.5% of them chew khat, and 1.9% of the participants smoke tobacco products at least once in the last three months. Regarding life time use of substances 78%, 17.2%, and 7.6% of the participants consume alcohol, khat, and tobacco, respectively.

Fifty-three (6.8%) participants had reported comorbid medical illness, where 20 (2.6%) had HIV/AIDS, 8 (1%) had hypertension, 6 (0.8%) had diabetic mellitus, 5 (0.6%) had renal disease, and the remaining ones had other disorders.

Regarding social support, 278 (35.7%) had poor social support, 345 (44.3%) of the participants had intermediate social support, and 156 (20%) of participants had strong social support.

TABLE 2: Bivariate and multivariate analysis of depression among adults of Ebinat town, Northwest Ethiopia, 2015.

Variable	Category	Depression Yes	Depression No	COR 95% CI	AOR 95% CI
Sex	Male	45	371	1	1
	Female	91	272	2.75 (1.86–4.07)	**2.45 (1.40–4.29)****
Age	18–24	25	209	1	1
	25–34	46	252	1.52 (0.90–2.56)	1.82 (0.95–3.45)
	35–44	30	101	2.48 (1.38–4.44)	3.44 (1.45–8.18)
	45–54	10	44	1.90 (0.85–4.23)	2.04 (0.69–6.07)
	55 & above	25	37	5.64 (2.97–10.87)	**5.21 (1.89–14.37)****
Marital status	Widowed & divorced	47	59	7.45 (4.45–12.47)	**2.60 (1.28–5.27)****
	Single	53	247	2.00 (1.27–3.16)	**2.10 (1.08–4.06)***
	Married	36	337	1	1
Educational status	Unable to read & write	53	151	2.45 (1.60–3.75)	0.67 (0.31–1.41)
	Primary	30	121	1.73 (1.06–2.84)	1.04 (0.54–1.99)
	Secondary & above	53	371	1	1
Occupation	Employed	54	409	1	1
	Nonemployed	82	234	2.65 (1.817–3.87)	0.73 (0.41–1.28)
Social support	Poor	99	179	10.23 (4.82–21.74)	**7.40 (3.16–17.32)*****
	Moderate	29	316	1.70 (0.75–3.80)	1.83 (0.76–4.40)
	Strong	8	148	1	1
Current tobacco use (smoking)	Yes	6	9	3.25 (1.13–9.29)	**5.67 (1.47–21.47)***
	No	130	634	1	1
Comorbid medical illness	Yes	35	23	9.34 (5.30–16.46)	**7.22 (3.51–14.88)*****
	No	101	620	1	1
Living circumstance	Alone	64	140	3.105 (2.11–4.56)	**2.58 (1.50–4.44)****
	Other	0	14		
	Family	72	489	1	1
Wealth index	Lower	47	94	3.76 (2.245–6.31)	2.19 (1.14–4.23)*
	Medium	59	323	1.37 (0.85–2.20)	0.83 (0.46–1.50)
	Higher	30	226	1	1

Note. *$p < 0.05$, **$p < 0.01$, and ***$p < 0.001$. COR = crude odds ratio at 95% confidence interval; AOR = adjusted odds ratio at 95% confidence interval.

Among participants, 136 had score of ≥5 in PHQ-9 which makes the prevalence of depression 17.5% (mild depression 10.7%, moderate depression 4.2%, moderately severe depression 1.9%, and severe depression 0.6%).

Age, wealth index, sex, marital status, occupation, educational status, social support, current tobacco smoking, having comorbid illness, and living circumstance were associated with depression in bivariate analysis.

However, older age, lower wealth index, being divorced and widowed, being female, poor social support, having comorbid illness, tobacco smoking, and living alone were significantly associated with depression in multivariate analysis (Table 2).

4. Discussion

The study showed that the prevalence of depression was 17.5%. The finding of this study was in line with the finding in urban India which was 15.1% and a study conducted in 18 countries (14.6%) [6, 9]. The prevalence was lower than studies done in Pakistan (45.98%) and Uganda (29.3%) [10, 12]. However, it was higher than the studies done in USA (9%), Canada (4.8%), Korea (11%), Malaysia (10.3%), Estonia (11.1%), and South Africa (9.7%) [7, 8, 11, 16, 18].

People in the age group of 55 years and above had 5.21 times more odds to develop depression than people less than 25 years. The possible reasons may be inability to perform daily activities, sedentary life style, and occurrence of concomitant medical illness. The finding was supported by studies done in Korea, USA, and Ethiopia [13, 14, 16]. The odds of having depression among participants with low income were 2.19 times more as compared with their counterparts. The finding was consistent with the Korean study [16]. Participants who were currently not married (divorced and widowed) were 2.6 times more likely to have depression as compared with participants who were married.

Females were 2.45 times more likely to be depressed as compared with males. This may be due to having fluctuating hormone levels that are associated with symptoms of depression. This result is supported by studies done in USA, Pakistan, Nigeria, South Africa, Uganda, and Ethiopia [6, 11–13, 16]. Depression was more common among participants who have poor social support as compared with individuals who have good social support. The finding was supported by a study done in Japan [17].

Comorbid medical illnesses were significantly associated with depression. The possible explanation may be that medical illness can cause tremendous life changes which may limit mobility and independency, interferes with doing enjoyable activities, and consequently decreases self-confidence that results in depressive symptoms. The result was supported by other studies done in Malaysia and Ethiopian [13, 18]. The odds of having depression for participants who smoke tobacco were 5.67 times more than those who did not smoke tobacco. This finding was supported by a study conducted in Australia [20].

5. Conclusion

The prevalence of depression in Ethiopia is as common as the other lower and middle income countries. The study also revealed that female gender, being currently not married, poor social support, low wealth index, tobacco smoking, older age, having comorbid illness, and living alone were significantly associated with depression. So depression is a significant public health problem that requires a great emphasis and some factors like smoking habit are modifiable.

Competing Interests

The authors declare that they have no competing interests.

Authors' Contributions

Getasew Legas Molla conceived the original idea, was involved in proposal writing, designed the study, and participated in all implementation stages of the project. He analyzed the data and drafted and finalized the write-up of the paper. Haregwoin Mulat Sebhat was involved in proposal writing and participated in all stages of the project implementation and write-up of the paper. Zebiba Nasir Hussen was involved in proposal writing and participated in all stages of the project implementation and write-up of the paper. Amsalu Belete Mekonen was involved in proposal writing and participated in all stages of the project implementation and write-up of the paper. Wubalem Fekadu Mersha was involved in proposal writing and participated in all stages of the project implementation and write-up of the paper. Tesfa Mekonen Yimer was involved in proposal writing and participated in all stages of the project implementation and write-up of the paper. All authors read and approved the final paper.

Acknowledgments

The research was funded by Amanuel Mental Specialized Hospital.

References

[1] J. S. Benjamin and A. S. Verginal, *Kaplan & Sadok's Synopsis of Psychiatry Behaviour Science/Clinical Psychiatry*, 10th edition, 2007.

[2] World Health Organization, *Depression: A Global Crisis. World Mental Health Day, October 10 2012*, World Federation for Mental Health, Occoquan, Va, USA, 2012.

[3] J.-P. Lépine and M. Briley, "The increasing burden of depression," *Neuropsychiatric Disease and Treatment*, vol. 7, supplement 1, pp. 3–7, 2011.

[4] A. J. Ferrari, F. J. Charlson, R. E. Norman et al., "Burden of depressive disorders by country, sex, age, and year: findings from the global burden of disease study 2010," *PLoS Medicine*, vol. 10, no. 11, Article ID e1001547, 2013.

[5] S. Moussavi, S. Chatterji, E. Verdes, A. Tandon, V. Patel, and B. Ustun, "Depression, chronic diseases, and decrements in health: results from the World Health Surveys," *The Lancet*, vol. 370, no. 9590, pp. 851–858, 2007.

[6] E. Bromet, L. H. Andrade, I. Hwang et al., "Cross-national epidemiology of DSM-IV major depressive episode," *BMC Medicine*, vol. 9, article 90, 2011.

[7] S. B. Patten, L. W. Jian, J. V. A. Williams et al., "Descriptive epidemiology of major depression in Canada," *Canadian Journal of Psychiatry*, vol. 51, no. 2, pp. 84–90, 2006.

[8] A. Aluoja, M. Leinsalu, J. Shlik, V. Vasar, and K. Luuk, "Symptoms of depression in the Estonian population: prevalence, sociodemographic correlates and social adjustment," *Journal of Affective Disorders*, vol. 78, no. 1, pp. 27–35, 2004.

[9] S. Poongothai, R. Pradeepa, A. Ganesan, and V. Mohan, "Prevalence of depression in a large urban south Indian population—the Chennai urban rural epidemiology study (Cures-70)," *PLoS ONE*, vol. 4, no. 9, Article ID e7185, 2009.

[10] A. A. Muhammad Gadit and G. Mugford, "Prevalence of depression among households in three capital cities of Pakistan: need to revise the mental health policy," *PLoS ONE*, vol. 2, no. 2, article e209, 2007.

[11] M. Tomlinson, A. T. Grimsrud, D. J. Stein, D. R. Williams, and L. Myer, "The epidemiology of major depression in South Africa: results from the South African Stress and Health study," *South African Medical Journal*, vol. 99, no. 5, part 2, pp. 367–373, 2009.

[12] E. Kinyanda, P. Woodburn, J. Tugumisirize, J. Kagugube, S. Ndyanabangi, and V. Patel, "Poverty, life events and the risk for depression in Uganda," *Social Psychiatry and Psychiatric Epidemiology*, vol. 46, no. 1, pp. 35–44, 2011.

[13] S. Hailemariam, F. Tessema, M. Asefa, H. Tadesse, and G. Tenkolu, "The prevalence of depression and associated factors in Ethiopia: findings from the National Health Survey," *International Journal of Mental Health Systems*, vol. 6, article 23, 2012.

[14] Control CfD, "Current depression among adults—United States, 2006 and 2008," *MMWR Morbidity and Mortality Weekly Report*, vol. 59, no. 38, pp. 1229–1235, 2010.

[15] D. S. Hasin, R. D. Goodwin, F. S. Stinson, and B. F. Grant, "Epidemiology of major depressive disorder: results from the National Epidemiologic Survey on Alcoholism and Related Conditions," *Archives of General Psychiatry*, vol. 62, no. 10, pp. 1097–1106, 2005.

[16] D. H. Oh, S. A. Kim, H. Y. Lee, J. Y. Seo, B.-Y. Choi, and J. H. Nam, "Prevalence and correlates of depressive symptoms in Korean adults: results of a 2009 Korean community health survey," *Journal of Korean Medical Science*, vol. 28, no. 1, pp. 128–135, 2013.

[17] Y. Koizumi, S. Awata, S. Kuriyama et al., "Association between social support and depression status in the elderly: results of a 1-year community-based prospective cohort study in Japan," *Psychiatry and Clinical Neurosciences*, vol. 59, no. 5, pp. 563–569, 2005.

[18] S. F. Kader Maideen, S. Mohd Sidik, L. Rampal, and F. Mukhtar, "Prevalence, associated factors and predictors of depression among adults in the community of Selangor, Malaysia," *PLoS ONE*, vol. 9, no. 4, Article ID e95395, 2014.

[19] L. Gu, J. Xie, J. Long et al., "Epidemiology of major depressive disorder in Mainland China: a systematic review," *PLoS ONE*, vol. 8, no. 6, Article ID e65356, 2013.

[20] J. L. Rich, J. M. Byrne, C. Curryer, J. E. Byles, and D. Loxton, "Prevalence and correlates of depression among Australian women: a systematic literature review, January 1999- January 2010," *BMC Research Notes*, vol. 6, article 424, 2013.

[21] D. P. Chapman, G. S. Perry, and T. W. Strine, "The vital link between chronic disease and depressive disorders," *Preventing Chronic Disease*, vol. 2, no. 1, 2005.

[22] T. Ohira, H. Iso, S. Satoh et al., "Prospective study of depressive symptoms and risk of stroke among Japanese," *Stroke*, vol. 32, no. 4, pp. 903–908, 2001.

[23] T. Bitew, "Prevalence and risk factors of depression in Ethiopia: a review," *Ethiopian Journal of Health Sciences*, vol. 24, no. 2, pp. 161–169, 2014.

[24] B. Gelaye, M. A. Williams, S. Lemma et al., "Validity of the patient health questionnaire-9 for depression screening and diagnosis in East Africa," *Psychiatry Research*, vol. 210, no. 2, pp. 653–661, 2013.

9

Enhanced Early Neuronal Processing of Food Pictures in Anorexia Nervosa: A Magnetoencephalography Study

Lauren R. Godier,[1] Jessica C. Scaife,[1] Sven Braeutigam,[1,2] and Rebecca J. Park[1]

[1]*Oxford Brain-Body Research into Eating Disorders, Department of Psychiatry, University of Oxford, Oxford OX3 7JX, UK*
[2]*Oxford Centre for Human Brain Activity, Department of Psychiatry, University of Oxford, Oxford OX3 7JX, UK*

Correspondence should be addressed to Lauren R. Godier; lauren.godier@psych.ox.ac.uk

Academic Editor: Veit Roessner

Neuroimaging studies in Anorexia Nervosa (AN) have shown increased activation in reward and cognitive control regions in response to food, and a behavioral attentional bias (AB) towards food stimuli is reported. This study aimed to further investigate the neural processing of food using magnetoencephalography (MEG). Participants were 13 females with restricting-type AN, 14 females recovered from restricting-type AN, and 15 female healthy controls. MEG data was acquired whilst participants viewed high- and low-calorie food pictures. Attention was assessed with a reaction time task and eye tracking. Time-series analysis suggested increased neural activity in response to both calorie conditions in the AN groups, consistent with an early AB. Increased activity was observed at 150 ms in the current AN group. Neuronal activity at this latency was at normal level in the recovered group; however, this group exhibited enhanced activity at 320 ms after stimulus. Consistent with previous studies, analysis in source space and behavioral data suggested enhanced attention and cognitive control processes in response to food stimuli in AN. This may enable avoidance of salient food stimuli and maintenance of dietary restraint in AN. A later latency of increased activity in the recovered group may reflect a reversal of this avoidance, with source space and behavioral data indicating increased visual and cognitive processing of food stimuli.

1. Introduction

Anorexia Nervosa (AN) is a severely debilitating psychiatric disorder characterized by the relentless pursuit of thinness, leading to severe emaciation. It is associated with low rates of recovery [1] and has the highest mortality rate of any psychiatric disorder [2]. AN is extremely challenging to treat [3], and a lack of evidence-based treatments [4] has increased interest in investigating the neurobiological mechanisms underlying AN [5, 6].

Neuroimaging evidence suggests that food stimuli are aberrantly processed in AN. Increases in activity in the ventral limbic stream of emotional processing have been reported in response to food images in AN compared to controls [7–10]. This network is involved in the identification of emotionally salient stimuli and affective states [11, 12], suggesting food stimuli have emotional significance to individuals with AN. Furthermore, our group has previously shown an increased neural response to both rewarding and aversive food taste stimuli even after recovery from AN, suggesting increased salience attribution is given to food stimuli in these individuals [13].

Motivationally and emotionally relevant stimuli are suggested to lead to greater attentional processing [14]. Indeed, an attentional bias for food stimuli is reported in AN, using behavioral tasks such as the Emotional Stroop Task, Visual Dot Probe tasks, and Startle Reflex paradigms [15, 16]. However, evidence from eye tracking indicates that, despite initial attentional engagement, individuals with AN allocate less overall attention to food pictures compared to healthy controls, indicating an initial attentional bias may be followed by avoidance in these individuals [17]. These temporally distinct attentional processes in AN cannot be fully captured by functional Magnetic Resonance Imaging (fMRI), which has low temporal resolution and requires further investigation.

Electrophysiological measures of neural processing, such as electroencephalography (EEG) and magnetoencephalography (MEG), provide a real-time measure of neural activity and as such can map precisely the temporal dynamics of attentional processes. Event-Related Potentials (ERP) at different latencies are suggested to reflect different aspects of the information processing stream. For example, ERP measures of attention found at an early latency (100–300 ms after stimulus; e.g., N100/P100) are suggested to reflect early sensory processing and attentional orienting/selection processes [18]. ERPs in the midrange (200–300 ms after stimulus; e.g., early posterior negativity, EPN/N200/P200) are associated with emotional arousal and selective processing of emotional stimuli [19, 20]. Lastly, ERPs in the later range (300 ms and above after stimulus; e.g., late positive potential, LPP/P300) reflect the incentive salience or motivated attention towards a stimulus [18, 21]. Despite neuroimaging and behavioral evidence of the increased salience of food stimuli in AN, there are a few EEG studies investigating the neural processing of food stimuli in AN, with inconsistent results [22–24], and no published MEG studies to date. With this in mind, the current study aimed to extend the investigation of the temporal dynamics of the neural processing of food stimuli in individuals with AN using MEG, in conjunction with a reaction time task and eye tracking.

There is also evidence to suggest that individuals with AN process high- and low-calorie food stimuli differently, which may underpin the underconsumption of high-calorie food and overconsumption of low-calorie food that characterizes AN. In a behavioral study, our group found that individuals with AN consciously desire and implicitly "want" low-calorie foods more than high-calorie foods. This is consistent with differences in the neural response to high- versus low-calorie foods in AN in reward and emotion processing regions in AN [25, 26]. Moreover, in a recent fMRI study, we found differential hyperactivation of the lateral frontal pole in AN versus healthy controls in response to high-calorie compared to low-calorie food pictures (unpublished data). The frontal pole serves as a supervisory attentional control centre [27, 28]. As such, hyperactivation during the high-calorie food pictures may reflect that, even in their malnourished state, individuals with AN feel the need to resist the biological drive to eat when energy-dense foods threaten their extreme dietary control [29].

In light of these results, we chose to investigate the neural response to both high- and low-calorie food pictures in AN. Participants included both individuals currently ill and recovered from AN, as this enables investigation of both state and trait differences in the processing of food stimuli in AN. It was hypothesized that high- and low-calories food pictures would be experienced as highly salient for both individuals currently ill and recovered from AN reflected by increased neural processing after stimulus for both high- and low-calorie food pictures in comparison to healthy controls. This was hypothesized to be further reflected by group differences in the behavioral reaction time and eye-tracking measures. We also predicted a difference would be seen in the neural response to high-calorie compared to low-calorie foods in the AN groups, reflecting previous fMRI results and behavioral differences in the implicit and explicit motivation for high- and low-calorie foods in AN.

2. Methods

2.1. Participants. Forty-two participants were recruited for 3 experimental groups; current AN (AN-C) (n = 13), recovered from AN (AN-R) (n = 14), and healthy controls (HC) (n = 15). General exclusion criteria included age <18 or >60, insufficient English language comprehension, male sex, left-handedness, and any contraindication to having a Magnetic Resonance Imaging (MRI) scan (head injury, neurological or any other severe medical illness, pregnancy, and metal implants of any kind). Ethical permission for this study was obtained from the South Central-Oxford A Research Ethics Committee.

2.1.1. AN-C Group. Inclusion criteria for the AN-C group included a current diagnosis of restrictive AN according to the Diagnostic and Statistical Manual of Mental Disorders, 4th edition (DSM-IV). Participants with a history or current diagnosis of binge/purge type AN or Bulimia Nervosa (BN) were excluded. Four participants were on both antidepressant (Selective Serotonin Reuptake Inhibitors [SSRI] or Serotonin Noradrenaline Reuptake Inhibitors [SNRI]) and atypical antipsychotic medication, and two were taking just antidepressant (SSRI) medication. Seven participants currently met the criteria for a mood disorder, 7 met the criteria for current Generalized Anxiety Disorder (GAD), and two met the criteria for current Obsessive Compulsive Disorder (OCD). Three participants reported previous but not current episodes of depression and 1 participant reported a previous episode of Posttraumatic Stress Disorder (PTSD).

2.1.2. AN-R Group. Inclusion criteria for the AN-R group included a past diagnosis of restrictive AN according to the DSM-IV. Participants with a history of binge/purge type AN or BN were excluded. In addition, participants must have maintained a body mass index (BMI) between 18.5 and 25 for the previous 12 months (assessed by self-report) and score within 1 SD of the Eating Disorder Examination (EDE) and Eating Disorder Examination-Questionnaire (EDE-Q) global mean scores for young women and not met current criteria for any DSM-IV disorder as assessed by the Structured Clinical Interview for the DSM-IV (SCID). Whilst none of the AN-R participants currently met criteria for depression, 12 had previously met the criteria for depression, and 5 were currently taking antidepressant medication. In addition, 3 participants had previously met the criteria for GAD and 1 for OCD.

2.1.3. HC Group. Inclusion criteria for the HC group included a current BMI between 18.5 and 25, no first-degree relative with a current or past ED diagnosis, no current or past diagnosis of a DSM-IV disorder, and scores within 1 SD of the EDE and EDE-Q mean scores for young women.

2.2. Procedures. Participants were initially screened by email to ensure they met the criteria for the study and then invited to a screening session at the Department of Psychiatry, University of Oxford. After informed consent was taken, participants were screened for current DSM-IV Axis-I disorders and given a battery of questionnaires to complete (described below).

Participants subsequently attended two more sessions in order to complete the MEG scan at the Oxford Centre for Human Brain Activity (OHBA) and the Oxford Centre for Magnetic Resonance Imaging (OCMR) for a Magnetic Resonance Imaging (MRI) structural scan. Participants were asked not to eat for 8 hours prior to the MEG scan. Previous studies have suggested that food deprivation may increase the activation of the appetitive motivational system [30]. As such, we predict it is in the fasted state that psychopathological processes will be most naturalistic for those with current AN. Subsequent to the MEG scan, participants completed subjective ratings of a number of food pictures they had seen in the scanner.

2.3. Measures. The SCID [31] was used to screen for Axis-I disorders. Eating disorder (ED) symptoms were measured using the global mean scores on the EDE [32], EDE-Q [33], and Self-Starvation Scale (SS) [34]. The Clinical Impairment Assessment (CIA) [35] was used to assess the severity of ED-related psychosocial impairment. Depression symptoms were measured using the Beck Depression Inventory (BDI-II) [36]. Anxiety symptoms were measured using the State Trait Anxiety Scale (STAI) [37]. Impulsivity was measured using the Barratt Impulsiveness Scale (BIS) [38]. Compulsivity was measured using the Obsessive Compulsive Inventory Revised (OCI-r) [39] and the Yale-Brown-Cornell Eating Disorder Scale Self-Report Questionnaire (YBC-EDs-SRQ) [40]. Participants also completed the Sensitivity to Punishment and Reward Questionnaire (SRSPQ) [41]. Verbal IQ was assessed using the National Reading Test (NART) [42]. Height and weight were taken to calculate BMI, and participants in the AN groups provided information regarding duration of illness, lowest BMI, treatments received, age of onset, and duration of recovery if applicable. To assess subjective states before the MEG scan, participants completed a series of 100 mm visual analogue scales (VAS) assessing in the moment mood (happiness, sadness, and anxiety), appetite related variables (hunger, thirst, fullness, and desire to eat), and ED-related variables (current body image, fear of gaining weight).

2.4. MEG Scan. MEG data was acquired using an Elekta VectorView™ MEG system at OHBA. The system provides a total of 306 channels; however, only data from the 204 gradiometers were considered here. The gradiometers are most sensitive to nearby (cortical) sources, where the local root-mean-square (RMS) value calculated over the two channels at each detector site and the global RMS value calculated over all channels are measures of the local and global brain activity, respectively. Accordingly, global RMS curve showed neuronal activity as a function of time, whereas local RMS maps illustrate the distribution of neuronal activity over the head at a given point in time.

On arrival, participants were screened for any contraindications to MEG and completed the VAS measures. They were then asked to sit in the scanner briefly to check for any artefacts in the MEG signal. Prior to the scan, two electrodes were placed next to the left eye to record electrooculogram (EOG) data, two electrodes were placed on the wrist to record electrocardiogram (ECG) data, and a grounding coil was placed in the centre of the forehead. Standard Elekta-Neuromag HPI (Head Position Indicator) was used for coregistration with MRI and head tracking during scan. Binocular eye-tracking data was recorded by means of an EyeLink 1000 (SR Research) device, which was set up and calibrated once the participants were in the scanner.

2.5. Food Pictures Task. Whilst in the MEG scanner, participants completed a simple food pictures task. Stimuli were 40 high-resolution (1034 × 768), standardized digital color photographs of foods divided equally into high-calorie and low-calorie categories. These images were provided by L. Charbonnier of the Image Sciences Institute, UMC Utrecht, and created as part of the Full4Health project (http://www.full4health.eu/), funded by the European Union Seventh Framework Program (FP7/2007–2013) under Grant agreement no. 266408. See supplementary materials (in Supplementary Material available online at http://dx.doi.org/10.1155/2016/1795901) for an example of the high- and low-calorie food pictures viewed by participants. The food pictures were presented via the Presentation software package and projected onto a screen via a Panasonic DLP based projector PT-D7700E (viewing distance 1.2 m, screen size 54.5 × 43 cm, resolution 1280 × 1024, and frequency 60 Hz). The order of the pictures was randomized and repeated three times. Each picture was on screen for 4000 ms, with an interstimulus interval of 1300 ± 500 ms, during which a fixation cross was shown centrally. During each food picture, a small black square appeared centrally between 500 and 1500 ms after stimulus onset. Participants were required to respond by pressing a button as soon as they saw the black square, and these reaction times were recorded via a fORP 932 interface box system. The task took approximately 10 minutes to complete.

Previous research from our group suggests that, despite no significant difference in explicit "liking" responses for high- and low-calorie foods, individuals with AN show increased "wanting" (incentive salience) for low-calorie foods compared to high-calorie foods, with the inverse pattern to that seen in controls [43]. For that reason, participants in this study were instructed to inwardly think about how much they wanted to eat each of the foods shown at that moment in time, although it is acknowledged that it was not possible to ensure that participants followed this instruction.

2.6. Subjective Rating of Food Pictures. To investigate group differences in subjective ratings of high- and low-calorie food pictures, participants subsequently rated 12 of the food pictures seen in the scanner (6 high-calorie and 6 low-calorie) on a 10-point VAS scale on the following two questions:

(1) How pleasant would it be to eat this food right now? (0: not pleasant, 10: very pleasant).

(2) How much do you want to eat this food right now? (0: not at all, 10: very much so).

2.7. MRI Structural Scan. An MRI structural scan was performed at the OCMR using a 3-Tesla Siemens Trio scanner with a 32-channel head coil. High-resolution T1-weighted images were acquired for subject alignment, using an MPRAGE sequence (174 × 192 × 192 matrix, voxel resolution 1 mm^3, TR = 2040 ms, TE = 4.7 ms, inversion time, and TI = 900 ms).

2.8. Data Analysis. Reaction time, subjective ratings, VAS scales, and questionnaire data were analyzed in the IBM Statistical Package for Social Sciences (SPSS) using between-subject analysis of variance (ANOVA). Reaction time data from three participants in the AN-C group was missing due to equipment failure during the experiment. The threshold for statistical significance was set at $p < 0.05$ for all analyses.

2.8.1. Eye-Tracking Analysis. Right eye data (x and y deflection, pupil size) were analyzed using a measure of the variation in the raw data (span) calculated as the difference between the maximum and minimum of values (position measure 11.2.3) [44]. Eye-tracking data from one participant in the AN-R group had to be excluded due to high levels of eye-blink interference in the data. Correlations between eye-tracking data and MEG data were carried out using Spearman's Rho in SPSS. The threshold for statistical significance was set at $p < 0.05$ for all analyses. Results are reported as X-span, Y-span, and P-Span to reflect x and y deflection and pupil size, respectively.

2.8.2. MEG Analysis

(1) Acquisition. Measurements were performed using a Neuromag-306 VectorView system. The data were sampled at 1000 Hz (0.03–330 Hz antialias filter; external artefact correction using Maxfilter™) and corrected for variations in head position before using MaxMove™. Physiological artefacts were identified from the recorded EOG and ECG and removed from the raw data using a projection method based on principal components (in-house software, algorithm similar to the spatial confound, and sensor data correction routines provided by SPM8; see also [45]). Remaining artefacts were manually excluded from the raw data (<2% of data). For averaging and subsequent analysis, data epochs from −0.3 to 2.5 s relative to stimulus onset were calculated separately for high- and low-calorie trials, band-pass filtered (1–30 Hz), and normalized to unit baseline (−0.1 to 0 s).

(2) Time-Series Analysis. Statistical differences in event-related fields (ERFs) between the conditions of interest across participants were analyzed employing a time-dependent measure $P(t)$, the details of which have been fully specified elsewhere [46]:

$$P(t) = \text{probability}\left(\chi^2\right), \quad \chi^2 = -2\sum_{i=1}^{N} \ln\left[f_i(t)\right]. \quad (1)$$

N denotes the number of channels. For each channel, $f_i(t)$ denotes a nonparametric statistical test applied to evoked fields of interest. For each significant interval ($P(t) < 0.01$), the spatial distribution of the significant difference was given by f_i. Correspondence between the spatial distribution of the significant difference and the spatial distribution of ERFs (using grand-average power maps = root-mean-square of the two gradiometers in a pair) was explored. Two different nonparametric tests (f) were used in the formula above. A nonparametric ANOVA (3 groups × 2 conditions) served as the main statistical test followed by Mann-Whitney U post hoc tests for between group analyses.

The ANOVA was based on standard algorithms applied to rank-transformed data. This is a well-known and validated technique commonly used to fit nonnormal data into framework of conventional statistical theory [47]. Note that $P(t)$ is a measure of the difference between brain signals (magnetic fields) which are related to but not necessarily the same as the difference between neuronal activities (here, squared readings). For simplification and robustness, significance (peaks of P) was further considered only if it was concomitant with a change in power (i.e., RMS signal; also tested with nonparametric statistics). Thus, the data presented here are indicative of both a change in dynamics (signal) and strengths of activity. As a consequence, some significant peaks (measure P) were not further analyzed because the simultaneous change in activity was not clear. Furthermore, latencies of above 500 ms were excluded due to potential interference from participants' button press response to the black square, which appeared 500–1500 ms after stimulus.

(3) Source Analysis. Source estimates were obtained for all subjects using S-Loretta inversion based on individual structural images. The head volume was approximated with overlapping spheres fitted to the local curvature. Voxel-based t-tests were used for statistical comparisons across groups. All source calculations were performed with Brainstorm 3.2 [48], which is documented and freely available for download online under the GNU general public license. The threshold for statistical significance was set at $p < 0.05$. The source analysis has certain limitations. Notably, it was not possible to establish significance after correcting for multiple comparisons (over voxels) due to strong intersubject variability in these data, which is most likely explained by the complex nature of stimuli used. Also, a lack of statistical power might account here for relatively weak source results. Note that the time-series analysis utilizes only data measured without interpolation typically required for source analysis (where thousands of voxel values are derived from hundreds of channel readings). Therefore, results in source space were restricted to times at which significance was established in signal space.

2.8.3. Correlations with MEG Time-Series Data. Correlations were investigated between MEG time-series data and reaction times, subjective ratings, eye-tracking data, and questionnaire measures of ED symptomology (EDE, EDE-Q, CIA, and SS) using Spearman's Rho in SPSS. Due to neuroimaging evidence of increased activity in regions associated with

TABLE 1: Demographic and psychological characteristics stratified by group.

Variable	AN-C (n = 13)		AN-R (n = 14)		HC (n = 15)		Significance (p value)	Post hoc (p < 0.05)
	Mean	SD	Mean	SD	Mean	SD		
Age	31.2	5.3	27.1	6.5	23.7	5.4	0.018	AN-C > HC
BMI	15.7	1.9	20.9	1.6	21.4	1.9	<0.001	AN-C < AN-R, HC
NART	114.0	7.5	114.6	6.8	109.1	7.3	0.087	—
Lowest BMI	13.0	1.2	13.8	1.2	—	—	0.571	—
Duration of illness	11.0	5.7	5.7	4.2	—	—	0.252	—
Age of onset	21.7	6.1	16.5	2.1	—	—	<0.001	AN-C > AN-R
EDE	3.1	1.4	0.74	0.6	0.24	0.2	<0.001	AN-C > AN-R, HC
EDE-Q	3.4	1.7	0.95	0.8	0.50	0.3	<0.001	AN-C > AN-R, HC
SS	52.8	28.7	5.3	8.4	0.27	0.8	<0.001	AN-C > AN-R, HC
BIS	56.5	12.5	61.6	9.7	56.0	11.8	0.363	—
CIA	29.5	13.4	7.9	6.5	1.9	2.3	<0.001	AN-C > AN-R, HC
OCI-r	20.8	15.8	10.8	6.4	5.7	6.8	0.002	AN-C > AN-R, HC
BDI	29.6	18.1	6.4	6.4	3.4	4.6	<0.001	AN-C > AN-R, HC
SPSRQ Punishment	15.5	5.9	12.1	4.7	8.4	4.0	0.001	AN-C > HC
SPSRQ Reward	8.1	4.3	8.9	4.3	9.3	3.4	0.707	—
STAI state	50.1	13.0	34.4	5.4	26.5	6.5	<0.01	AN-C > AN-R > HC
STAI trait	60.7	12.9	45.2	10.6	32.00	9.4	<0.001	AN-C > AN-R > HC
YBC-EDS-SRQ, current	16.4	8.2	3.8	3.9	0	0	<0.001	AN-C > AN-R, HC
YBC-EDS-SRQ, past	24.6	5.3	23.8	5.3	0	0	<0.001	AN-C, AN-R > HC

BMI: body mass index; NART: National Adult Reading Test; EDE: Eating Disorder Examination; EDE-Q: Eating Disorder Examination-Questionnaire; SS: Self-Starvation Scale; BIS: Barratt Impulsiveness Scale; CIA: Clinical Impairment Assessment; OCI-r: Obsessive Compulsive Inventory Revised; BDI: Beck Depression Inventory; YBC-EDS-SRQ: Yale-Brown-Cornell Eating Disorder Scale Self-Report Questionnaire; STAI: State Trait Anxiety Inventory; — indicates no significant difference between groups.

cognitive control and response inhibition, correlations were also carried out with questionnaire measures of impulsivity and compulsivity (BIS, OCI-r, and YBC-EDS-SRQ). MEG time-series data for each participant was extracted by averaging activity over the peak intervals at $p = 0.01$ for time points of interest. Due to the focus on group differences in the current study, correlations were carried out separately for each experimental group.

3. Results

Participant demographics and psychological characteristics can be seen in Table 1.

3.1. VAS Scales. VAS scale scores for each experimental group can be seen in the supplementary materials. There were significant group differences in happiness ($F[2, 41] = 3.679$, $= 0.034$), hunger ($F[2, 41] = 6.465$, $p = 0.004$), desire to eat ($F[2, 41] = 6.503$, $p = 0.004$), and fear of fatness ($F[2, 41] = 16.03$, $p < 0.001$). Bonferroni corrected post hoc analysis indicated significantly higher happiness, hunger, and desire to eat in the HC compared to AN-C group ($p < 0.05$). Fear of fatness followed a pattern of AN-C > AN-R > HC ($p < 0.05$).

3.2. Behavioral Results

3.2.1. Subjective Food Picture Ratings. Subjective ratings of pleasantness and wanting for high- and low-calorie food pictures stratified by experimental groups can be seen in the supplementary materials. There were a significant Calorie ∗ Group interaction in pleasantness ratings ($F[2, 39] = 5.916$, $p = 0.006$) and a significant main effect of group ($F[2, 39] = 10.44$, $p > 0.001$). This was driven by higher pleasantness ratings for both high- and low-calorie food pictures in the HC group compared to the AN-C and AN-R group ($p < 0.05$). There was also a significant main effect of calorie condition, indicating that all groups rated the high-calorie pictures as more pleasant than the low-calorie pictures ($F[1, 39] = 39.239$, $p < 0.001$). There was no significant Group ∗ Calorie interaction ($F[2, 39] = 2.630$, $p = 0.085$) or main effect of group ($F[2, 39] = 1.161$, $p = 0.364$) in wanting ratings for food pictures. This suggests there was no difference between groups on ratings of wanting for high- or low-calorie food pictures. There was however a main effect of calorie category, with all groups indicating higher wanting for high-calorie compared to low-calorie food pictures ($F[1, 39] = 14.824$, $p < 0.001$).

3.2.2. Reaction Times. Reaction times to high- and low-calorie food pictures across experimental groups can be seen in the supplementary materials. There was no significant group effect ($F[5, 72] = 2.087$, $p = 0.131$), calorie condition effect ($F[1, 72] = 1.669$, $p = 0.201$), or Group ∗ Calorie condition interaction ($F[2, 72] = .128$, $p = 0.880$) in reaction times to the food pictures.

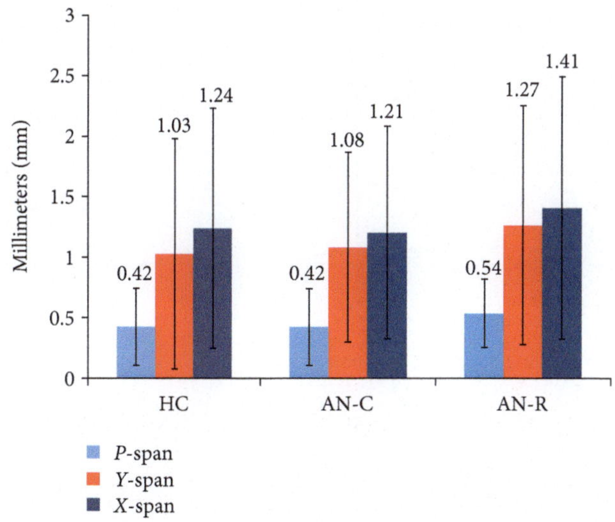

FIGURE 1: The main effect of group on P-span, Y-span, and X-span. P-span scores reflect pupil dilation (in mm) after stimulus onset. Y-span and X-span scores reflect movement horizontally and vertically (mm) from the central point of the picture. A significant main effect of group was found for all three measures ($p < 0.05$). Post hoc Bonferroni corrected t-tests indicated this was driven by increased scores on all three measures in the AN-R compared to the AN-C and HC groups ($p < 0.05$). AN-C: acute Anorexia Nervosa group, AN-R: recovered Anorexia Nervosa group, and HC: healthy control group.

3.2.3. Eye Tracking. X-span, Y-span, and P-span scores for each group can be seen in the supplementary materials. Significant group differences were found in the exploration of food pictures in general (both high and low conditions versus baseline). Group differences are shown in Figure 1 for the three measures of eye movement: X-span ($F[2, 2130] = 8.487$, $p < 0.001$), Y-span ($F[2, 2130] = 13.143$, $p < 0.001$), and P-span ($F[2, 2130] = 31.185$, $p < 0.001$). X- and Y-span denote movement of the eye from the central position of the black star on the x- and y-axis. P-span denotes change in pupil size. Bonferroni corrected post hoc analyses suggested significantly higher scores in the AN-R group compared to both the AN-C and HC groups in X-span, Y-span, and P-span ($p < 0.05$). There was also a main effect of calorie condition on X-span ($F[1, 2130] = 20.472$, $p < 0.001$), Y-span ($F[1, 2130] = 13.791$, $p < 0.001$), and P-span ($F[1, 2130] = 3.847$, $p = 0.05$), suggesting all participants explored high-calorie food pictures more than low calorie food pictures. There were no significant Group $*$ Calorie condition interactions (X-span: $F[2, 2130] = 0.270$, $p = 0.763$; Y-span: $F[2, 2130] = 0.458$, $p = 0.663$; P-span: $F[2, 2130] = 0.555$, $p = 0.574$).

3.3. MEG Results

3.3.1. Time-Series Analysis. Time-series analysis of the MEG data indicated a significant main effect of group in response to all food pictures (high- and low-calorie conditions) compared to baseline (see Figure 2, middle panel). Post hoc analyses (Mann-Whitney U tests) identified two significant time points of interest at which group differences reached a significance of $p < 0.01$: 150 ms and 320 ms. A significant increase in neuronal activity at 150 ms over posterior regions of the brain was observed in the AN-C group, compared to both the AN-R and HC groups. A significant increase in neuronal activity at 320 ms was also observed in the AN-R group, compared to both the AN-C and HC groups, over occipital regions of the brain. No significant main effect of calorie condition or Group $*$ Calorie condition interaction was found. Figure 2 shows the amplitude of neural activity over time collapsed across calorie conditions in each experimental group (top panel), the significance of the main effect of group over time (middle panel), and the significance of the Mann-Whitney U test group comparisons over time (bottom panel). Figure 3 shows the amplitude of neural activity across the experimental groups in signal space at 140–160 ms and 310–330 ms after stimulus (collapsed across calorie conditions).

3.3.2. Source Analysis. As explained in Section 2, the source analysis is somewhat limited and the results should be treated with care. We feel, however, that the clinical data here is worth presenting given the novelty of approach.

(1) Source Analysis of Neural Response at 150 ms. As a significant difference in neural activity at this time point was identified between the AN-C and HC group and the AN-C and AN-R group, differences in source space were investigated in Brainstorm using between-group t-tests. As the AN-C group showed increased neural activity compared to the HC and AN-R group, the focus of the source space analysis was also limited to regions of increased activation. Figure 4 shows the regions of increased activation in the AN-C compared to the HC group at 150 ms after stimulus (shown in red; $p = 0.005$). These regions were identified as the left precentral gyrus (Brodmann area 10), right frontopolar cortex (Brodmann area 10), and right superior frontal gyrus (Brodmann area 6).

Figure 5 shows the regions with increased activation in the AN-C compared to the AN-R group at 150 ms after stimulus (shown in red; uncorrected, $p = 0.005$). These regions were identified as the bilateral inferior parietal lobule (IPL; left supramarginal gyrus, Brodmann area 40; right angular gyrus, Brodmann area 39), the right middle temporal gyrus (ITG; Brodmann area 38), the right inferior frontal gyrus (IFG; Brodmann area 44), and the right frontopolar cortex (Brodmann area 10).

(2) Source Analysis of Neural Response at 320 ms. As a significant difference in neural activity at this time point was identified between the AN-R and AN-C group and the AN-R and HC group, differences in source space were investigated in Brainstorm using between-group t-tests. Significant regions emerged only when uncorrected for multiple comparisons. As the AN-R group showed increased neural activity compared to the HC and AN-C group, the focus of the source space analysis was also limited to regions of increased activation. Figure 6 shows regions with increased activation in the AN-R compared to the HC group at 320 ms after stimulus (shown in red, $p = 0.005$). These regions were identified as the right inferior temporal gyrus (Brodmann area 20), the

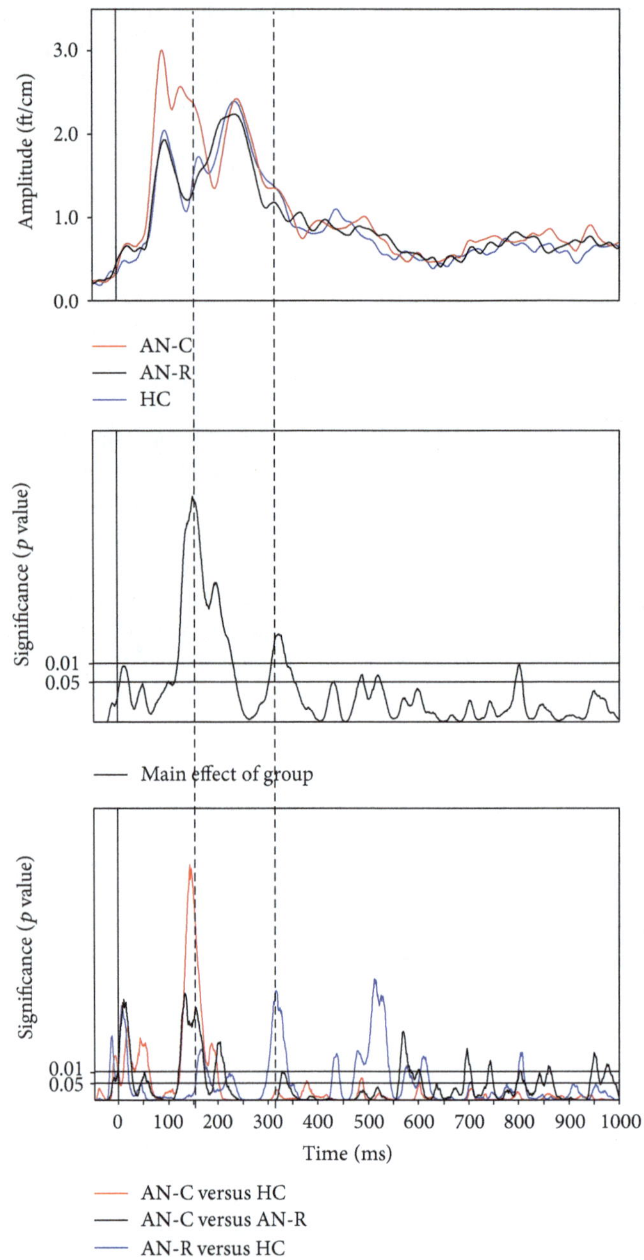

Figure 2: Group differences in neural activity. The top panel shows the mean amplitude (ft/cm) of neural activity after stimulus (collapsed across food categories) across the experimental groups. The middle panel illustrates the significance levels over time of the ANOVA main effect of group. The bottom panel illustrates the significance levels of post hoc Mann-Whitney U test analyses of group differences in mean amplitude of neural activity (collapsed across food categories) shown in the top panel. Note: ------ denotes the two peaks of interest: 150 and 320 milliseconds after stimulus, in which group comparisons were significant to the $p < 0.01$ level (see Methods for justification of peak selection). AN-C: acute Anorexia Nervosa group, AN-R: recovered Anorexia Nervosa group, and HC: healthy control group.

right superior parietal lobule (SPL; Brodmann area 7), and the left frontopolar cortex (Brodmann area 10).

Figure 7 shows regions with increased activation in the AN-R compared to the AN-C group at 320 ms after stimulus (shown in red, $p = 0.005$). These regions were identified as the right SPL (Brodmann area 7), the left frontopolar cortex (Brodmann area 10), the left occipital cortex (Brodmann area 18), and right occipital cortex (Brodmann area 19).

3.4. Correlations with MEG Time-Series Data. As no significant differences were found in the neural response to high- and low-calorie food stimuli, correlations were carried out

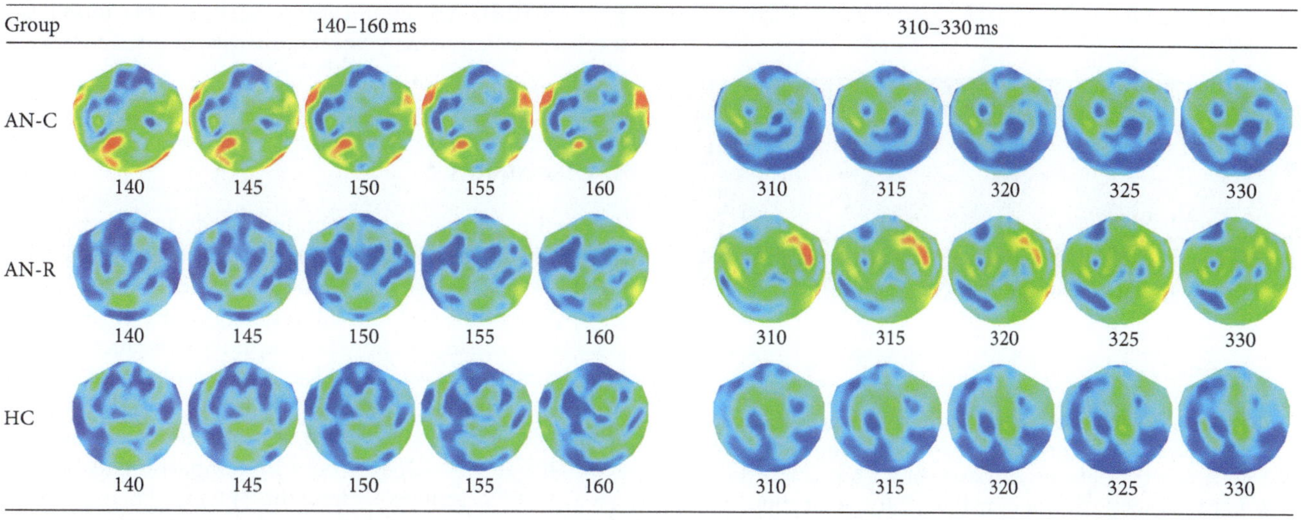

FIGURE 3: Mean amplitude of neural activity (ft/cm) for the two peak times of interest shown in sensor space (gradiometers) for each experimental group. Neural activity is shown with 10 milliseconds either side of the 150 and 320 milliseconds peaks after stimulus (all food pictures versus baseline). The scale used was 0–5 ft/cm with the exception of the 310–330 milliseconds' time period in the AN-R group, for which a scale of 0–3 ft/cm was used for visualisation purposes. AN-C: acute Anorexia Nervosa group, AN-R: recovered Anorexia Nervosa group, and HC: healthy control group.

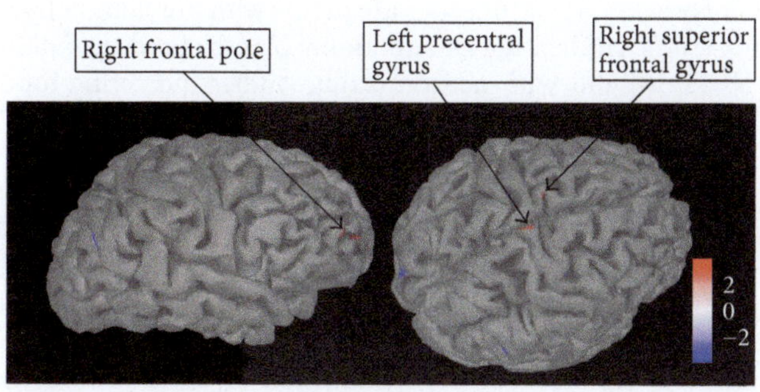

FIGURE 4: Regions showing significantly higher activation in the AN-C compared to HC group at 150 ms after stimulus. The figure shows the regions showing significantly higher activation in a t-test comparing the AN-C and HC group (shown in red) at 150 ms after stimulus (all food pictures versus baseline). Regions were identified by eye and are uncorrected for multiple comparisons ($p = 0.005$). Scale shown represents the t-value. AN-C: current Anorexia Nervosa group, HC: healthy control group.

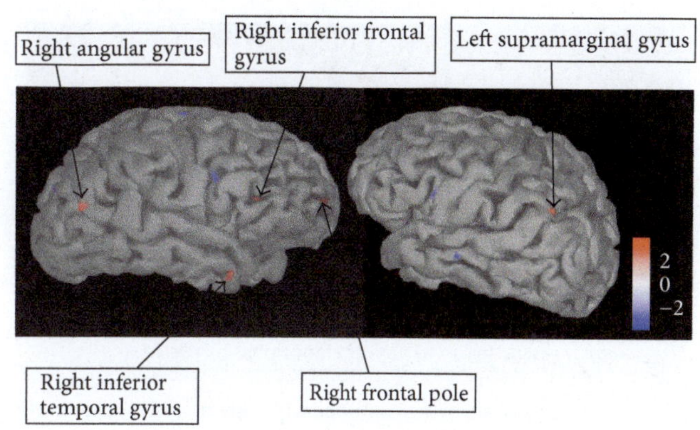

FIGURE 5: Regions showing significantly higher activation in the AN-C compared to AN-R group 150 ms after stimulus. Regions showing significantly higher activation in a t-test comparing the AN-C and AN-R group (shown in red) at 150 ms after stimulus (all food pictures versus baseline). Regions were identified by eye and are uncorrected for multiple comparisons ($p = 0.005$). Scale shown represents the t-value. AN-C: current Anorexia Nervosa group, AN-R: recovered Anorexia Nervosa group.

with the average neural response to *all* food stimuli at each time point of interest. MEG time-series data was averaged over the peak intervals at $p = 0.01$ for the two significant time points (120–180 ms, 300–340 ms).

3.4.1. Correlations with Neural Response at 150 ms. No significant correlation was found with the reaction time data or subjective food picture ratings at this time point in any of the experimental groups. A significant negative correlation was found in the AN-C group with both Y-span ($r = -0.736$, $p = 0.004$) and P-span ($r = -0.676$, $p = 0.011$). No significant correlation was found with eye-tracking measures in the AN-R and HC groups.

No significant correlation was found with measures of ED symptoms at the time point in any of the experimental groups. A significant correlation was found in the HC group with overall BIS scores ($r = 0.517$, $p = 0.048$) and the BIS nonplanning impulsivity subscale ($r = 0.625$, $p = 0.013$). In the AN-C group, a significant negative correlation was found with the BIS nonplanning impulsivity subscale ($r = -0.593$, $p = 0.033$). No significant correlation was found with any measures of impulsivity or compulsivity in the AN-R group.

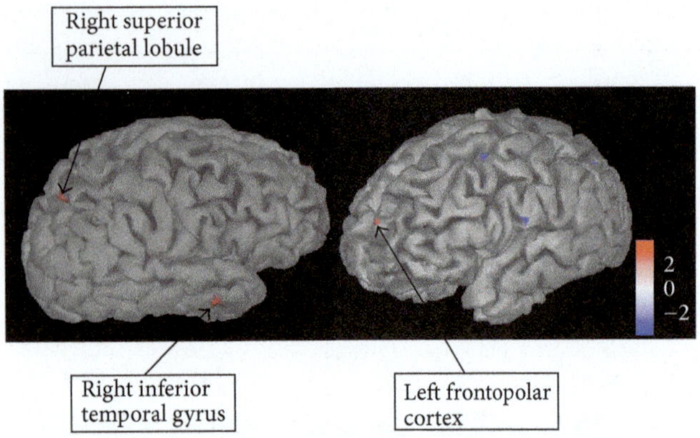

FIGURE 6: Regions showing significantly higher activation in the AN-R compared to HC group at 320 ms after stimulus. Regions showing significantly higher activation in a t-test comparing the AN-R and HC group (shown in red) at 320 ms after stimulus (all food pictures versus baseline). Regions were identified by eye and are uncorrected for multiple comparisons ($p = 0.005$). Scale shown represents the t-value. AN-R: recovered Anorexia Nervosa group, HC: healthy control group.

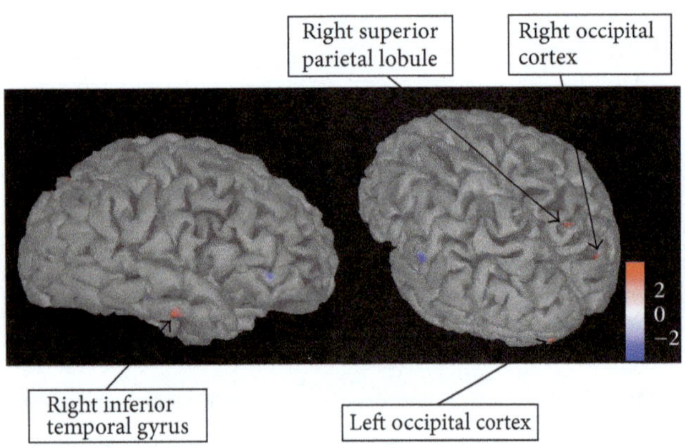

FIGURE 7: Regions showing significantly higher activation in the AN-R compared to AN-R group at 320 ms after stimulus. Regions showing significantly higher activation in a t-test comparing the AN-R and AN-C group (shown in red) at 320 ms after stimulus (all food pictures versus baseline). Regions were identified by eye and are uncorrected for multiple comparisons ($p = 0.005$). Scale shown represents the t-value. AN-R: recovered Anorexia Nervosa group, AN-C: current Anorexia Nervosa group.

3.4.2. Correlations with Neural Response at 320 ms. No significant correlation was found with the reaction time data at this time point in any of the experimental groups. A significant correlation was found in the AN-R group with P-span ($r = 0.599$, $p = 0.031$). A significant negative correlation was found in the AN-C group with Y-span ($r = -0.610$, $p = 0.027$). A significant correlation was found in the HC group with pleasantness ratings of food stimuli ($r = 0.590$, $p = 0.021$), a correlation not found in the AN groups.

No significant correlation was found with measures of ED symptoms in any of the experimental groups. A significant negative correlation was found in the AN-R group with the BIS nonplanning impulsivity subscale ($r = -0.584$, $p = 0.028$). No significant correlation was found with measures of impulsivity or compulsivity in the AN-C or HC group.

4. Discussion

To our knowledge, this is the first study to investigate the neural processing of food stimuli in AN using MEG. Using a time-series analysis, we found a significant main effect of group at two time points of interest in response to both calorie conditions versus baseline: 150 ms and 320 ms after stimulus. Significantly increased neural activity was observed at 150 ms in the AN-C group, compared to both the AN-R and HC groups. In addition, increased neural activity was observed at 320 ms in the AN-R group, in comparison to both the AN-C and HC groups. Despite this enhanced neural activity, both AN groups rated the food pictures as significantly less pleasant than the HC group. Contrary to our hypothesis, we found no significant differences in the neural response to high- versus low-calorie food pictures in any of the groups.

This early increase in neural activity confirms our hypothesis of enhanced early processing of food pictures in AN compared to HCs, which is also seen at a slightly later latency after recovery. These findings are in line with previous behavioral studies indicating an attentional bias for food stimuli in AN [15, 16] and with neuroimaging studies indicating food stimuli are aberrantly salient for individuals with AN [7–10, 13, 49–51].

The absence of nonfood picture stimuli in this study means we cannot rule out the possibility of enhanced neural processing of pictorial stimuli in general in AN. However, our findings show parallels with other electrophysiological studies of food stimuli processing in AN, which have also indicated enhanced early processing of food pictures using EEG [22, 23]. Blechert et al. [23] reported enhanced neural activity at 200–300 ms (the Early Positive Negativity; EPN) after stimulus to both high- and low-calorie food pictures in acute AN, compared to enhanced activity for high-calorie foods only observed in HCs, suggesting a generalized bias towards food stimuli in AN [23]. Furthermore, Novosel et al. [22] reported an increased P300 response to food stimuli, but not to emotional or neutral stimuli in individuals with AN compared to HCs [22]. These results are consistent with the motivated guidance of attention towards disorder-related stimuli in AN, which may allow preferential processing of these stimuli at a later stage [23]. However, both of these studies also reported a significant difference in the response to high- and low-calorie pictures in AN, a differentiation which was not observed in the current study. This may be due to methodological differences between these studies and the current paradigm, such as the inclusion of neutral or nonfood stimuli or insufficient statistical power in picking up subtle differences, due to small sample size.

The different latencies of increased neural activity in the AN-C and AN-R groups may reflect enhanced processing at different stages in the information processing stream. The earlier increase in neural activity found in the AN-C group is at a latency associated with early sensory processing and attentional orienting/selection processes [18]. An increase in activity at 100 ms after stimulus has been shown in response to fearful and threatening stimuli in those with high trait anxiety [52, 53]. As such, these results may reflect an increased threat response, or increased vigilance, very early in the neural processing of food stimuli in individuals with AN. This supports suggestion that individuals with AN show hypersensitivity towards food stimuli, which may enable subsequent avoidance of these stimuli and maintenance of dietary restraint [13]. The later latency of enhanced neural activity in the AN-R is consistent with increased emotional processing of stimuli [19, 20]. Indeed, an increase in activity around 300 ms has been reported in response to emotional pictures (appetitive or aversive) [54, 55], suggesting food stimuli are experienced as emotionally significant even after recovery from AN. It could be hypothesized that recovery from AN requires that food is no longer avoided as in the acute state, but it may still hold increased emotional salience for these individuals, resulting in increased emotional processing at this latency.

The results of the time-series analysis are further supported by an analysis of group differences in source space. It should be emphasized that group differences in source space were only observed when uncorrected for multiple comparisons, which is likely due to low statistical power. However, the regions identified are consistent with both hypersensitivity and increased cognitive control in response to food pictures, previously suggested in neuroimaging and electrophysiological studies in AN [13, 22, 23, 50, 51]. Increased neural activity at 150 ms after stimulus in the AN-C group was observed in the primary motor cortex (precentral gyrus), previously suggested to reflect an increased appetitive response to food pictures in AN [50]. Furthermore, increased activity in the AN-R group at 320 ms was observed in the SPL and ITG, suggesting increased visual and spatial processing of food stimuli even after recovery [56, 57].

Increased activation of the frontal pole, responsible for complex decision-making and cognitive control [58], was observed in both the AN-C group at 150 ms and the AN-R group at 320 ms, compared to the HC group. This finding mirrors that of our recent fMRI study using a parallel food pictures paradigm, in which we found differential activation of the frontal pole to high-calorie foods in AN; the opposite of that was found in controls (unpublished data). Activation of the frontal pole in both acute and recovered AN may represent trait-related activation of regions associated with higher-order cognitive processing in response to food. This is supported by a significant negative correlation in both AN groups, between neural activity at 150 ms, and the BIS nonplanning impulsivity subscale. This suggests that, in both AN groups, higher neural activity at 150 ms after stimulus was associated with a tendency to plan ahead and to think about future consequences. Whilst speculative, this may reflect the activation of higher-order cognitive control processes to downregulate increased attention for food stimuli and enable subsequent avoidance of food in AN.

The different latencies of increased neural activity between the AN-C and AN-R groups were also reflected by group differences in source space. At 150 ms, the AN-C group showed increased activation in regions associated with attention and response inhibition (IPL, frontal pole, and IFG) [59–61], although again this was only observed when uncorrected for multiple comparisons. Activation of these regions again suggests a possible state-related enhancement of both attention and response inhibition towards food stimuli in acute AN compared to recovery. Furthermore, at 320 ms, the AN-R group showed increased activation in regions consistent with increased visual processing of food stimuli [56, 57]. This is further supported by eye-tracking data, indicating significantly increased exploration of food stimuli in the AN-R group, compared to the AN-C and HC groups. Furthermore, neural activity at 320 ms was positively correlated with the *P*-span eye-tracking measure in the AN-R group. These results raise the possibility that this increase in neural activity in the AN-R group represents an increase in the visual P300 component. Modulation of this component is related to motivation/emotional properties of visual stimuli [21], and it has been associated with overfocused attention and hyperaroused cognitive processes [62]. As such, it is possible that food stimuli are associated with an increase in emotional and cognitive processing in recovery, in contrast with the AN-C group, for which increased activity at 150 ms was negatively correlated with measures of eye tracking. Whilst speculative, it could be hypothesized that increased cognitive/emotional processing of food stimuli following recovery represents a reversal of avoidance of food seen in the acute state of AN.

4.1. Limitations. Some methodological limitations are of note. As with many studies in this area, the sample size used was fairly small; however, we did isolate a sample of purely restrictive AN. Many neuroimaging studies in AN have included both restrictive and binge/purge AN subtypes and as such are unable to control for the possibility of within-group variability in neural activity, which may be related to important differences in psychopathology between subtypes of AN. However, future research may benefit from larger sample sizes enabling the inclusion and comparison of both AN subtypes. In addition, a number of participants had comorbid anxiety or depression diagnoses and were taking serotonergic antidepressants and/or antipsychotic medications. Antidepressant and antipsychotic medications have been shown to alter neural activity measured by MEG [63, 64], and so the effects of these medications, or indeed comorbid diagnoses, on our results cannot be ruled out.

An important limitation of the experimental paradigm was that it did not include nonfood pictures as a control condition, and as such we cannot rule out the possibility that individuals with AN would show an increased neural response to viewing pictures in general. In addition, significant differences in source space were only observed when uncorrected for multiple comparisons, which is likely due to low statistical power. As such, these results should be interpreted with caution, and replication is needed with a larger sample size and the inclusion of nonfood stimuli for comparison. However, previous studies corroborate our findings in source space [13, 22, 23, 50, 51] and show individuals with AN do not differ from healthy individuals in neural response to nonfood images [22, 23].

4.2. Conclusions. In conclusion, we observed early enhanced activity for both high- and low-calorie foods in individuals with acute AN, compared to HCs. This finding is consistent with an early attentional bias for food stimuli in AN, which appears to occur at a later latency in recovery. Whilst uncorrected for multiple comparisons, source space analysis indicated increased activity in regions associated with attention and cognitive control in the AN groups. This is consistent with previous neuroimaging and electrophysiological studies and may enable identification and subsequent avoidance of salient food stimuli and the maintenance of dietary restraint in AN. The later latency of increased activity in the AN-R group may reflect a reversal of this avoidance, with increased visual and cognitive processing of food stimuli in this group.

Competing Interests

The authors declare that there is no conflict of interests regarding the publication of this paper.

Acknowledgments

This work was funded by an MRC Confidence in Concept grant and an HEFCE Clinical Lecturer Award granted to Rebecca J. Park. Lauren R. Godier is funded by an MRC PhD studentship.

References

[1] N. D. Berkman, K. N. Lohr, and C. M. Bulik, "Outcomes of eating disorders: a systematic review of the literature," *International Journal of Eating Disorders*, vol. 40, no. 4, pp. 293–309, 2007.

[2] J. Arcelus, A. J. Mitchell, J. Wales, and S. Nielsen, "Mortality rates in patients with anorexia nervosa and other eating disorders: a meta-analysis of 36 studies," *Archives of General Psychiatry*, vol. 68, no. 7, pp. 724–731, 2011.

[3] C. M. Bulik, "The challenges of treating anorexia nervosa," *The Lancet*, vol. 383, no. 9912, pp. 105–106, 2014.

[4] National Institute for Health and Care Excellence, *Eating Disorders. Core Interventions in the Treatment and Management of Anorexia Nervosa, Bulimia Nervosa and Related Eating Disorders. CG09*, National Institute for Health and Care Excellence, London, UK, 2004.

[5] W. H. Kaye, C. E. Wierenga, U. F. Bailer, A. N. Simmons, A. Wagner, and A. Bischoff-Grethe, "Does a shared neurobiology for foods and drugs of abuse contribute to extremes of food ingestion in anorexia and bulimia nervosa?" *Biological Psychiatry*, vol. 73, no. 9, pp. 836–842, 2013.

[6] W. H. Kaye, J. L. Fudge, and M. Paulus, "New insights into symptoms and neurocircuit function of anorexia nervosa," *Nature Reviews Neuroscience*, vol. 10, no. 8, pp. 573–584, 2009.

[7] R. Uher, M. J. Brammer, T. Murphy et al., "Recovery and chronicity in anorexia nervosa: brain activity associated with differential outcomes," *Biological Psychiatry*, vol. 54, no. 9, pp. 934–942, 2003.

[8] R. Uher, T. Murphy, M. J. Brammer et al., "Medial prefrontal cortex activity associated with symptom provocation in eating disorders," *The American Journal of Psychiatry*, vol. 161, no. 7, pp. 1238–1246, 2004.

[9] A. A. B. Joos, B. Saum, L. T. van Elst et al., "Amygdala hyperreactivity in restrictive anorexia nervosa," *Psychiatry Research—Neuroimaging*, vol. 191, no. 3, pp. 189–195, 2011.

[10] K. R. Kim, J. Ku, J.-H. Lee, H. Lee, and Y.-C. Jung, "Functional and effective connectivity of anterior insula in anorexia nervosa and bulimia nervosa," *Neuroscience Letters*, vol. 521, no. 2, pp. 152–157, 2012.

[11] M. L. Phillips, W. C. Drevets, S. L. Rauch, and R. Lane, "Neurobiology of emotion perception I: the neural basis of normal emotion perception," *Biological Psychiatry*, vol. 54, no. 5, pp. 504–514, 2003.

[12] J. L. Stein, L. M. Wiedholz, D. S. Bassett et al., "A validated network of effective amygdala connectivity," *NeuroImage*, vol. 36, no. 3, pp. 736–745, 2007.

[13] F. A. Cowdrey, R. J. Park, C. J. Harmer, and C. McCabe, "Increased neural processing of rewarding and aversive food stimuli in recovered anorexia nervosa," *Biological Psychiatry*, vol. 70, no. 8, pp. 736–743, 2011.

[14] M. M. Bradley, D. Sabatinelli, P. J. Lang, J. R. Fitzsimmons, W. King, and P. Desai, "Activation of the visual cortex in motivated attention," *Behavioral Neuroscience*, vol. 117, no. 2, pp. 369–380, 2003.

[15] V. Aspen, A. M. Darcy, and J. Lock, "A review of attention biases in women with eating disorders," *Cognition and Emotion*, vol. 27, no. 5, pp. 820–838, 2013.

[16] S. J. Brooks, A. Prince, D. Stahl, I. C. Campbell, and J. Treasure, "A systematic review and meta-analysis of cognitive bias to food stimuli in people with disordered eating behaviour," *Clinical Psychology Review*, vol. 31, no. 1, pp. 37–51, 2011.

[17] K. E. Giel, M. Teufel, H.-C. Friederich, M. Hautzinger, P. Enck, and S. Zipfel, "Processing of pictorial food stimuli in patients with eating disorders—a systematic review," *International Journal of Eating Disorders*, vol. 44, no. 2, pp. 105–117, 2011.

[18] J. T. Coull, "Neural correlates of attention and arousal: insights from electrophysiology, functional neuroimaging and psychopharmacology," *Progress in Neurobiology*, vol. 55, no. 4, pp. 343–361, 1998.

[19] H. T. Schupp, T. Flaisch, J. Stockburger, and M. Junghöfer, "Emotion and attention: event-related brain potential studies," in *Progress in Brain Research*, S. Anders and D. Wildgruber, Eds., pp. 31–51, Elsevier, New York, NY, USA, 2006.

[20] J. K. Olofsson, S. Nordin, H. Sequeira, and J. Polich, "Affective picture processing: an integrative review of ERP findings," *Biological Psychology*, vol. 77, no. 3, pp. 247–265, 2008.

[21] G. Hajcak, A. Macnamara, and D. M. Olvet, "Event-related potentials, emotion, and emotion regulation: an integrative review," *Developmental Neuropsychology*, vol. 35, no. 2, pp. 129–155, 2010.

[22] A. Novosel, N. Lackner, H.-F. Unterrainer et al., "Motivational processing of food cues in anorexia nervosa: a pilot study," *Eating and Weight Disorders*, vol. 19, no. 2, pp. 169–175, 2014.

[23] J. Blechert, B. Feige, A. Joos, A. Zeeck, and B. Tuschen-Caffier, "Electrocortical processing of food and emotional pictures in anorexia nervosa and bulimia nervosa," *Psychosomatic Medicine*, vol. 73, no. 5, pp. 415–421, 2011.

[24] C. Nikendei, H.-C. Friederich, M. Weisbrod et al., "Event-related potentials during recognition of semantic and pictorial food stimuli in patients with anorexia nervosa and healthy controls with varying internal states of hunger," *Psychosomatic Medicine*, vol. 74, no. 2, pp. 136–145, 2012.

[25] Z. R. Ellison, J. Foong, R. Howard, E. Bullmore, S. Williams, and J. Treasure, "Functional anatomy of calorie fear in anorexia nervosa," *The Lancet*, vol. 352, no. 9135, p. 1192, 1998.

[26] Y. Rothemund, C. Buchwald, P. Georgiewa et al., "Compulsivity predicts fronto striatal activation in severely anorectic individuals," *Neuroscience*, vol. 197, pp. 242–250, 2011.

[27] P. W. Burgess, I. Dumontheil, and S. J. Gilbert, "The gateway hypothesis of rostral prefrontal cortex (area 10) function," *Trends in Cognitive Sciences*, vol. 11, no. 7, pp. 290–298, 2007.

[28] J. M. Orr, H. R. Smolker, and M. T. Banich, "Organization of the human frontal pole revealed by large-scale DTI-based connectivity: implications for control of behavior," *PLoS ONE*, vol. 10, no. 5, Article ID e0124797, 2015.

[29] R. J. Park, B. D. Dunn, and P. J. Barnard, "Schematic models and modes of mind in anorexia nervosa I: a novel process account," *International Journal of Cognitive Therapy*, vol. 4, no. 4, pp. 415–437, 2011.

[30] B. I. Mauler, A. O. Hamm, A. I. Weike, and B. Tuschen-Caffier, "Affect regulation and food intake in bulimia nervosa: emotional responding to food cues after deprivation and subsequent eating," *Journal of Abnormal Psychology*, vol. 115, no. 3, pp. 567–579, 2006.

[31] American Psychiatric Association, *Diagnostic and Statistical Manual of Mental Disorders*, American Psychiatric Association, Washington, DC, USA, 4th edition, 2000.

[32] C. G. Fairburn, Z. Cooper, and M. O'Connor, "Eating disorder examination," in *Cognitive Behaviour Therapy and Eating Disorders*, Guildford Press, New York, NY, USA, 2008.

[33] C. G. Fairburn and S. Beglin, "Eating disorder examination questionnaire (EDE-Q 6.0)," in *Cognitive Behaviour Therapy and Eating Disorders*, C. Fairburn, Ed., pp. 309–313, Guildford Press, New York, NY, USA, 2008.

[34] L. R. Godier and R. J. Park, "A novel measure of compulsive food restriction in anorexia nervosa: validation of the Self-Starvation Scale (SS)," *Eating Behaviors*, vol. 17, pp. 10–13, 2015.

[35] K. Bohn and C. G. Fairburn, "The clinical impairment assessment questionnaire (CIA 3.0)," in *Cognitive Behaviour Therapy and Eating Disorders*, C. G. Fairburn, Ed., Guildford Press, New York, NY, USA, 2008.

[36] A. T. Beck, R. A. Steer, R. Ball, and W. F. Ranieri, "Comparison of Beck depression inventories -IA and -II in psychiatric outpatients," *Journal of Personality Assessment*, vol. 67, no. 3, pp. 588–597, 1996.

[37] C. D. Spielberger, R. L. Gorsuch, R. Lushene, P. R. Vagg, and G. A. Jacobs, *Manual for the State-Trait Anxiety Inventory*, Consulting Psychologists Press, Palo Alto, Calif, USA, 1983.

[38] J. H. Patton, M. S. Stanford, and E. S. Barratt, "Factor structure of the Barratt Impulsiveness Scale," *Journal of Clinical Psychology*, vol. 51, no. 6, pp. 768–774, 1995.

[39] E. B. Foa, J. D. Huppert, S. Leiberg et al., "The obsessive-compulsive inventory: development and validation of a short version," *Psychological Assessment*, vol. 14, no. 4, pp. 485–496, 2002.

[40] D. L. Bellace, R. Tesser, S. Berthod et al., "The yale-brown-cornell eating disorders scale self-report questionnaire: a new, efficient tool for clinicians and researchers," *International Journal of Eating Disorders*, vol. 45, no. 7, pp. 856–860, 2012.

[41] R. Torrubia, C. Ávila, J. Moltó, and X. Caseras, "The Sensitivity to Punishment and Sensitivity to Reward Questionnaire (SPSRQ) as a measure of Gray's anxiety and impulsivity dimensions," *Personality and Individual Differences*, vol. 31, no. 6, pp. 837–862, 2001.

[42] H. E. Nelson, *The National Adult Reading Test (NART)*, NFER-Nelson, Windsor, UK, 1982.

[43] F. A. Cowdrey, G. Finlayson, and R. J. Park, "Liking compared with wanting for high- and low-calorie foods in anorexia nervosa: aberrant food reward even after weight restoration," *American Journal of Clinical Nutrition*, vol. 97, no. 3, pp. 463–470, 2013.

[44] K. Holmqvist, N. Nyström, R. Andersson, R. Dewhurst, H. Jarodzka, and J. Van de Weijer, *Eye Tracking—A Comprehensive Guide to Methods and Measures*, Oxford University Press, New York, NY, USA, 2011.

[45] P. Berg and M. Scherg, "A multiple source approach to the correction of eye artifacts," *Electroencephalography and Clinical Neurophysiology*, vol. 90, no. 3, pp. 229–241, 1994.

[46] S. Braeutigam, S. P. R. Rose, S. J. Swithenby, and T. Ambler, "The distributed neuronal systems supporting choice-making in real-life situations: differences between men and women when choosing groceries detected using magnetoencephalography," *European Journal of Neuroscience*, vol. 20, no. 1, pp. 293–302, 2004.

[47] W. J. Conover and R. L. Iman, "Rank transformations as a bridge between parametric and nonparametric statistics," *The American Statistician*, vol. 35, no. 3, pp. 124–129, 1981.

[48] F. Tadel, S. Baillet, J. C. Mosher, D. Pantazis, and R. M. Leahy, "Brainstorm: a user-friendly application for MEG/EEG analysis," *Computational Intelligence and Neuroscience*, vol. 2011, Article ID 879716, 13 pages, 2011.

[49] S. Santel, L. Baving, K. Krauel, T. F. Münte, and M. Rotte, "Hunger and satiety in anorexia nervosa: fMRI during cognitive processing of food pictures," *Brain Research*, vol. 1114, no. 1, pp. 138–148, 2006.

[50] S. J. Brooks, O. G. ODaly, R. Uher et al., "Differential neural responses to food images in women with bulimia versus anorexia nervosa," *PLoS ONE*, vol. 6, no. 7, article e22259, 2011.

[51] S. J. Brooks, O. O'Daly, R. Uher et al., "Thinking about eating food activates visual cortex with reduced bilateral cerebellar activation in females with anorexia nervosa: an fMRI study," *PLoS ONE*, vol. 7, no. 3, Article ID e34000, 2012.

[52] W. Li, R. E. Zinbarg, and K. A. Paller, "Trait anxiety modulates supraliminal and subliminal threat: brain potential evidence for early and late processing influences," *Cognitive, Affective and Behavioral Neuroscience*, vol. 7, no. 1, pp. 25–36, 2007.

[53] W. Li, R. E. Zinbarg, S. G. Boehm, and K. A. Paller, "Neural and behavioral evidence for affective priming from unconsciously perceived emotional facial expressions and the influence of trait anxiety," *Journal of Cognitive Neuroscience*, vol. 20, no. 1, pp. 95–107, 2008.

[54] A. Mini, D. Palomba, A. Angrilli, and S. Bravi, "Emotional information processing and visual evoked brain potentials," *Perceptual and Motor Skills*, vol. 85, no. 1, pp. 143–152, 1996.

[55] D. Palomba, A. Angrilli, and A. Mini, "Visual evoked potentials, heart rate responses and memory to emotional pictorial stimuli," *International Journal of Psychophysiology*, vol. 27, no. 1, pp. 55–67, 1997.

[56] S. H. Creem and D. R. Proffitt, "Defining the cortical visual systems: 'what', 'where', and 'how'," *Acta Psychologica*, vol. 107, no. 1–3, pp. 43–68, 2001.

[57] M. Critchely, *The Parietal Lobes*, Hafner Publishing Company, New York, NY, USA, 1st edition, 1953.

[58] E. D. Boorman, T. E. J. Behrens, M. W. Woolrich, and M. F. S. Rushworth, "How green is the grass on the other side?

frontopolar cortex and the evidence in favor of alternative courses of action," *Neuron*, vol. 62, no. 5, pp. 733–743, 2009.

[59] M. F. S. Rushworth, A. Ellison, and V. Walsh, "Complementary localization and lateralization of orienting and motor attention," *Nature Neuroscience*, vol. 4, no. 6, pp. 656–661, 2001.

[60] V. Singh-Curry and M. Husain, "The functional role of the inferior parietal lobe in the dorsal and ventral stream dichotomy," *Neuropsychologia*, vol. 47, no. 6, pp. 1434–1448, 2009.

[61] A. R. Aron, T. W. Robbins, and R. A. Poldrack, "Inhibition and the right inferior frontal cortex," *Trends in Cognitive Sciences*, vol. 8, no. 4, pp. 170–177, 2004.

[62] P. Mavrogiorgou, G. Juckel, T. Frodl et al., "P300 subcomponents in obsessive-compulsive disorder," *Journal of Psychiatric Research*, vol. 36, no. 6, pp. 399–406, 2002.

[63] M. A. Mendez, P. Zuluaga, R. Hornero et al., "Complexity analysis of spontaneous brain activity: effects of depression and antidepressant treatment," *Journal of Psychopharmacology*, vol. 26, no. 5, pp. 636–643, 2012.

[64] M. Korostenskaja and S. Kähkönen, "What do ERPs and ERFs reveal about the effect of antipsychotic treatment on cognition in schizophrenia?" *Current Pharmaceutical Design*, vol. 15, no. 22, pp. 2573–2593, 2009.

10

The Relation between Psychiatric Diagnoses and Constipation in Hospitalized Patients

Janique G. Jessurun,[1,2] Peter N. van Harten,[1,3] Toine C. G. Egberts,[2,4] Ysbrand J. Pijl,[1] Ingeborg Wilting,[2,4] and Diederik E. Tenback[1]

[1] *GGz Centraal Psychiatric Center, Innova, 3818 EW Amersfoort, Netherlands*
[2] *Division of Pharmacoepidemiology & Clinical Pharmacology, Utrecht Institute for Pharmaceutical Sciences, Faculty of Science, Utrecht University, 3584 CG Utrecht, Netherlands*
[3] *Department of Psychiatry and Neuropsychology, Maastricht University, 6211 LK Maastricht, Netherlands*
[4] *Department of Clinical Pharmacy, University Medical Center Utrecht, 3584 CX Utrecht, Netherlands*

Correspondence should be addressed to Janique G. Jessurun; janiquejessurun@gmail.com

Academic Editor: Jogin Thakore

Objective. Constipation is a prevalent problem in patients with psychiatric disorders; it reduces quality of life and may lead to severe complications. The prevalence distribution of constipation across all psychiatric diagnoses in patients with severe mental illness (SMI) has hardly been studied. The aim of this study is to estimate the association between psychiatric disorders and constipation in SMI inpatients. *Methods.* The strength of the association between constipation (based on use of laxatives) and DSM-IV psychiatric diagnosis was studied in a cross-sectional study with "adjustment disorders" as the reference group. The association was analyzed using logistic regression. *Results.* Of the 4728 patients, 20.3% had constipation. In the stratum of patients older than 60 years, all psychiatric categories except for substance related disorders were significantly associated with a higher prevalence of constipation (odds ratios ranging from 3.38 to 6.52), whereas no significant associations were found in the stratum of patients between 18 and 60 years (odds ratios ranging from 1.00 to 2.03). *Conclusion.* In the elderly, all measured psychiatric diagnoses are strongly associated with an increased prevalence of constipation. Physicians should be extra alert for constipation in SMI patients, independent of specific psychiatric diagnoses.

1. Introduction

Constipation is a prevalent symptom in the psychiatric population, with a reported two-year period prevalence of 36.3% in schizophrenic patients [1] and 57.7% in depressive patients [2]. In addition, an incidence rate of 15 per 100 person-years has been observed in patients with severe mental illness (SMI) [3]. Although constipation is a frequent problem in the psychiatric population, there is little attention for it in research. This is in contrast with the clinical consequences of constipation that can cause or aggravate many common digestive symptoms and complaints and may even lead to severe complications such as fecal impaction, bowel perforation, paralytic ileus, and death [4] and is associated with a decreased quality of life in a similar degree as depression and diabetes [5]. In addition, SMI patients usually face delay in diagnosis and treatment of somatic comorbidity [6, 7]. A recent study has shown that only 18.5% of constipated psychiatric inpatients reported the presence of constipation to their psychiatrists [8]. The burden of the disease makes early recognition and treatment of constipation of clinical importance.

Dementia and depression are considered possible secondary causes of constipation [9]. In addition, anxiety and depression have been widely associated with functional gastrointestinal disorders, especially irritable bowel syndrome [10–12]. When diagnosing depression, constipation is usually taken into consideration, however, not with other psychiatric diagnoses. Despite the high incidence of constipation in psychiatric patients and the high burden of the disease,

Table 1: The association between psychiatric diagnoses and constipation (stratified for age).

Psychiatric diagnoses	18 to 60 years ($n = 3433$)		60 years and older ($n = 1295$)	
	Period prevalence of constipation (% (n/N))	Adjusted odds ratio (95% confidence interval)[a]	Period prevalence of constipation (% (n/N))	Adjusted odds ratio (95% confidence interval)[a]
Adjustment disorders	6.0% (16/267)	1.00 (reference)	5.7% (5/87)	1.00 (reference)
Schizophrenia and other psychotic disorders	16.1% (170/1054)	1.52 (0.83 to 2.78)	49.8% (142/285)	5.72 (2.01 to 16.28)*
Depressive disorders	12.5% (65/518)	1.28 (0.70 to 2.33)	40.9% (110/269)	4.94 (1.77 to 13.73)*
Personality disorders	17.2% (94/548)	1.68 (0.92 to 3.08)	47.1% (32/68)	5.20 (1.68 to 16.12)*
Delirium, dementia, and amnestic and cognitive disorders	13.2% (21/159)	1.42 (0.68 to 2.99)	34.6% (92/266)	4.45 (1.58 to 12.50)*
Alcohol-related disorders	13.8% (29/210)	1.56 (0.78 to 3.13)	18.7% (29/155)	3.59 (1.21 to 10.68)*
Bipolar disorders and other mood disorders	19.4% (48/247)	1.60 (0.91 to 3.15)	40.2% (35/87)	3.38 (1.08 to 10.57)*
Anxiety disorders	10.7% (17/159)	1.14 (0.53 to 2.45)	32.7% (17/52)	4.18 (1.28 to 13.66)*
Pervasive developmental disorders	12.8% (12/94)	2.03 (0.84 to 4.90)	100% (1/1)	NE
Rest group	9.7% (7/72)	1.00 (0.36 to 2.82)	45.0% (9/20)	6.52 (1.58 to 27.00)*

[a]All categories were adjusted for gender, age, the use of antipsychotics, mood stabilizers, antidepressants, calcium supplements, iron supplements, diuretics, NSAIDs, opioids, lithium, sympathicomimetics, anticholinergics, and benzodiazepines.
*Significant at a 5% level.
NE = not estimable.

the distribution across all psychiatric diagnoses in the severe mentally ill has hardly been studied. The aim of this study is to assess the association between (primary) psychiatric diagnoses and constipation in psychiatric inpatients.

2. Materials and Methods

A cross-sectional study was performed at GGz Centraal "Zon en Schild," a psychiatric center located in the Netherlands. Patients of 18 years and older hospitalized during 2007 and 2010, for whom a psychiatric diagnosis was available, were included. When patients were admitted multiple times during this observation period, data of the longest admission were taken into account. All data were obtained from the Electronic Healthcare Information System and from the Pharmacotherapeutical Response and Inventory Management system. The medical staff, according to DSM-IV criteria, entered diagnoses. Laxative use was taken as a proxy for constipation. Patients receiving at least one prescription for a laxative were considered having constipation.

The following potential confounders were evaluated [9]: gender, age, prescriptions for antidepressants, mood stabilizers (lithium, carbamazepine, lamotrigine, and valproic acid), benzodiazepines, antipsychotics, antispasmodics, motility inhibitors, anti-Parkinson drugs, hypnotics, antiepileptics, sympathicomimetics, antidiarrheal drugs, diuretics, calcium channel blockers, calcium supplements, iron supplements, antihistamines, opioids, nonsteroidal anti-inflammatory drugs, and comorbid somatic disorders including diabetes and hypothyroidism. Logistic regression analyses were used to evaluate the strength of the association between the psychiatric diagnoses and constipation. The patients being diagnosed with "adjustment disorders" were taken as the reference group; that is, the risk was set at 1, because (i) this kind of mental disorder is usually of short duration and a result of a specific stressor [13] and (ii) the disorder is relatively mild compared to other mental disorders [14]. Each covariate that univariately changed the odds ratios of the psychiatric diagnoses with more than 10% was incorporated into the final multivariate model. In addition, all analyses were checked for multicollinearity and interaction tests were performed across different age categories (18 to 60 years and 60 years or older). All data analyses were performed using SPSS version 18. This study was not subject to medical ethical review since (i) no data were collected in the course of a study, (ii) the patients did not have to change their behavior in any way, and (iii) all data were anonymous.

3. Results

A total of 5027 psychiatric patients were eligible. For 299 patients, no psychiatric diagnosis was available. Therefore, the final study population consisted of 4728 patients of which 959 patients (20.3%) had constipation. The results of the logistic regression analyses are presented in Table 1. Analysis of the categories "additional codes," "other disorders in childhood," "substance related disorders," and "attention deficit disorders and disruptive behavior disorders" did not render representative results because of small numbers (less than 10 events). The interaction test between age and psychiatric diagnoses was significant ($p < 0.05$). Therefore, a stratified analysis was performed. For patients older than 60 years, all psychiatric diagnoses were significantly associated with an increased risk for constipation with odds ratios ranging from 3.38 to 6.52. However, in patients aged between 18 and 60 years, psychiatric categories were not significantly associated with an increased risk of constipation with odds ratios ranging from 1.00 to 2.03.

4. Discussion

This study shows that, in the elderly, all measured psychiatric diagnoses are significantly associated with constipation in comparison with patients with adjustment disorder. Among the young and middle-aged SMI patients, the strength of associations was much less and not statistically significant. The results of this first study on the association between psychiatric diagnosis and constipation are in contrast with clinical handbooks and previous studies that irritable bowel syndrome/constipation is more or less specifically related to depression and anxiety disorders [10–12]. Clinical handbooks do not report about the relationship between other psychiatric diagnoses and constipation [15].

Psychiatric disorders may be associated with constipation due to an effect of the disease itself and/or due to other associated factors. Patients with SMI generally have an unhealthy lifestyle (characterized by a poor diet, poor fluid intake, and inactivity) [16]. This may contribute to the occurrence of constipation [9]. No studies have been performed in psychiatric inpatients comparing the degrees to which these unhealthy lifestyle factors occur amongst the different psychiatric diagnoses and different ages. The results show statistically significant strong associations in the elderly but not in the young and middle aged. It can be hypothesized that these unhealthy lifestyle factors occur more frequently in elderly patients with psychiatric disorders [17], which may partially explain the results of this study. Another possible explanation for the results of the study is a differential use of psychotropic drugs in the elderly, as psychotropics are associated with the occurrence of constipation [3, 9]. Psychotropics with anticholinergic activities are widely believed to cause constipation to a different degree than psychotropics without anticholinergic activities; however, conflicting results have been reported [3]. Of the elderly patients and younger patients, respectively, 75.3% and 74.9% used psychotropics (i.e., antidepressants, antipsychotics, and/or mood stabilizers). The average duration of psychotropic drug use was much longer and the total defined daily doses were higher in those ageing 60 years or more. There is a possibility that physiological factors, such as colonic motility, anorectal physiology, cognitive impairment, and impaired rectal sensation, become more prevalent with increasing age. In addition, it is known that several comorbidities, which are associated with altered autonomic functioning (such as diabetes), become more prevalent with increasing age. It is also likely that the prevalence of past abdominal surgeries (which are associated with constipation) increases with age.

One limitation of this study is that there were no data regarding several potential risk factors like a high body mass index (BMI), poor diet, low physical activity, low socioeconomic status, and smoking status [9, 18]. However, all hospitalized patients receive a similar diet in this institution. Furthermore, diabetes, age, and psychotropic use (covariates in the analysis) are related to BMI and physical inactivity [19, 20].

A second limitation is the use of laxatives as a proxy for constipation. This has probably led to an underestimation of the incidence as SMI patients usually face delay in diagnosis and treatment of somatic comorbidity [6, 7]. Another possibility for underestimation is the use of over-the-counter laxatives. However, most inpatients have a low income and prefer to ask for a prescription for laxatives instead of buying laxatives themselves.

A third limitation may be the choice of the control group. However, the group of inpatients with adjustment disorders was chosen, because this group is far more comparable to the group of inpatients with other psychiatric diagnosis than healthy controls that are not admitted and do not have a psychiatric diagnosis. Average duration of hospitalization, duration of psychotropic drug use, and the average of total defined daily doses were much shorter/lower in the patients with adjustment disorders. The period prevalence of constipation was 6% in this group, which is lower than the reported prevalence of 15% in the Dutch general population [21]. These findings suggest a useful and valid reference group.

Finally, it is important to note the cross-sectional nature of the study, not enabling making conclusions regarding causation.

Although conclusions with regard to causation are limited, constipation is prevalent in patients with SMI and associated with a decreased quality of life. In addition, constipation may lead to severe complications and SMI patients usually face delay in diagnosis and treatment of somatic comorbidity [6, 7]. Thus, the burden of constipation makes early recognition and treatment of constipation of clinical importance. This study shows the importance of alertness on constipation in all elderly SMI patients. Possible solutions on reducing the incidence and complications of constipation could be creating more awareness and thereby earlier recognition of constipation and stimulating healthier lifestyle. Treatment options of constipation include lifestyle modifications, the use of laxatives, and cessation/dose-reduction of contributing medication [9].

5. Conclusion

In elderly psychiatric inpatients, all measured psychiatric diagnoses are significantly associated with an increased prevalence of constipation. Physicians should be extra alert for constipation in this population. This alertness should not be limited to specific diagnostic groups or specific psychotropics.

Conflict of Interests

The authors declare no conflict of interests.

References

[1] M. De Hert, L. Dockx, C. Bernagie et al., "Prevalence and severity of antipsychotic related constipation in patients with schizophrenia: a retrospective descriptive study," *BMC Gastroenterology*, vol. 11, article 17, 2011.

[2] M. I. Afridi, M. A. Siddiqui, and A. Ansari, "Gastrointestinal somatization in males and females with depressive disorder," *Journal of the Pakistan Medical Association*, vol. 59, no. 10, pp. 675–679, 2009.

[3] J. G. Jessurun, P. N. van Harten, T. C. G. Egberts, B. J. Pijl, I. Wilting, and D. E. Tenback, "The effect of psychotropic medications on the occurrence of constipation in hospitalized psychiatric patients," *Journal of Clinical Psychopharmacology*, vol. 33, no. 4, pp. 587–590, 2013.

[4] M. De Hert, H. Hudyana, L. Dockx et al., "Second-generation antipsychotics and constipation: a review of the literature," *European Psychiatry*, vol. 26, no. 1, pp. 34–44, 2011.

[5] A. Wald, C. Scarpignato, M. A. Kamm et al., "The burden of constipation on quality of life: results of a multinational survey," *Alimentary Pharmacology and Therapeutics*, vol. 26, no. 2, pp. 227–236, 2007.

[6] M. J. Oud and B. Meyboom-de Jong, "Somatic diseases in patients with schizophrenia in general practice: their prevalence and health care," *BMC Family Practice*, vol. 10, article 32, 2009.

[7] M. Phelan, L. Stradins, and S. Morrison, "Physical health of people with severe mental illness," *The British Medical Journal*, vol. 322, no. 7284, pp. 443–444, 2001.

[8] T. Koizumi, H. Uchida, T. Suzuki et al., "Oversight of constipation in inpatients with schizophrenia: a cross-sectional study," *General Hospital Psychiatry*, vol. 35, no. 6, pp. 649–652, 2013.

[9] G. Lindberg, S. S. Hamid, P. Malfertheiner et al., "World Gastroenterology Organisation global guideline: constipation—a global perspective," *Journal of Clinical Gastroenterology*, vol. 45, no. 6, pp. 483–487, 2011.

[10] W. E. Whitehead, O. Palsson, and K. R. Jones, "Systematic review of the comorbidity of irritable bowel syndrome with other disorders: what are the causes and implications?" *Gastroenterology*, vol. 122, no. 4, pp. 1140–1156, 2002.

[11] S. Howell, R. Poulton, A. Caspi, and N. J. Talley, "Relationship between abdominal pain subgroups in the community and psychiatric diagnosis and personality. A birth cohort study," *Journal of Psychosomatic Research*, vol. 55, no. 3, pp. 179–187, 2003.

[12] G. Fond, A. Loundou, N. Hamdani et al., "Anxiety and depression comorbidities in irritable bowel syndrome (IBS): a systematic review and meta-analysis," *European Archives of Psychiatry and Clinical Neuroscience*, vol. 264, no. 8, pp. 651–660, 2014.

[13] S. Gur, H. Hermesh, N. Laufer, M. Gogol, and R. Gross-Isseroff, "Adjustment disorder: a review of diagnostic pitfalls," *Israel Medical Association Journal*, vol. 7, no. 11, pp. 726–731, 2005.

[14] M. J. Friedman, P. A. Resick, R. A. Bryant, J. Strain, M. Horowitz, and D. Spiegel, "Classification of trauma and stressor-related disorders in DSM-5," *Depression and Anxiety*, vol. 28, no. 9, pp. 737–749, 2011.

[15] B. J. Sadock, V. A. Sadock, P. Ruiz, and H. I. Kaplan, *Kaplan & Sadock's Comprehensive Textbook of Psychiatry*, Lippincott Williams & Wilkins, 9th edition, 2009.

[16] D. P. J. Osborn, I. Nazareth, and M. B. King, "Physical activity, dietary habits and Coronary Heart Disease risk factor knowledge amongst people with severe mental illness: a cross sectional comparative study in primary care," *Social Psychiatry and Psychiatric Epidemiology*, vol. 42, no. 10, pp. 787–793, 2007.

[17] P. Gallagher and D. O'Mahony, "Constipation in old age," *Best Practice and Research: Clinical Gastroenterology*, vol. 23, no. 6, pp. 875–887, 2009.

[18] C. Gratziou, "Respiratory, cardiovascular and other physiological consequences of smoking cessation," *Current Medical Research and Opinion*, vol. 25, no. 2, pp. 535–545, 2009.

[19] D. E. Tenback, F. Van Kessel, J. Jessurun, Y. J. Pijl, E. R. Heerdink, and P. N. van Harten, "Risk factors for inactivity in patients in long-term care with severe mental illness," *Tijdschrift voor Psychiatrie*, vol. 55, no. 2, pp. 83–91, 2013.

[20] R. Dent, A. Blackmore, J. Peterson et al., "Changes in body weight and psychotropic drugs: a systematic synthesis of the literature," *PLoS ONE*, vol. 7, no. 6, Article ID e36889, 2012.

[21] L. A. S. van Kerkhoven, T. Eikendal, R. J. F. Laheij, M. G. H. van Oijen, and J. B. M. J. Jansen, "Gastrointestinal symptoms are still common in a general Western population," *The Netherlands Journal of Medicine*, vol. 66, no. 1, pp. 18–22, 2008.

11

Mass Psychogenic Illness: Demography and Symptom Profile of an Episode

Binoy Krishna Tarafder,[1] Mohammad Ashik Imran Khan,[2] Md. Tanvir Islam,[3] Sheikh Abdullah Al Mahmud,[4] Md. Humayun Kabir Sarker,[5] Imtiaz Faruq,[5] Md. Titu Miah,[6] and S. M. Yasir Arafat[7]

[1] *Department of Medicine, Faridpur Medical College, Faridpur, Bangladesh*
[2] *Pulmonology, Bangabandhu Sheikh Mujib Medical University, Bangladesh*
[3] *Internal Medicine, Bangabandhu Sheikh Mujib Medical University, Bangladesh*
[4] *Pediatrics, Sheikh Sayera Khatun Medical College, Gopalganj, Bangladesh*
[5] *Sheikh Sayera Khatun Medical College, Gopalgang, Bangladesh*
[6] *Medicine, Dhaka Medical College Hospital, Dhaka, Bangladesh*
[7] *Department of Psychiatry, Bangabandhu Sheikh Mujib Medical University, Bangladesh*

Correspondence should be addressed to S. M. Yasir Arafat; arafatdmc62@gmail.com

Academic Editor: Nicola Magnavita

Background. Mass psychogenic illness has been a recurrent phenomenon in Bangladesh over recent times. *Objectives.* This study was aimed at investigating the demographic characteristics and symptom profile of an outbreak of mass psychogenic illness occurring in a girls' high school. *Methods and Materials.* In 14 April 2013, a total of 93 students of a girls' high school suddenly developed various symptoms following intake of tiffin cake which resulted in panic and hospital admission. A descriptive, cross-sectional observational survey was done to define various characteristics of the outbreak. *Results.* No organic explanation for the reported illnesses was found. 93 female students were included who were hospitalized during the incident. Trigger factor was found in 98% of students. Most of the students were 13 years old. Average interval between exposure to the trigger and onset of symptoms was 151.5 minutes. Commonest symptoms were abdominal pain (83%), headache (73%), chest pain (69%), body ache (63%), nausea (69%), and generalized weakness and fatigue (61%). Hospital stay following the incident was about 12 hours on average. *Conclusion.* To avoid unnecessary panic in the community a prompt, coordinated response is important in resolving widespread community anxiety surrounding these episodes.

1. Introduction

Mass psychogenic illness (MPI) is a not a very rare phenomenon anymore. It is probably more common than the reported incidences and imposes a significant financial burden and unexpected management difficulties for the emergency department [1]. Affected schools or occupational sites are often closed for days or weeks [2]. It can be defined as "the rapid spread of illness signs and symptoms affecting members of a cohesive group, originating from a nervous system disturbance involving excitation, loss, or alteration of function, whereby physical complaints that are exhibited unconsciously have no corresponding organic etiology" [3]. Outbreak of mass psychogenic illness often starts with an environmental trigger such as a bad smell, a sound, a suspicious looking substance, or something else that makes people in a group believe that they have been exposed to a danger and they start to experience symptoms of illness [4, 5]. An index case sometimes has organic problem. It has unique characteristics—symptoms without any plausible organic cause, transient and benign, occurring in a segregated group, presence of extraordinary anxiety, spread via sight, sound, or oral communication; the spread moves down the age scale, more affecting the females [6]. Common symptoms are nausea, dizziness, fainting, headache, abdominal pain, hyperventilation, cough, fatigue, drowsiness, weakness, watery eyes, chest pain, vomiting, and so forth [6–9]. Investigators failed to conclude regarding any predisposing factor of an episode, but psychological factors, environmental factors, different stressors, conflicts, lower education, lower socioeconomic status, minority race, and history of abuse or trauma may be involved [10–19]. Responders of emergency management and the initial media reports of unexplained illness are believed to amplify the phenomenon by spreading threatening information and lead more people to report symptoms [20]. Brief duration of illness, sudden onset without specific time, place, or person, and lack of opportunity for controlled experiment have made it a difficult field for the researchers. This study was aimed at reporting the demographic characteristics and symptom profile of an outbreak of mass psychogenic illness occurring in a girls' high school at Gopalganj in Bangladesh in April 2013.

2. The Episode

The incidence occurred in a girls' high school in the morning of 14 April 2013 after serving tiffin to the students like every other day. Few students of class five started feeling unwell within few minutes of taking the tiffin while playing in the playground. They were brought to the headmaster's room immediately. As the news spread among other students, some of the other students also started to feel sick. They were brought to the emergency department of nearby hospital. Subsequently some of the students who carried the sick students to hospital also felt unwell. Most of the students complained of bad odor or bad taste of the cake. All affected students were admitted. Treatment was given after a triage done by the hospital consultants. Counseling was done repeatedly to the sick students. Assurance and reassurance were also given to the parents and relatives. Within a short period of time media men and more anxious relatives rushed to the hospital. The situation was getting worse and local administration along with police department got involved to control the situation. Political leaders, social workers, and many curious people also came. Reports of a mysterious illness were being broadcasted in all the major television channels. Rumor of death of two to three students further worsened the situation. Situation was gradually controlled with the combined efforts of the doctors, nurses, other hospital staff, administrative personnel, and police. Some students feeling well left the hospital. Before evening, many students recovered and were discharged. Some students needed to stay in hospital up to the next day and few up to the following day. Some students became ill again after returning home and needed readmission. Three students were referred to the nearest tertiary care hospital because of deep concern of the relatives whose anxiety could not be alleviated by existing facilities. The supplied cake was considered as the environmental trigger of the episode and sample of cake was sent for microbiological and toxicological examination.

3. Materials and Methods

This cross-sectional observational survey was done in 250 Bedded General Hospital, Gopalganj, from 14 to 20 April 2013 to describe the characteristics of the outbreak, timeline of events, symptoms experienced, risk factors, and community perception of the event. An ethical clearance was taken from the concerned authority for the purpose of the study considering an emergency.

Diagnosis was confirmed by an internist, pediatrician. In some cases, relevant investigations were done to exclude organic causes. A detailed questionnaire was prepared promptly after the episode. All the students who were admitted with the illness during this period were included in the study. Those who came to hospital out of fear of illness and having no symptoms were excluded. Information was gathered from the sick students on their recovery and from their attending guardians by face to face interview. Help from the teachers, guardians, and administrative and health personnel was received during data collection and managing the hospital rush during the episode. Data were managed and analyzed by Statistical Package for Social Science (SPSS, V 16) version 16 and Microsoft Excel 2007 version.

4. Results

In the study, total 93 students were included who were hospitalized following the incident. Age distribution of the students showed that most students (34%) were 13 years old. Next commonest age group was 14 years (28%) and 12 years (15%), respectively (Table 1).

Average interval between exposure to the trigger and onset of symptoms was 151.5 minutes. About 27% of students developed symptoms within 45–60 minutes following exposure and 26% developed symptoms after 60–90 minutes. Some students (15%) developed symptoms very rapidly (within 0–15 minutes).

The trigger factor of the outbreak was consumption of the cake which was found in 98% of the ill students. An abnormal smell or taste or both were noticed in the supplied cake by 88% of students, whereas 5.4% of students felt ill spontaneously while playing in the ground. 20% of the students felt ill by only seeing other ill students in the school. During transfer of the sick students, 63% of students who volunteered and came in direct contact with the ill students felt sick. 11% of students felt sick while watching television telecast of the incident. All students reported exam ahead within one month (Table 2).

Affected students had various symptoms. Commonest symptoms were abdominal pain (83%), headache (73%), body ache (63%), nausea (69%), generalized weakness and fatigue (61%), and chest pain (69%). Among other complaints, 58% felt burning sensation of body, 45% complained of dizziness, and 31% had dry mouth (Table 3).

Around 53% of the students left the hospital within 6 hours of admission. About 24% left the hospital between 7 and 12 hours, 16% between 13 and 24 hours, and 5% between 25 and 48 hours of admission. Only 2% required hospital

TABLE 1: Age distribution ($n = 93$).

Age in years	Number of students	Percentage
11	9	10%
12	14	15%
13	32	34%
14	26	28%
≥15	9	13%

TABLE 2: Exposure to probable trigger factor among students.

Probable Trigger Factor	Percentage of Students
Consumption of cake	98%
Noticed abnormal smell or taste or both in the cake	88%
Came to school without taking breakfast	84%
Felt ill while handling ill students to transfer to hospital	63%
Felt ill by only seeing other felt ill in the school	20%
Became ill while watching television telecast of the incidence at home	11%
Felt ill spontaneously while playing	05%

TABLE 3: Symptoms profile of ill students ($n = 93$).

Symptoms	No of students	Percentage
Abdominal pain	77	82.8%
Headache	68	73.1%
Body ache	59	63.4%
Nausea	64	68.8%
Chest pain	64	68.8%
Generalized weakness & fatigue	57	61.3%
Burning body	54	58.1%
Dizziness	42	45.2%
Dry mouth	29	31.2%
Hyperventilation	23	24.7%
Breathlessness	18	19.4%
Throat burning	15	16.1%
Crying & shouting	15	16.1%
Muscle cramp	13	14.0%
Salivation	10	10.8%
Vomiting	8	8.6%
Pseudo seizure	7	7.5%
Cold extremity	6	6.5%
Sweating	5	5.4%
Unconsciousness	4	4.3%
Limb weakness	3	3.2%
Visual disturbance	2	2.2%

stay up to 49–72 hours (Figure 1). Hospital stay following the incident was 12.3 hours on average. A relapse of the attack needing readmission was present in 18% of students.

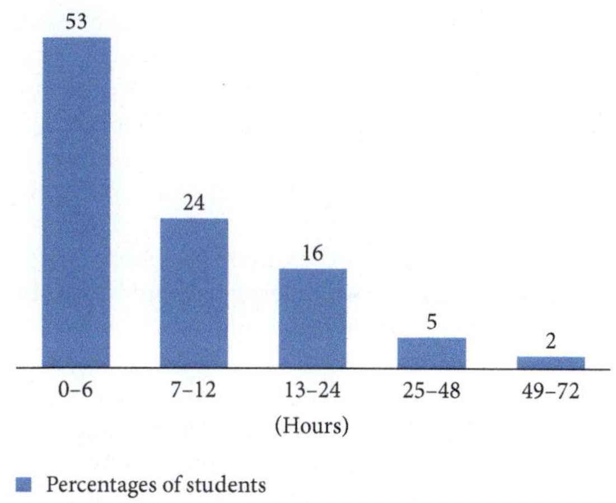

FIGURE 1: Duration of hospital stay of the respondents of the episode.

5. Discussion

Every year, an estimated four to six separate outbreaks of mass psychogenic illness reach public attention, but the actual frequency is not known [21]. Our reported episode gives a classical example of mass psychogenic illness with an identifiable triggering factor, rapid onset of illness, rapid recovery, and absence of any organic illness. Age distribution of the students shows that most students were 13 years old. This distribution is consistent with the characteristics of mass psychogenic illness and also the current published reports [6]. Various studies published between 1973 and 1993 show that schools are very common place for mass psychogenic illness accounting for more than 50% of the events [22].

Among the admitted 93 students, 98% took the cake which was supplied and 88% noticed either bad taste or bad smell or both. This had acted as an environmental trigger factor to initiate the episode. In many reported episodes the trigger factors are found and were like tiffin biscuits, following vaccination, bad environmental smell, and so forth [2, 23, 24]. A clear index case is often the source of symptoms from whom the symptoms spread to others [25, 26]. The index case may or may not be suffering from organic illness. In this incidence we could not clearly identify the index case, but five girls initially became ill spontaneously and they were not suffering from any previous organic diseases. The result of sample of cake sent for microbiological examination did not prove any association with toxic or infectious agent. Also, teachers and other students who took the same cake at the same time did not experience any abnormal symptom. Preliminary investigations did not indicate any organic illness in our subjects.

Onset of symptoms following exposure to environmental trigger is rapid in mass psychogenic illness. In our study, average time of onset following trigger exposure was 151.5 minutes. The onset was very rapid in some students. Most of the students started to show symptoms within the period of 45–90 minutes after the trigger. This may be due to the fact that they were helping during transportation of fellow ill students to the hospital and coming in direct contact and got ill. Contagion is increased by being close to affected and unaffected persons, reassembly of the group such as being put in the same ward in a hospital, and "line of sight" transmission [2, 27]. Some students were found to be affected very lately. Another factor might have been the intensive media attention which heightened the collective anxiety and contributed to the second cluster of cases.

A very rapid spread of symptoms which frequently includes hyperventilation or syncope with minimal physical findings often occurs in groups under physical or psychological stress. Unnecessary dramatic and prolonged media coverage on the issue frequently enhances such outbreaks [28–33]. In our outbreak, exam schedule was ahead within one month for all students which might have acted as stressor and significant number (84%) of ill students came to school without taking breakfast which might have acted to precipitate the outbreak. Commonest symptoms in our study were abdominal pain (83%), headache (73%), body ache (63%), nausea (69%), generalized weakness and fatigue (61%), and chest pain (69%). Among other complaints, 58% felt burning body, 45% complained of dizziness, 31% had dry mouth which is consistent with other studies [8, 9, 18, 24, 25].

Around 53% of the students left the hospital within six hours of admission. Recovery is rapid in MPI. In our study, average hospital stay was 12.3 hours, but some students (2%) had to remain in hospital even for 3 days. Recurrent attack has been described in some studies [23, 25]. In our study, 18% students experienced recurrence of symptoms and needed readmission. Once the diagnosis is determined, reassuring patients is the primary therapy. Separating them can be beneficial. Most patients experience rapid resolution of symptoms once they are removed from the environment in which the outbreak started [6].

There may exist a relation of MPI episode and exposer of low level environmental toxins as reported in studies [34], but in this reported episode there was no association to be noted and mentioned as it was duly searched for the possible and assessable causes based on clinical, laboratory investigations and microbiological examination and all outcomes revealed nothing contributory regarding the episode.

A teamwork of internists, pediatricians, hospital administrators, and nurses was key to the successful handling of the situation. The idea that the outbreak was psychogenic is very clear but because of intense anxiety in the parents, investigations were undertaken to rule out any organic cause. With any approach to mass psychogenic illness, the goal should be to restore the community to normal functioning as quickly as possible. In our study we found that most of the guardians (82.8%) thought the outbreak was due to unknown poisoning from the cake. The rest of them thought it was some other illness. None believed it as any supernatural act. In a study done in various districts of Bangladesh in 2007, 15% of affected students believed that supernatural act is responsible for such outbreak but no study was found to reflect the perception of the guardians at the time of outbreak [24]. Prompt public identification of episodes of mass psychogenic illness has been advocated as an important step in terminating them, but such an approach can be problematic in practice [9, 20]. Prompt recognition, coordinated investigations, effective stress coping strategy, and environmental modifications are essential in alleviation of the widespread anxiety surrounding an episode of mass psychogenic illness [19]. Awareness of the characteristics of mass psychogenic illness is crucial for physicians and other healthcare personnel who respond to such outbreaks [1].

6. Conclusion

Mostly adolescents are endangered in mass psychogenic illness with typically medically unexplained somatic complains creating an emergency. In dealing with a mass psychogenic illness, a prompt, coordinated response is important in resolving widespread community anxiety surrounding these episodes.

Competing Interests

The authors declare that they have no competing interests.

Authors' Contributions

Binoy Krishna Tarafder, Sheikh Abdullah Al Mahmud, Md. Humayun Kabir Sarker, and Imtiaz Faruq contributed to concept and design of the study. Binoy Krishna Tarafder and Md. Tanvir Islam contributed to the data management. Md. Humayun Kabir Sarker, Imtiaz Faruq, and Md. Titu Miah contributed materials/analysis tools. Binoy Krishna Tarafder, Mohammad Ashik Imran Khan, Md. Tanvir Islam, and S. M. Yasir Arafat did the paper preparation.

Acknowledgments

The authors are grateful to the parents and local community people who communicated with the researchers during the episode.

References

[1] S. Balaratnasingam and A. Janca, "Mass hysteria revisited," *Current Opinion in Psychiatry*, vol. 19, no. 2, pp. 171–174, 2006.

[2] T. F. Jones, A. S. Craig, D. Hoy et al., "Mass psychogenic illness attributed to toxic exposure at a high school," *The New England Journal of Medicine*, vol. 342, no. 2, pp. 96–100, 2000.

[3] R. E. Bartholomew and S. Wessely, "Protean nature of mass sociogenic illness. From possessed nuns to chemical and biological terrorism fears," *British Journal of Psychiatry*, vol. 180, no. 4, pp. 300–306, 2002.

[4] R. H. Pastel, "Collective behaviors: mass panic and outbreaks of multiple unexplained symptoms," *Military Medicine*, vol. 166, no. 12, supplement, pp. 44–46, 2002.

[5] G. W. Small, D. T. Feinberg, D. Steinberg, and M. T. Collins, "A sudden outbreak of illness suggestive of mass hysteria in schoolchildren," *Archives of Family Medicine*, vol. 3, no. 8, article 711, 1994.

[6] T. F. Jones, "Mass psychogenic illness: role of the individual physician," *American Family Physician*, vol. 62, no. 12, pp. 2649–2653, 2000.

[7] E. Weir, "Mass sociogenic illness," *Canadian Medical Association Journal*, vol. 172, no. 1, p. 36, 2005.

[8] L. P. Boss, "Epidemic hysteria: a review of the published literature," *Epidemiologic Reviews*, vol. 19, no. 2, pp. 233–243, 1997.

[9] R. E. Bartholomew, *Rethinking the Dancing Mania*, vol. 24.4 of *The Committee for Skeptical Inquiry*, 2000, http://www.csicop.org/si/show/rethinking_the_dancing_mania.

[10] R. H. Pastel, "Fear of radiation in US military medical personnel," *Military Medicine*, vol. 166, no. 12, pp. 80–82, 2001.

[11] A. J. Barsky, E. J. Orav, and D. W. Bates, "Distinctive patterns of medical care utilization in patients who somatize," *Medical Care*, vol. 44, no. 9, pp. 803–811, 2006.

[12] K. Kroenke, R. L. Spitzer, J. B. Williams et al., "Physical symptoms in primary care. Predictors of psychiatric disorders and functional impairment," *Archives of Family Medicine*, vol. 3, no. 9, article 774, 1994.

[13] D. Watson and L. A. Clark, "Negative affectivity: the disposition to experience aversive emotional states," *Psychological Bulletin*, vol. 96, no. 3, pp. 465–490, 1984.

[14] T. K. J. Craig, A. P. Boardman, K. Mills, O. Daly-Jones, and H. Drake, "The South London Somatisation Study. I: longitudinal course and the influence of early life experiences," *The British Journal of Psychiatry*, vol. 163, no. 5, pp. 579–588, 1993.

[15] J. I. Escobar, M. A. Burnam, M. Karno, A. Forsythe, and J. M. Golding, "Somatization in the community," *Archives of General Psychiatry*, vol. 44, no. 8, pp. 713–718, 1987.

[16] M. Swartz, D. Blazer, L. George, and R. Landerman, "Somatization disorder in a community population," *The American Journal of Psychiatry*, vol. 143, no. 11, pp. 1403–1408, 1986.

[17] K. Kroenke and R. L. Spitzer, "Gender differences in the reporting of physical and somatoform symptoms," *Psychosomatic Medicine*, vol. 60, no. 2, pp. 150–155, 1998.

[18] F. Haque, S. K. Kundu, M. S. Islam et al., "Outbreak of mass sociogenic illness in a school feeding program in Northwest Bangladesh, 2010," *PLoS ONE*, vol. 8, no. 11, Article ID e80420, 2013.

[19] N. Magnavita, "Industrial mass psychogenic illness: the unfashionable diagnosis," *British Journal of Medical Psychology*, vol. 73, no. 3, pp. 371–375, 2000.

[20] J. E. Broderick, E. Kaplan-Liss, and E. Bass, "Experimental induction of psychogenic illness in the context of a medical event and media exposure," *American Journal of Disaster Medicine*, vol. 6, no. 3, pp. 163–172, 2011.

[21] G. W. Small, "Psychiatry: mass hysteria," *Western Journal of Medicine*, vol. 142, no. 5, pp. 682–683, 1985.

[22] B. B. Beyene, A. Teka, and R. Luce, "Outbreak of mass psychogenic illness at a high school, Amhara Region, Ethiopia, April, 2010," *International Journal of Medicine and Medical Sciences*, vol. 1, no. 10, pp. 157–161, 2014.

[23] S. Kharabsheh, H. Al-Otoum, J. Clements et al., "Mass psychogenic illness following tetanus-diphtheria toxoid vaccination in Jordan," *Bulletin of the World Health Organization*, vol. 79, no. 8, pp. 764–770, 2001.

[24] ICDDRB, "Outbreak of mass sociogenic illness in students in secondary schools in Bangladesh during July-August 2007," *Health and Science Bulletin*, vol. 6, no. 2, pp. 6–12, 2008.

[25] M. R. Amin, S. Mahmood, S. F. Rabbi, A. A. Hossain, and H. M. Sharif, "Mass psychogenic illness among learners at Jaforabad High School, in Hathazari, Chittagong, Bangladesh," *Journal of Dhaka Medical College*, vol. 18, no. 2, pp. 105–111, 2009.

[26] R. Philen, T. Mckinley, E. Kilbourne, and R. G. Parrish, "Mass sociogenic illness by proxy: parentally reported epidemic in an elementary school," *The Lancet*, vol. 334, no. 8676, pp. 1372–1376, 1989.

[27] B. S. Selden, "Adolescent epidemic hysteria presenting as a mass casualty, toxic exposure incident," *Annals of Emergency Medicine*, vol. 18, no. 8, pp. 892–895, 1989.

[28] G. W. Small, M. W. Propper, E. T. Randolph, and S. Eth, "Mass hysteria among student performers: social relationship as a symptom predictor," *The American Journal of Psychiatry*, vol. 148, no. 9, pp. 1200–1205, 1991.

[29] P. Robinson, M. Szewczyk, L. Haddy, P. Jones, and W. Harvey, "Outbreak of itching and rash. Epidemic hysteria in an elementary school," *Archives of Internal Medicine*, vol. 144, no. 10, pp. 1959–1962, 1984.

[30] S. Araki and T. Honma, "Mass psychogenic systemic illness in school children in relation to the Tokyo photochemical smog," *Archives of Environmental Health*, vol. 41, no. 3, pp. 159–162, 1986.

[31] A. S. David and S. C. Wessely, "The legend of Camelford: medical consequences of a water pollution accident," *Journal of Psychosomatic Research*, vol. 39, no. 1, pp. 1–9, 1995.

[32] A. Hefez, "The role of the press and the medical community in the epidemic of 'mysterious gas poisoning' in the Jordan West Bank," *The American Journal of Psychiatry*, vol. 142, no. 7, pp. 833–837, 1985.

[33] P. Vasterman, C. J. Yzermans, and A. J. E. Dirkzwager, "The role of the media and media hypes in the aftermath of disasters," *Epidemiologic Reviews*, vol. 27, pp. 107–114, 2005.

[34] H. S. Faust and L. B. Brilliant, "Is the diagnosis of 'mass hysteria' an excuse for incomplete investigation of low-level environmental contamination?" *Journal of Occupational Medicine*, vol. 23, no. 1, pp. 22–26, 1981.

Common Mental Disorders among Occupational Groups: Contributions of the Latent Class Model

Kionna Oliveira Bernardes Santos,[1] Fernando Martins Carvalho,[2] and Tânia Maria de Araújo[3]

[1] *Physical Therapy Department, Federal University of Bahia (UFBA), Avenida Reitor Miguel Calmon s/n, Vale do Canela, 40.110-100 Salvador, BA, Brazil*
[2] *Department of Preventive and Social Medicine, Federal University of Bahia (UFBA), Avenida Reitor Miguel Calmon s/n, Vale do Canela, 40.110-100 Salvador, BA, Brazil*
[3] *Health Department, State University of Feira de Santana (UEFS), Avenida Transnordestina, s/n Novo Horizonte, 44036-900 Feira de Santana, BA, Brazil*

Correspondence should be addressed to Kionna Oliveira Bernardes Santos; kionna.bernardes@ufba.br

Academic Editor: Nicola Magnavita

Background. The Self-Reporting Questionnaire (SRQ-20) is widely used for evaluating common mental disorders. However, few studies have evaluated the SRQ-20 measurements performance in occupational groups. This study aimed to describe manifestation patterns of common mental disorders symptoms among workers populations, by using latent class analysis. *Methods.* Data derived from 9,959 Brazilian workers, obtained from four cross-sectional studies that used similar methodology, among groups of informal workers, teachers, healthcare workers, and urban workers. Common mental disorders were measured by using SRQ-20. Latent class analysis was performed on each database separately. *Results.* Three classes of symptoms were confirmed in the occupational categories investigated. In all studies, class I met better criteria for suspicion of common mental disorders. Class II discriminated workers with intermediate probability of answers to the items belonging to anxiety, sadness, and energy decrease that configure common mental disorders. Class III was composed of subgroups of workers with low probability to respond positively to questions for screening common mental disorders. *Conclusions.* Three patterns of symptoms of common mental disorders were identified in the occupational groups investigated, ranging from distinctive features to low probabilities of occurrence. The SRQ-20 measurements showed stability in capturing nonpsychotic symptoms.

1. Introduction

Common mental disorders (CMDs) are a group of nonspecific symptoms, without any clinical classification relating to psychosocial, occupational, and social context factors. The name CMD encompasses nonpsychotic symptoms, characterized by insomnia, fatigue, irritability, forgetfulness, difficulty in concentrating, and somatic complaints that can coexist in the presence of other comorbidities and define a state of emotional transitory vulnerability, with incapacitating characteristics [1].

The global prevalence of common mental disorders was estimated as 17.6% during the last 12-month period [2]. The World Health Organization [3] has proposed the Self-Reporting Questionnaire (SRQ) as a screening instrument for mental disorders in developing countries, in population-based surveys on individuals who use primary healthcare services [4]. SRQ has undergone structure modifications from its initial composition of 30 items to 20 items relating to psychosomatic symptoms [5]. From the 1980s until today, the validity of SRQ-20 measurements has been evaluated in specific population groups and among healthcare service users [3, 4, 6–10]. However, few studies have evaluated the performance of SRQ-20 measurements in occupational groups [11, 12].

Despite the small number of validation studies about SRQ-20 measurements among workers, this questionnaire has been frequently used in the screening for mental disorders in the labor force [13–18]. The interpretation of the SRQ-20 score is hampered by the wide variation in the cut-off points for diagnostic suspicion, cultural differences, and the diverse work contexts that hinder the analysis of the patterns of symptoms among different occupational groups [3, 19, 20].

Studies [17, 18] have associated common mental disorders with work process characteristics like instability and job dissatisfaction, low wages, earning by productivity, hard work, and job supervision. These conditions trigger a set of signs and symptoms that mostly correspond to CMD and, regardless of the activity performed, reveal a sense of sadness, reduced ability to enjoy daily activities, and decreased concentration and decision-making [21].

Evaluation of measurements used for screening for CMDs in occupational contexts represents a methodological advance for psychiatric epidemiology. The current concept of validity requires the construction of a structured argument and the production of evidence for supporting or refuting interpretations suggested by the scores of a specific instrument [22]. Even with the technical and methodological advances in the analyses, limitations on the screening instruments for evaluations of the main dimensions that compose common mental disorders still remain.

This study aimed to describe manifestation patterns of common mental disorders symptoms among workers populations, by using latent class analysis.

2. Methods

This study involves four cross-sectional design surveys conducted on populations of workers that were selected through specific sampling procedures.

Study 1: Informal Workers. This epidemiological survey used systematic sampling to select 1,458 open market traders, street dealers, and motorcycle taxi drivers in Feira de Santana, Bahia, in 2008.

Study 2: Teachers. This survey is a census on 4,496 teachers at the 365 kindergarten and elementary schools of the public network of Salvador, Bahia, in 2006 [13].

Study 3: Healthcare Workers. This survey was a multicenter study with primary healthcare workers from four municipalities from the State of Bahia (Feira de Santana, Jequié, Santo Antônio de Jesus, and a health district in Salvador). A proportional random stratified sample has selected 2,448 workers, from 2012 to 2013.

Study 4: Urban Workers. This survey was a random sample of 1,557 individuals, representing workers over 15 years of age, stratified according to subdistricts of the urban zone of Feira de Santana City, in 2007.

In all four studies, common mental disorders were evaluated using the Self-Reporting Questionnaire (SRQ-20).

Latent class analysis was used. This method underlies a wide analytical spectrum based on structural equation models, and it is used when evaluation of a measurement and classification model based on a group of answers and exploration of possible associations is desired. Latent class models refer to situations in which the variable and its indicator are categories [23]. The latent class model is often considered to be analogous to factor analysis for categorical data, because of the possibility of data reduction. However, factor analysis takes the structure of the variables and their correlations into consideration, while latent class analysis evaluates the structure of the cases through the latent taxonomic structure, which therefore relates it to cluster analysis [3, 23, 24].

The traditional latent class model has limited psychometric analyses on instruments that evaluate multidimensional events such as common mental disorders, given that this model does not allow explicit distinction of the dimensional structure [25]. Despite not being appropriate for evaluating the dimensional structure, this technique has become indicated in subjective component descriptions because it is used to analyze representations of multiple variables simultaneously [26].

Latent class analysis was performed on each database separately, following the theoretical assumption that the mental disorders would conform to four dimensions [8, 12]. Initially, extraction of four latent classes was requested. To evaluate the adequacy of the number of classes extracted from the CMD cases gathered, the Vuong-Lo-Mendell-Rubin test, adjusted Lo Mendell Rubin (LRT) test, and parametric bootstrap likelihood ratio test were used. These tests compared a model with K classes and a model with $(K-1)$ classes. In the present study, the criterion of concordance of the three tests was used for acceptance of the number of classes, and p values < 0.05 were taken to be statistically significant.

Latent class analysis is based on the assumption of local independence, which assumes that, in the latent class model, the variables manifested are independent of one another within the latent classes. For this reason, the local dependence of the items in each database was evaluated. The items were combined in pairs and Pearson's chi-square (χ^2) and residual z-score were calculatedfor all the data in the adjustment model (for all possible pair combinations). When over 50% of the z-scores were over 1.96 or below -1.96 and when Pearson's chi-square value was over 50,000, local dependence was considered to be present. To adjust the local dependence, the item fusion method was used [27].

Item fusion was used in accordance with clinical judgment. Thus, in studies 1 and 2, out of the 20 items of SRQ-20, 12 items with local dependence were evaluated and were fused into single items: Q7 ("poor digestion") and Q19 ("stomach problems") were named "somatization/digestive"; Q8 ("not thinking clearly") and Q12 ("difficulty in decision-making") were considered to be "unsafe behavior"; Q9 ("unhappy") and Q10 ("crying more than normally") were classified as "unhappy." Items Q11 ("not enjoying activities") and Q13 ("work suffering") were grouped under "work suffering"; Q14 ("not feeling life is useful") and Q16 ("feeling worthless") were considered to be "feeling useless"; Q18 ("always feeling tired") and Q20 ("easily tired") received the name "tiredness."

In study 3, out of the 20 items evaluated, eight presented local dependence: Q7/Q19, Q8/Q12, Q9/Q10, and Q18/Q20. In study 4, conditional dependence was found for six items of SRQ-20: Q9/Q10, Q14/Q16, and Q18/Q20. In both of these studies, the same names as described in relation to studies 1 and 2 were used.

Entropy measurements were then evaluated to indicate class separation quality. Values over 0.80 were considered to be excellent for class discrimination [28].

After the quantity and quality of the classes extracted had been analyzed using the methods mentioned above, the classes were evaluated descriptively according to the numbers and proportions of workers participating in each class. The conditional probabilities that items would belong in each class were evaluated, and the affirmative responses for each item forming part of the questionnaire were taken into consideration. Since this method allows items to simultaneously belong to more than one class, the subgroups forming the CMD construct were judged based on items presenting higher conditional probability in the preestablished classes.

Finally, the conditional probabilities were presented in charts. The x-axis presented the questionnaire items and the y-axis presented the probability of answering "yes" to a certain item, considering that it belonged to a certain class. For this analysis, the MPLUS software, version 7, was used [29].

The reliability of the latent classes was evaluated by means of the latent class reliability coefficient (LCRC) test, as estimated using the analysis method of Mokken's scale [30, 31]. This scaling procedure is indicated for dichotomous and/or polytomous items. Mokken's estimate, which is a group of reliability statistics comprising Molenaar Sijtsma (MS) statistics, Guttman's lambda 2, and the latent class reliability coefficient (LCRC), was calculated using the R software of the Foundation for Statistical Computing.

The four studies mentioned in our paper were approved by Ethical Committees, before they have been carried out. All participants involved in the four studies signed the consent form for participation. The present study was also approved by an Ethical Committee (CAAE 18723813.9.0000.5030).

3. Results

The informal workers evaluated in study 1 were characterized by low education level (95.9%), with equal distribution according to sex and predominance of the age groups < 30 years and 30–45 years. Study 2, which evaluated teachers, involved a predominantly female population (92.0%) aged 30–45 years, with high prevalence of technical/tertiary education level (82.1%). The healthcare workers of study 3 were mostly female (80.6%), aged 30–45 years (44.7%), and the largest proportions had elementary and technical/tertiary education levels (42.9% and 41.3%, resp.). The urban workers evaluated in study 4 presented a higher percentage of females (54.7%), with predominance of the age groups < 30 years and 30–45 years; 55.9% had technical/tertiary education level (Table 1).

The latent class analysis followed the established statistical criteria for acceptance of the number of classes extracted and revealed that three classes had been extracted for all the studies. The entropy values used for evaluating class separation reached values that were either high (from 0.78 to 0.80) or close to the reference value for excellence (higher than 0.80).

TABLE 1: Sociodemographic characteristics of the populations of the four studies.

Study: population (N)	n	%
Study 1: informal workers (1,458)		
Sex		
Female	728	49.9
Age group		
<30 years	537	36.8
30 to 45 years	553	37.9
>45 years	368	25.2
Education level (1,438)		
Elementary	1,379	95.9
Technical/tertiary	9	0.6
Without qualification	50	3.5
Study 2: teachers (4,496)		
Sex (4,342)		
Female	3,994	92.0
Age group (4,302)		
<30 years	773	18.0
30 to 45 years	2,289	53.2
>45 years	1,240	28.8
Education level (4,398)		
Elementary	717	16.3
Technical/tertiary	3,609	82.1
Postgraduate	72	1.6
Study 3: healthcare workers (2,448)		
Sex (2,421)		
Female	1,951	80.6
Age group (2,395)		
<30 years	581	24.3
30 to 45 years	1,071	44.7
>45 years	743	31.0
Education level (2,419)		
Elementary	1,038	42.9
Technical/tertiary	1,000	41.3
Postgraduate	381	15.8
Study 4: urban workers (1,557)		
Sex (1,557)		
Female	851	54.7
Age group (1,557)		
<30 years	576	37.0
30 to 45 years	584	37.5
>45 years	397	25.5
Education level (1,269)		
Elementary	536	42.3
Technical/tertiary	710	55.9
Without qualification	23	1.8

Estimators evaluated using Mokken's method presented acceptable reliability values for the number of classes extracted in the latent class model, in all the studies. The latent class reliability coefficient (LCRC) was used as a parameter in this analysis. Studies 1 and 3 presented higher reliability

TABLE 2: Summary of the latent class analysis in four professional categories.

	Informal workers (N = 1,458) 5**		Teachers (N = 4,397) 162**		Healthcare workers (N = 2,448) 36**		Urban workers (N = 1,556) 14**	
	n	%	n	%	n	%	n	%
Class I	200	14.2	724	17.1	324	10.3	215	13.8
Class II	712	47.9	1736	38.7	923	38.5	642	41.3
Class III	546	37.9	1935	44.2	1286	51.2	699	44,9
Entropy	0.78		0.72		0.80		0.76	
VLMR[a] test*	0.00		0.00		0.00		0.00	
LMR-LRT[b] test*	0.00		0.00		0.00		000	
PB[c] test*	0.00		0.00		0.00		0.00	
			Latent class reliability estimators					
Molenaar Sijtsma	1.0		0.86		1.0		0.85	
Lambda	0.93		0.86		0.92		0.85	
LCRC[d]	0.93		0.86		0.91		0,84	

*p value.
**Number of imputed pattern observations.
[a]VLMR: Vuong-Lo-Mendell-Rubin.
[b]LMR-LRT: adjusted Lo Mendell Rubin (LRT) test.
[c]PB: parametric bootstrapped maximum likelihood.
[d]Latent class reliability coefficient.

indicators: 0.93 and 0.91, respectively. The lowest value was found in study 4: 0.84 (Table 2).

The worker distribution into classes, in the four studies, followed the same pattern: the lowest proportion in class I, followed in increasing proportions by classes 2 and 3.

In all the studies, class I concentrated on the workers with highest probability of positive responses to the items in SRQ-20 and revealed better criteria for suspecting common mental disorders. In particular, there were higher probabilities for item Q6 ("Do you feel nervous, tense or preoccupied?") and for the combined items Q18/20 ("feeling tired") and Q9/10 ("sadness"), which discriminated this class well (Figures 1 and 2).

Among the professional categories evaluated, study 2 (teachers) presented a higher proportion of workers grouped in class I (17.1%), followed by the informal workers of study 1 (13.4%). Healthcare workers were the category with the lowest percentage of workers in this class (10.3%).

Class II presented a positive response profile similar to what was found for class I, thus discriminating workers with intermediate levels of probability for responses to items belonging to the components of anxiety, sadness, and decreased energy that shape CMDs. Studies 1 and 4 presented higher proportion of workers in this class: 47.9% and 41.3%, respectively.

Class III was composed of subgroups of workers with low probability (under 10%) of responding positively to questions screening for CMDs. Healthcare workers (study 3) were the category with the highest proportion of workers in this class (51.2%) (Figure 2(a)).

In all the studies, Q17 ("Have you thought of ending your life?") was the item presenting least probability of a positive response among the classes extracted. The same pattern of low probability of an affirmative response was followed by item Q15 ("Have you lost interest in things?") (Figures 1 and 2).

4. Discussion

The latent class model did not allow isolation of items in specific dimensions. Instead, it revealed conditional positive response patterns associated with the extracted classes, thereby allowing discrimination of subgroups that had not been directly observable in the participating studies. The profiles showed variation in intensity, that is, high, intermediate, and low probabilities for positive responses to the questionnaire. Thus, it was possible to identify traits of the anxious/depressive components, represented by higher probabilities of positive responses given by the workers in relation to items Q6, Q9/10, and Q18/20.

The method has been used in healthcare research, especially in the field of psychiatry. The classes translate phenotypes of clinical and/or behavioral manifestations. However, difficulties in identifying the number of classes that best represents the phenomenon evaluated remain [24]. Despite the limitations imposed by the latent class method and cross-sectional study, the CMD manifestation patterns were similar among the professional categories evaluated.

Class III composite with workers with low probability of positive responses to SRQ-20 items was significant in all studies. This result showed the work context of the evaluated groups and reflects positive interference of autonomy in the workplace [17, 20].

The latent class reliability (LCR) estimator confirmed that the number of classes extracted represented the investigated populations, thus satisfactorily capturing the latent features

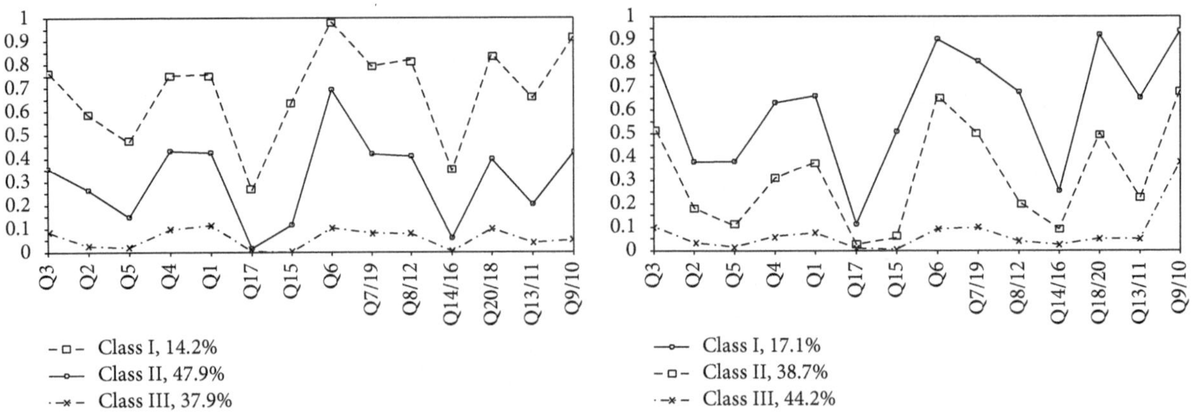

(a) Informal workers of Feira de Santana, 2008

(b) Teachers in the city of Salvador, 2006

FIGURE 1: Conditional probabilities of positive responses to SRQ-20 items according to latent class analysis between informal workers and teachers. Q3: sleeping problems; Q2: lack of appetite; Q5: shaking hands; Q4: being frightened; Q1: headaches; Q17: thinking of ending life; Q15: loss of interest in life; Q6: feeling nervous; Q7/19: "somatization/digestive"; Q8/12: "unsafe behavior"; Q14/16: "feeling useless"; Q18/20: "tiredness"; Q13/11: work suffering; Q9/10: "unhappy."

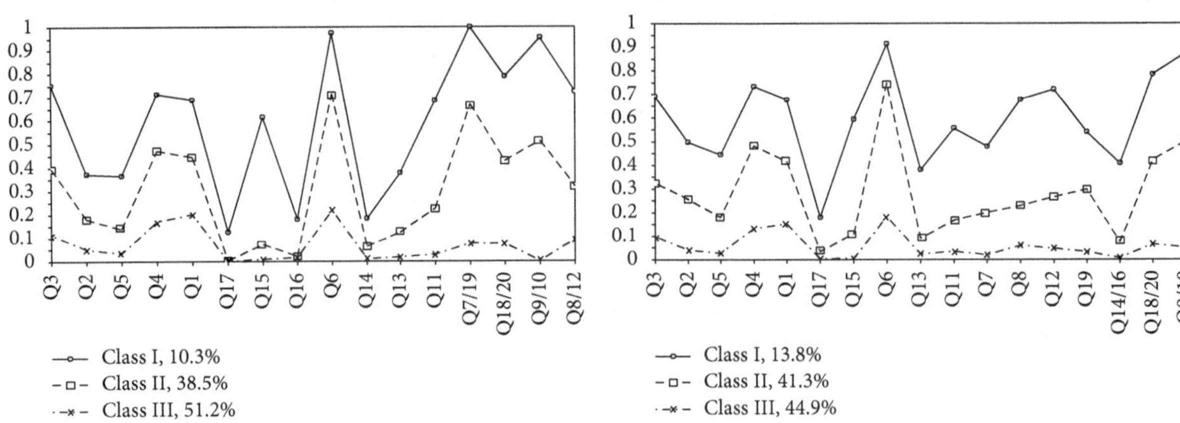

(a) Workers in primary healthcare in Bahia in 2013

(b) Urban workers of Feira de Santana in Bahia in 2007

FIGURE 2: Conditional probability of positive responses to SRQ-20 items according to latent class analysis between healthcare workers and urban workers. Q3: sleeping problems; Q2: lack of appetite; Q5: shaking hands; Q4: being frightened; Q1: headaches; Q17: thinking of ending life; Q15: loss of interest in life; Q6: feeling nervous; Q7: Is your digestion poor?; Q19: stomach problems; Q7/19: "somatization/digestive"; Q8: Do you have trouble thinking clearly?; Q12: difficulty in decision-making; Q8/12: "unsafe behavior"; Q14: not feeling life is useful; Q16: feeling worthless; Q14/16: "feeling useless"; Q18/20: "tiredness"; Q13: Is your daily work suffering?; Q11: not enjoying activities; Q9/10: "unhappy."

composing CMDs in the different groups evaluated. It is postulated that the method applied in the present study is less skewed in evaluating real reliability than the methods of Guttman's lambda 2, Molenaar Sijtsma (MS), and split-half reliability coefficient [32, 33]. The method of class reliability estimation allowed a more accurate analysis, because the terms were estimated with lower restriction, thus allowing evaluation of multidimensional instruments through considering the essential effects of tau-equivalence and double monotonicity.

The CMD evaluation in multidimensional categories incorporated advances in investigations on mental illness of occupational scope. The screening to obtain homogeneous groups for research and the action strategies established for maintaining mental health were methodological advances in this field. However, there is no consensus on the most appropriate type of multivariate analysis for multidimensional model evaluation, given that any statistical model translates a simplified picture of reality [1]. Scores from instruments evaluating subjective content will reflect the underlying construct with higher or lower precision, but never perfectly. Therefore, validity is considered to be an inferred property from measurements produced by the instrument and needs to be established for each intended evaluation context [22].

The CMDs screened by SRQ-20 reflect transient symptoms and capture recent changes to consider the work environment [33]. However, the persistence of symptoms denotes depressive behavior profiles and anxious somatoform scope and is associated with high burden of disability, missed work, and comorbidities among workers.

5. Conclusions

Three patterns of symptoms of common mental disorders were identified in the occupational groups investigated, ranging from distinctive features to low probabilities of occurrence. The SRQ-20 measurements showed stability in capturing nonpsychotic symptoms. Although most workers present low probability of presenting common mental disorders, the symptom patterns encompassing sadness, anxiety, and energy expenditure were very frequent in all occupational groups.

Competing Interests

The authors declare that they have no competing interests.

Acknowledgments

Fernando Martins Carvalho received a research fellowship grant by the Brazilian National Research Council (CNPq).

References

[1] D. Goldberg and P. Huxley, *Common Mental Disorders: A Bio-Social Model*, Tavistock, London, UK, 1992.

[2] Z. Steel, C. Marnane, C. Iranpour et al., "The global prevalence of common mental disorders: a systematic review and meta-analysis 1980–2013," *International Journal of Epidemiology*, vol. 43, no. 2, pp. 476–493, 2014.

[3] T. W. Harding, M. V. De Arango, J. Baltazar et al., "Mental disorders in primary health care: a study of their frequency and diagnosis in four developing countries," *Psychological Medicine*, vol. 10, no. 2, pp. 231–241, 1980.

[4] D. M. Gonçalves, A. T. Stein, and F. Kapczinski, "Performance of the Self-Reporting Questionnaire as a psychiatric screening questionnaire: a comparativestudy with Structured Clinical Interview for DSM-IV-TR," *Cadernos de Saude Publica*, vol. 24, no. 2, pp. 380–390, 2008.

[5] World Health Organization, *WHO Expert Committee on Mental Health: User's Guide to Self-Reporting Questionnaire (SRQ)*, World Health Organization, Geneva, Switzerland, 1994.

[6] M. Scazufca, P. R. Menezes, H. Vallada, and R. Araya, "Validity of the self reporting questionnaire-20 in epidemiological studies with older adults: results from the Sao Paulo Ageing & Health Study," *Social Psychiatry and Psychiatric Epidemiology*, vol. 44, article 247, 2009.

[7] S. Chen, G. Zhao, L. Li, Y. Wang, H. Chiu, and E. Caine, "Psychometric properties of the Chinese Version of the Self-Reporting Questionnaire 20 (SRQ-20) in community settings," *International Journal of Social Psychiatry*, vol. 55, no. 6, pp. 538–547, 2009.

[8] E. Iacoponi and J. De Jesus Mari, "Reliability and factor structure of the Portuguese version of Self-Reporting Questionnaire," *International Journal of Social Psychiatry*, vol. 35, no. 3, pp. 213–222, 1989.

[9] B. Sen, G. Wilkinson, and J. J. Mari, "Psychiatric morbidity in primary health care. A two-stage screening procedure in developing countries: choice of instruments and cost-effectiveness," *British Journal of Psychiatry*, vol. 151, pp. 33–38, 1987.

[10] J. J. Mari and P. Williams, "A comparison of the validity of two psychiatric screening questionnaires (GHQ-12 and SRQ-20) in Brazil, using relative operating characteristic (ROC) analysis," *Psychological Medicine*, vol. 15, no. 3, pp. 651–659, 1985.

[11] S. R. P. Fernandes and N. Almeida-Filho, "Validação do SRQ-20 em amostra de trabalhadores em informática," *Revista Brasileira de Saude Ocupacional*, no. 89, pp. 105–112, 1998.

[12] K. O. B. Santosi, T. M. de Araújo, and N. F. de Oliveira, "Factor structure and internal consistency of the self-reporting questionnaire (SRQ-20) in an urban population," *Cadernos de Saude Publica*, vol. 25, no. 1, pp. 214–222, 2009.

[13] J. P. Cardoso, T. M. Araújo, F. M. Carvalho, N. F. Oliveira, and E. J. Reis, "Aspectos psicossociais do trabalho e dor musculoesquelética em professores," *Cadernos de Saúde Pública*, vol. 27, no. 8, pp. 1498–1506, 2011.

[14] R. E. C. Barbosa, A. Á. Assunção, and T. M. de Araújo, "Musculoskeletal disorders among healthcare workers in Belo Horizonte, Minas Gerais State, Brazil," *Cadernos de Saude Publica*, vol. 28, no. 8, pp. 1569–1580, 2012.

[15] M. A. Fernandes and M. H. Marziale, "Riscos ocupacionais e adoecimento de trabalhadores em saúde mental," *Acta Paulista de Enfermagem*, vol. 27, no. 6, pp. 539–547, 2014.

[16] R. A. Abbas, R. A. M. Hammam, S. S. El-Gohary, L. M. E. Sabik, and M. S. Hunter, "Screening for common mental disorders and substance abuse among temporary hired cleaners in egyptian governmental hospitals, Zagazig city, Sharqia governorate," *International Journal of Occupational and Environmental Medicine*, vol. 4, no. 1, pp. 13–26, 2013.

[17] A. B. Ludermir, "Associação dos transtornos mentais comuns com a informalidade das relações de trabalho," *Jornal Brasileiro de Psiquiatria*, no. 54, pp. 198–204, 2005.

[18] L. A. Porto, F. M. Carvalho, N. F. de Oliveira et al., "Association between mental disorders and work-related psychosocial factors in teachers," *Revista de Saude Publica*, vol. 40, no. 5, pp. 818–826, 2006.

[19] R. Araya, R. Wynn, and G. Lewis, "Comparison of two self administered psychiatric questionnaires (GHQ-12 and SRQ-20) in primary care in Chile," *Social Psychiatry and Psychiatric Epidemiology*, vol. 27, no. 4, pp. 168–173, 1992.

[20] T. Harpham, M. Reichenheim, R. Oser et al., "Measuring mental health in a cost-effective manner," *Health Policy and Planning*, vol. 18, no. 3, pp. 344–349, 2003.

[21] E. Seligmann-Silva, M. H. Bernardo, M. Maeno, and M. Kato, "O mundo contemporâneo do trabalho e a saúde mental do trabalhador," *Revista Brasileira de Saúde Ocupacional*, vol. 35, no. 122, pp. 187–191, 2010.

[22] D. A. Cook and T. J. Beckman, "Current concepts in validity and reliability for psychometric instruments: theory and application," *The American Journal of Medicine*, vol. 119, no. 2, pp. 166.e7–166.e16, 2006.

[23] L. M. Collins and S. T. Lanza, *Latent Class and Latent Transition Analysis: With Applications in the Social, Behavioral, and Health Sciences*, John Wiley & Sons, New York, NY, USA, 2010.

[24] A. K. Formann, "Latent class model diagnosis from a frequentist point of view," *Biometrics. Journal of the International Biometric Society*, vol. 59, no. 1, pp. 189–196, 2003.

[25] J. K. Vermunt and M. Jay, "Latent class analysis," in *The Sage Encyclopedia of Social Science Research Methods*, M. Lewis-Beck, A. Bryman, and T. F. Liao, Eds., pp. 549–553, Sage, Newbury Park, Calif, USA, 2004.

[26] R. Pilati and J. A. Laros, "Modelos de equações estruturais em psicologia: conceito e aplicações," *Psicologia: Teoria e Pesquisa*, no. 23, pp. 205–216, 2007.

[27] J. S. Uebersax, "Statistical modeling of expert ratings on medical treatment appropriateness," *The Journal of the American Statistical Association*, vol. 88, no. 422, pp. 421–427, 1993.

[28] V. Ramaswamy, W. S. Desarbo, D. J. Reibstein, and W. T. Robinson, "An empirical pooling approach for estimating marketing mix elasticities with PIMS data," *Marketing Science*, vol. 12, no. 1, pp. 103–124, 1993.

[29] L. K. Muthén and B. O. Muthén, *Mplus User's Guide*, Muthén & Muthén, Los Angeles, Calif, USA, 7th edition, 1998–2012.

[30] R. J. Mokken, *A Theory and Procedure of Scale Analysis*, Mouton/De Gruyter, Berlin, Germany, 1971.

[31] K. Sijtsma and I. M. Molenaar, *Introduction to Nonparametric Item Response Theory*, Sage, New York, NY, USA, 2002.

[32] L. A. van der Ark, D. W. van der Palm, and K. Sijtsma, "A latent class approach to estimating test-score reliability," *Applied Psychological Measurement*, vol. 35, no. 5, pp. 380–392, 2011.

[33] M. E. Reichenheim, C. L. Moraes, C. S. Lopes, and G. Lobato, "The role of intimate partner violence and other health-related social factors on postpartum common mental disorders: a survey-based structural equation modeling analysis," *BMC Public Health*, vol. 14, no. 1, pp. 427–436, 2014.

13

Exploring Complexity of Deliberate Self-Poisoning through Network Analysis

Leila R. Kalankesh,[1,2] Mostafa Farahbakhsh,[3] Rebecca A. Fein,[4,5] Nazila Moftian,[2] and Zahra Nasiry[2]

[1] *Tabriz Health Services Management Research Center, Tabriz, Iran*
[2] *School of Management and Medical Informatics, Tabriz University of Medical Sciences, Tabriz, Iran*
[3] *Tabriz Research Center of Psychiatry and Behavioral Sciences, Tabriz University of Medical Sciences, Tabriz, Iran*
[4] *Laboratory Informatics Institute, Smyrna, GA, USA*
[5] *National Alliance of Research Associates Programs (NARAP), Hartford, CT, USA*

Correspondence should be addressed to Leila R. Kalankesh; leila.kalankesh@gmail.com

Academic Editor: Rory O'Connor

The purpose of this research was to examine the complexity of circumstances that result in deliberate self-poisoning cases. For the purposes of this paper, the cases were patients that presented for care and were admitted to the specialty hospital in Northwest of Iran. The research examined the problems preceding deliberate self-poisoning and the interrelations among them by applying network analysis methods. The network was scored for degrees of centrality and betweenness centrality. Structural analysis of network also was conducted using block modelling. The results showed that family conflicts had the highest score for degree of centrality among women, while the highest score for degree of centrality among men belonged to those dealing with drug addiction. Analysis for degree of betweenness centrality revealed that drug addiction had the highest score among men, whereas the highest score for women on betweenness centrality was related to physical illness. Structural analysis of the network showed differences in role that various problems played in intentional self-poisoning. The findings from this research can be used by public health authorities to create prevention programs that address the problems leading to deliberate self-poisoning.

1. Introduction

Incidence rate of suicide attempt in Iran is estimated 91.65 per 100000 (82.2 in men and 115.79 in women) and it is more common in the 15–24 age group [1]. A common method for suicide attempt in both developed and developing countries is deliberate self-poisoning [2–4]. Intentional self-poisoning has also been reported as the most common method of self-harm among patients admitted to the hospital for self-harm incidents [5]. This is also true in Iran [6]. Suicide attempts are not accidents but are deliberate actions taken by individuals that are attempting to free themselves from the pressures that are caused by distressing life circumstances [7]. The importance of investigation on preceding factors and life stressors on attempting suicide has been highlighted [8, 9]. Circumstances that lead to suicide attempts can be classified into two different groups: social circumstances and medical circumstances. Examples of social circumstances are unemployment, divorce, poverty, loss of family members, family problems, and financial problems. Medical circumstances can include mental disorders (depression, bipolar disorder, schizophrenia, etc.) or physical disorders (for example, cancer and multiple sclerosis) [8, 10–12].

While some patients identified family problems as the precursor to the attempted suicide [13–16], others highlighted the link between the attempted suicide and life stressors [17] such as separation, financial problems, work-related problem, unemployment, change of residence place, physical diseases [18], or other health related issues [19] and surgeries [20–22]. Studies of attempting suicides including deliberate self-poisoning have reported factors such as mental disorders, financial and economic problems, unemployment, quarrel with spouse, family conflicts, physical illness and hopelessness, and substance abuse among cases from different parts of Iran [23–25].

It should be noted that suicide and suicide attempts are complex phenomena and often are the result of a complex set of circumstances in the patient's life [26–30] and complex matrix of different interacting variables [16]. Evidence shows the role of combination of risk factors in deliberate self-harm [31]. Comorbidities of multiple factors such as physical and mental problems have been reported among those attempting deliberate self-harm [32]. Some researchers have investigated interconnections among risk factors such as depression, health problems and status of the family support in suicidal ideation [33, 34]. Coexistence of risk factors has been found to increase the probability of attempted suicide compared with existence of only one factor [9, 35]. Understanding interconnection among different factors can be of great importance in formulating suicide prevention programs [36].

Network analysis, originally used for examining the relationship among social entities [37], can be used to perform quantitative analysis of complex systems. Recently this method has been deployed for comparing Diagnostic and Statistical Manual (DSM) and non-DSM symptoms of depression [38] and for explaining comorbidity pattern of mental disorders based on network of psychiatric symptoms derived from DSM-IV [39]. Network analysis method was first applied to examining interconnections between motives for completed suicide attempts using Japanese police statistics [40]. This method allows researchers to form a better understanding of the complexity of factors and problems preceding attempting suicide as it gives us the whole picture of interconnections among all factors contributing to it. Research for this paper examined interconnections among problems preceding deliberate self-poisoning among cases presented and admitted to the hospital (overall and in terms of gender) in the Northwest of Iran through applying network analysis methods.

2. Methods

2.1. Subjects and Data. A cross sectional study was carried out to assess the problems preceding intentional self-poisoning and their interconnection among cases admitted to the hospital in the Northwest of Iran. The study sample was all cases hospitalized with a diagnosis of deliberate self-poisoning in the second half of the solar year in Iranian calendar. Data were extracted from medical records of all cases ($n = 357$) presented and admitted to a teaching hospital (in Northwest Iran) with a diagnosis of deliberate self-poisoning during 6 months (between September 23, 2013, and March 21, 2014). Patients' records were studied to extract a set of preceding circumstances or problems reported by patients or their family and written in patient history record. List of these variables had been extracted through literature review and had been categorized and validated by the psychiatrist. The data collector was a specialist in field of Health Information Management who had experience of data abstraction from medical records. She was practically trained by psychiatrist on how to extract the data from the patient medical records for this research before starting the data collection.

2.2. Generating the Network and Its Measures. A network of the problems preceding intentional self-poisoning was constructed, and interconnections among the problems were depicted as a graph using network analysis methods. The constructed graph contains nodes and the edges between any two connected nodes. Each node represents a distinct problem preceding the intentional self-poisoning and the edge between two nodes represents their cooccurrence. The weight of each edge is determined by frequency of their cooccurrence. GEPHI software [41] was used for constructing and visualizing the network. In addition, centrality measures including degree centrality and betweenness centrality were computed and analyzed for the graph. Degree centrality measure refers to the number of direct connections that an individual node has to other nodes within a network. Increase in number of one factor necessarily may not result in high degree score. In fact, the degree measure of one factor in this paper indicates coexistence of this factor along with other factors. Factors (nodes in the network) with high degree centrality appear to be more important in the network compared with others.

Betweenness centrality measure represents the extent to which a node can act as an intermediary or the most travelled path to other nodes [42]. This measure is of particular interest because it measures the relative importance of a factor by measuring not how well connected it is but instead where it falls between other factors in the network. Any two factors or issues are connected by either a direct path or a path that travels via other factors. Factor with high betweenness score is one that lies along the shortest path relating other factors. Mediation of some of the factors by other factors in suicidal behavior has been reported in the literature [43–46]. The factors with the highest betweenness derive a lot of importance from their position in the network and their removal from the network will disrupt interconnections among other factors. Effective disruption of a network of contributing factors may prevent attempting suicide. It means control or removal of factors with high score of betweenness can be considered as the priority area in prevention strategies for attempted suicide. Example of using degree and betweenness measures in network analysis approach can be found in the literature for investigating the interconnections among contributing factors in other disciplines [40, 47, 48].

2.3. Block Modelling of the Network. Structure of the network was examined by the means of block modelling through applying CONCOR *(CONvergence of iterated CORrelations)* algorithm in UCINET (software for block modelling of network). In fact aim of this algorithm is to partition network data by splitting blocks based upon the CONvergence of iterated CORrelations (CONCOR) [49]. The idea of block modelling is to bring out some main features of the network by partitioning the nodes into categories of equivalent nodes. Nodes A and B are structurally equivalent if they relate to other nodes in the same way [50]. In other words, a block model is a representation for clustering objects into groups based upon patterns that occur in the relations among these objects. Two measures of intrablock density and interblock density are used for interpreting structure obtained from block modelling. High intrablock density indicates highly related factors while high interblock density reveals the significant correlation between a pairs of blocks. Average density score of the whole network was considered as the cut-off point for judging on significance of interblock and intrablock density scores. Density of network can be computed through dividing total number of connections in the network by total possible connection in that network [37, 51].

3. Results

3.1. Basic Characteristics of the Motives. About 57.4 percent of patients (205 cases) were female and 42.6% of them (152 cases) were male. Age of cases ranged between 13 and 84. Average age of the patient was 29.94 (SD = 14). About 18 percent of the cases were under age 20 years, 67% of them aged between 20 and 40 years, and 15 percent of them were over 40 years old. Job categories observed among the patients were housewife (28%), self-employed jobs (15%), middle school and high school pupils (9.34), unemployed (7.2), university students (5%), governmental jobs (2%), soldiers (1.2), and prisoners (0.2). No specified job was mentioned for about 8.5 percent of cases.

The most common substance the cases used for deliberate poisoning was Medicines (77.7%), followed by Pesticides (8%), Tramadol and Methadone (5.5%), Bleach (3.9%), non-specified substance (3.6%), Petrol (0.8%), and Alcohol (0.5%). In 107 cases, there was only one problem written and reported in their chart. 157 cases had more than one issue written in their records. Overall 579 factors were identified as problems preceding the deliberate self-poisoning and then they were classified into the 6 above-mentioned classes: family problems, health problems, economic problems, romantic problems, educational problems, and others. This categorization was conducted in accordance with the classes of issues recognized in the literature. Table 1 presents these issues in detail.

3.2. Network Visualization and Centrality Measures. The network constructed for visualizing the interconnection of the issues and circumstances preceding the intentional self-poisoning are depicted in Figure 1. Moreover, the centrality measures for each class of the problems are provided in Table 1.

3.3. Degree Centrality Measures of the Network. As Table 1 shows the class of health problems has the greatest degree (0.45) followed by the family problems (degree centrality of 0.37), meaning that these two classes of issues had the first and second highest number of connections with other categories. Among subclasses of family problems, family conflicts had the highest degree centrality (0.178) and among subcategories of health issues, drug addiction had the highest degree centrality (0.173) followed by other mental problems (0.125) and physical illness (0.102). In fact these are the issues highly connected with other problems.

By looking at degree centrality scores in terms of gender, it is noticeable that the issues in the class of family problems are more connected to others in women (degree centrality of 0.416) compared with men (0.302). In subcategories of family problems, the most highly connected issue is family conflicts among both men and women. However, degree centrality of this issue among women (0.241) is twice as much the score among men (0.126).

Health problems have approximately equal number of connections with other factors in both men (degree centrality of 0.45) and women (degree centrality of 0.448). In subclasses of health problems, three most highly connected factors to others among women are other mental problems (degree centrality of 0.152), physical illness (degree centrality of 0.131), and depression (degree centrality of 0.103) while these factors among men include drug addiction (degree centrality of 0.258), alcoholism (degree centrality of 0.147), and other mental problems (degree centrality of 0.107).

3.4. Betweenness Centrality Measures of the Network. As it can be seen from Table 1, the betweenness centrality measure was found to be equal for both health and family problems. Looking at subcategories of each class, the four highest betweenness centrality scores belong to other mental problems (0.185), depression (0.122) physical illness (0.118), and drug addiction (0.07), respectively.

Betweenness centrality score for family problems was found to be higher among women (0.167) compared with men (0.05). Moreover, when it comes to the subcategories of this class, family conflict had higher score of betweenness centrality among women (0.147) compared with men (0.09).

Higher score of betweenness centrality score was revealed for health problems among men (0.65) compared with women (0.25). In subcategories of health problems, betweenness scores of physical illness were found to be higher among women (0.172) than men (0.096), while the score of depression was found to be higher for men (0.135) compared with women (0.005).

Similarly the betweenness scores of drug addiction (0.196) and other mental problems (0.186) were higher for men compared with those among women.

3.5. Structure of Total Network. As Figure 2 illustrates, overall block modelling has categorized problems preceding the deliberate self-poisoning into 6 blocks. Numbers under and between the nodes refer to the intrablock and the interblock density scores, respectively. The most important problems characterized by the degree centrality score have been clustered into block 1 which has the highest intrablock density. Moreover, this block has connection with all other blocks in the network (with the interblock density score higher than the score of whole network (1 > 0.44)).

3.6. Structure of the Network among Women. The structure of problems proceeding the deliberate self-poisoning among women has been depicted in Figure 3. As it can be seen

TABLE 1: Pattern of problems preceding deliberate self-poisoning and their related centrality measures in the network.

Categories	Number (%)			Centrality measures					
				Total		Male		Female	
	Total	Male	Female	Degree	Betweenness	Degree	Betweenness	Degree	Betweenness
Health problems	276 (47.6)	146 (0.55)	130 (0.41)	0.45	0.183	0.448	0.65	0.449	0.25
Physical illness	49 (8.4)	13 (4.9)	36 (11.4)*	0.102	0.118	0.074	0.096	0.131	0.172
Depression	49 (8.4)	15 (5.6)	34 (10.8)*	0.097	0.122	0.086	0.135	0.103	0.005
Alcoholism	25 (4.3)	23 (8.6)*	2 (0.6)	0.087	0.003	0.147	0.009	0.017	0
Drug addiction	69 (11.9)	59 (22.2)*	10 (3.1)	0.173	0.070	0.258	0.196	0.059	0.074
Other mental problems**	67 (11.5)	30 (11.3)	37 (11.7)	0.125	0.185	0.107	0.186	0.152	0.119
Surgery	17 (2.9)	6 (2.2)	11 (3.5)	0.049	0.002	0.034	0.007	0.055	0.010
Family problems	212 (36.6)	66 (0.25)	146 (0.47)	0.37	0.183	0.302	0.05	0.416	0
Family conflicts	156 (26.9)	56 (21.1)	100 (31.8)*	0.178	0.057	0.126	0.090	0.241	0.147
Marital problems	22 (3.7)	4 (1.5)	18 (5.7)*	0.023	0.036	0.009	0	0.041	0.045
Divorce	15 (2.5)	4 (1.5)	11 (3.5)	0.045	0.008	0.034	0	0.069	0.029
Death of family member	5 (0.8)	0 (0)	5 (1.5)*	0.005	0	—	—	0.014	0.010
Physical violence	3 (0.5)	0 (0)	3 (0.9)	0.003	0	—	—	0.007	0
Other family problems	11 (1.8)	2 (0.7)	9 (2.8)	0.011	0.007	0.006	0	0.014	0.011
Economic problems	29 (5)	26 (0.098)	3 (0.01)	0.088	0	0.164	0	0.026	0
Financial problems	23 (3.9)	20 (7.5)*	3 (0.9)	0.047	0.044	0.067	0.057	0.017	0.003
Unemployment	2 (0.3)	2 (0.7)	0 (0)	0.005	0	0.003	0	—	—
Other economic problems	4 (0.6)	4 (1.5)*	0 (0)	0.003	0	0.006	0	—	—
Romantic problems	16 (2.7)	5 (1.8)	11 (3.5)	0.024	0.042	0.017	0	0.065	0
Educational problems	5 (0.8)	3 (1.1)	2 (0.6)	0.005	0	0.009	0	0.003	0
Others***	41 (7)	19 (7.1)	22 (7)	0.018	0.002	0.018	0.005	0.021	0
Total	579	265	314						

* refers to the statistical difference between men and women. **Category of "other mental problems" includes personality disorder, bipolar disorder, and schizophrenia.
***Category of "others" includes work place conflicts, failure in sport competition, conflict with friends, heavy conviction, and escape from military service.

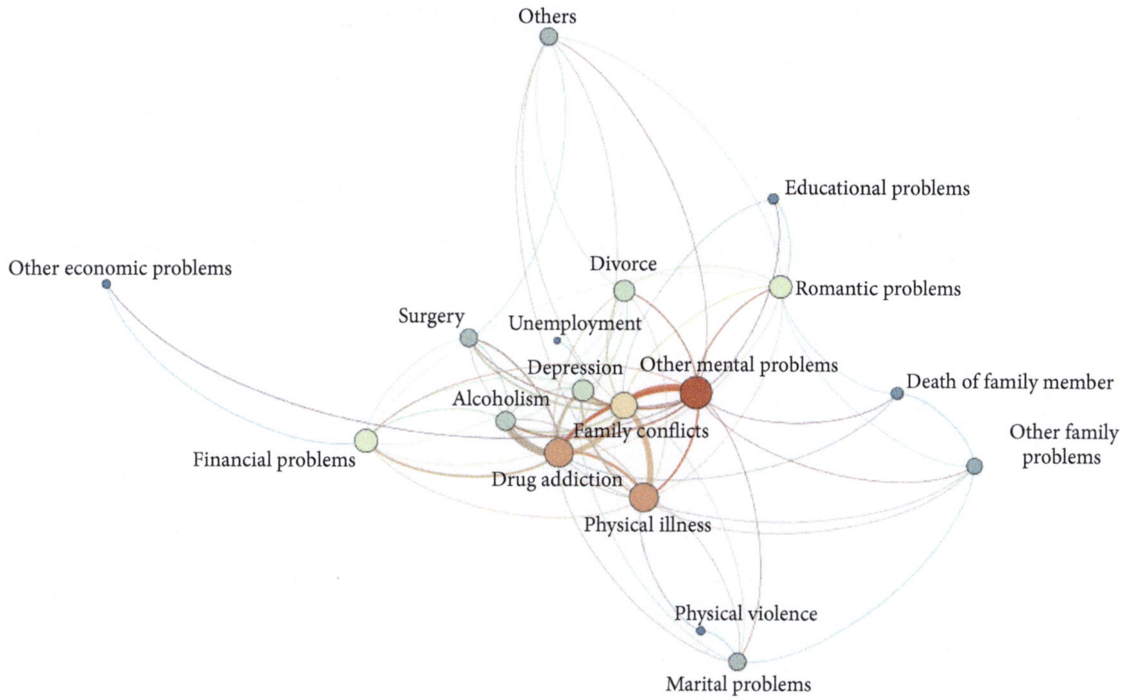

Figure 1: Network of issues preceding the deliberate self-poisoning.

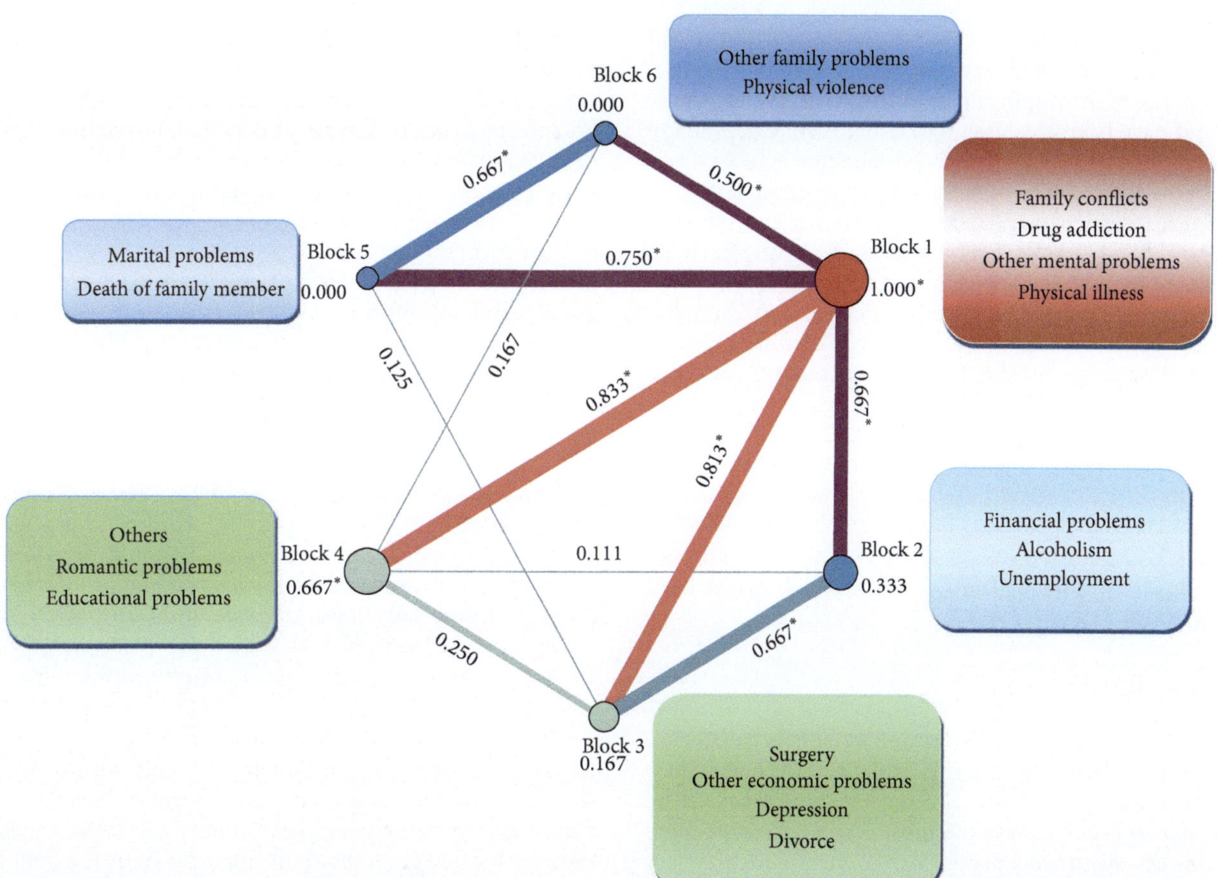

Figure 2: Block modelling in the network of problems preceding deliberate self-poisoning. *Density scores higher than the score of whole network.

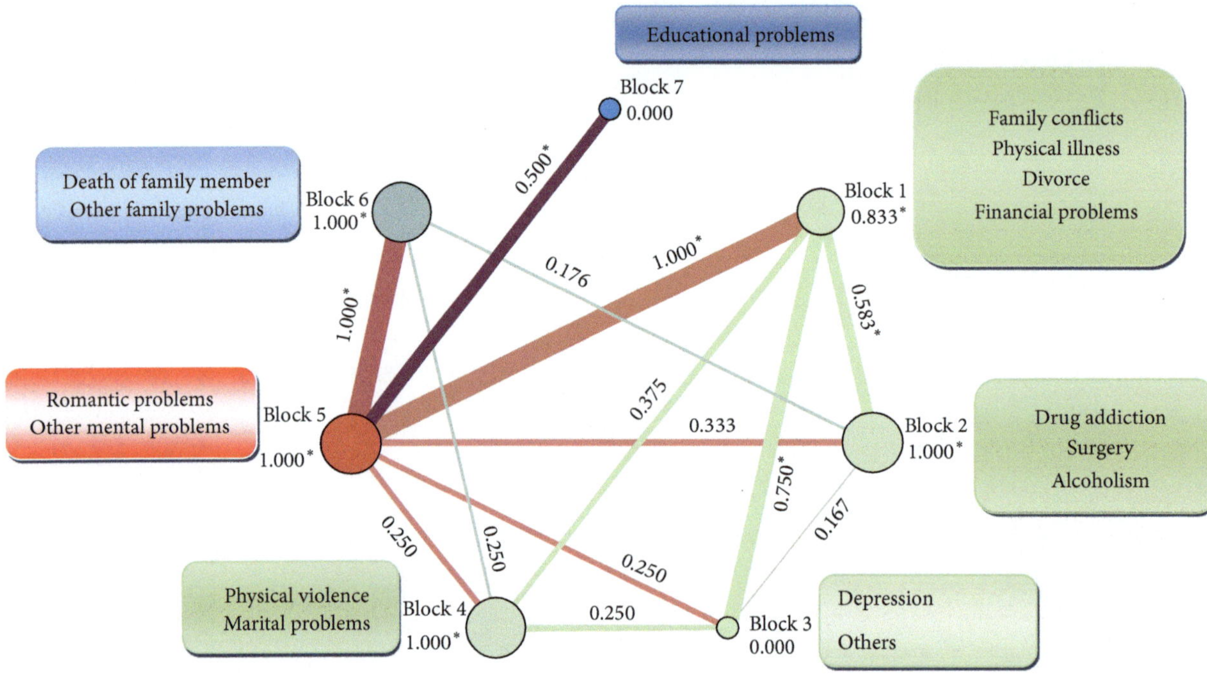

Figure 3: Block modelling in the network of problems preceding deliberate self-poisoning among women. *Density scores higher than the score of whole network.

from this figure, both family conflicts (as the first important problem in terms of the degree centrality score) and physical illness (as the third important problem in terms of degree centrality) have been clustered into block 1 while depression and other mental problems have been classified in block 3 and block 5, respectively. The highest score of interblock density can be observed between block 1 and block 5 and between block 5 and block 6, followed by interblock density between block 1 and block 3.

As Figure 4 shows the block modelling algorithm has clustered the most important problems identified among men into 4 separate blocks. Block 1 and block 5 have the intrablock density higher than the whole network. Drug addiction as the most important problem among men has been located in block 5 while both family conflict (as the second important problem) and other mental problems (as the third important problem) have been clustered together into block 1. Depression (as the fourth important issue) has been completely isolated from other issues and has been placed in block 3.

4. Discussion

This study revealed the pattern of problems preceding deliberate self-poisoning in terms of their importance, their interconnection, and their role. In terms of the main classes of factors, health problems are the most highly interconnected factor. In fact this main category has connection with every other category of factors in the network. This is in consistent with the results from Japanese study [40]. Inside the category of health problems three most interconnected issues are drug addiction, other mental problems, and physical illnesses. Cooccurrence of drug addiction with severe mental health problems has been highlighted in the literature [52]. Moreover, emphasis on importance of employment intervention on substance abuse treatment reveals interrelation between drug addiction and unemployment [53]. Interconnection between family conflicts or problems with drug abuse has been documented in the literature as well [54].

The second most interconnected issue is family problems. This differs from finding of Japanese study in which economic and livelihood problems have been found to be as the second interconnected issues in the network [40]. Previous studies have reported family conflicts among the common and important factors contributing to the intentional self-harm and attempting suicide in Iran and other countries [16, 55–57].

Overall three highest scores of betweenness centrality belong to other mental problems (including character disorder, schizophrenia, and bipolar disorder), depression, and physical illness, respectively. It means mental problems and physical illness have important role in interrelations among other factors. This implies that disrupting network through these factors can be very effective in preventing attempting suicide.

Based on analysis of the network in terms of gender, drug addiction was found to be the most highly connected issue in the network among men. Moreover, this issue in males played as an intermediary issue among other factors. This was indicative of its centrality and importance in the deliberate self-poisoning among men. According to the recent meta-analysis conducted on prevalence and pattern of drug use among Iranian adolescents, males are in considerably greater risk of drug use compared with females [58]. This finding

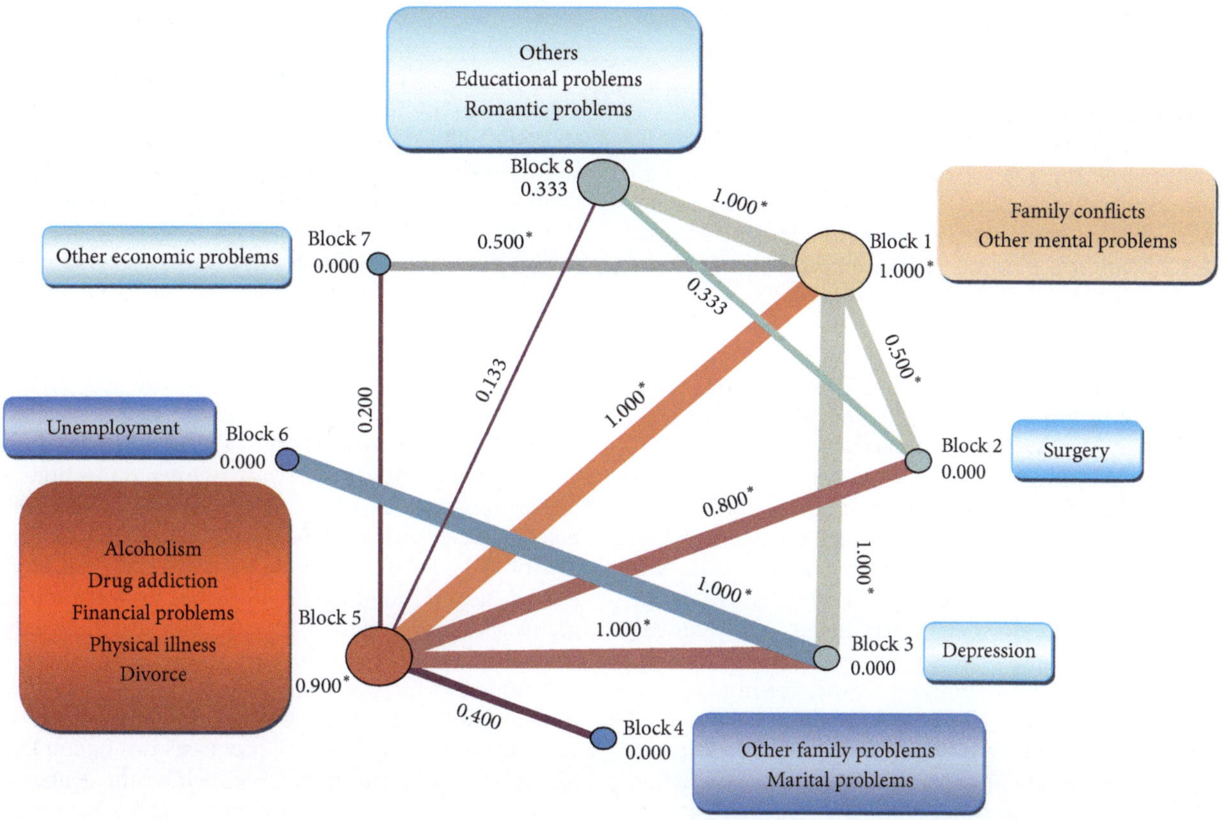

FIGURE 4: Block modelling in the network of problems preceding deliberate self-poisoning among men. *Density scores higher than the score of whole network.

was completely different from the result found in the study conducted on the completed suicide cases in Japan, in which drug abuse was not such an important factor among either men or women. This might be attributed to some extent to the differences in nature of completed suicide and the attempting suicide. Furthermore, the issue of drug addiction might be a problem specific to Iranian society with its own related individual or social problems; the Iranian community considers addiction the third biggest threat to their society after the inflation and unemployment [59]. Comorbidity of drug addiction with personality disorders has been reported in a study carried out in west part of Iran [60]. This implied that any successful intervention on drug addiction issues can break down the network and may result in the prevention of deliberate self-poisoning. This means intervention strategies for preventing deliberate self-poisoning among men should give priority to the issue of drug addiction as the main factor in attempted self-poisoning among men. Boys must be the main target of preventive programs in this aspect. Prevention initiatives including life skill training and parenting skill programs with focus on adolescents have been suggested in the literature since it is believed that the onset of substance use and abuse is during adolescents [61, 62].

When it comes to women, family conflicts were found to be the most connected with and the most critical issue preceding intentional self-poisoning. This finding was in line with the finding of a study from Karachi in which women had been found to attempt suicide more compared with men due to the family conflicts [63]. Families in Iranian community are witnessing a change in which interplay between tradition and modernity is happening [64]. This may influence women members of the family even more. Moreover, family member may belong to different generations who could not understand each other. This may result in family conflict. Evidence shows that some of the factors are gender-specific in attempting suicide. For example, financial problems and Alcohol use disorders have been reported as a risk factor specific to the males while weakness of connection with family has been highlighted to be specific to the females [65, 66].

Overall block modelling of the network was indicative of similar roles played by family conflicts, drug addiction, other mental problems, and physical illness in deliberate self-poisoning. These four issues have been clustered into block 1 with highest score of intrablock density. Meanwhile, these are issues with the highest score of degree centrality in the network. Issues located in this block constitute about 51% of all problems extracted. This implies that 51 percent of the problems have similar roles in deliberate self-poisoning. This reflects the importance of factors in this block. Financial problems, alcoholism, and unemployment have been clustered into block 2. Overall 8.5 percent of the problems are included in this cluster. Scores of interblock density of block 1 with other blocks imply the reinforcing effect of factors in this block on others.

Among men, the role of other mental problems and family conflicts was found to be similar in deliberate self-poisoning while the role of drug addiction was found to be different from the family conflicts and other mental problems. This factor has been clustered inside block 5 which includes alcoholism, physical illness, divorce, and financial problems. This can reflect the similar roles played with these five factors in deliberate self-poisoning. Block 1 and block 5 are the distinguished blocks of the model as their intrablock and interblock density measure is high. This reveals the high importance of factors clustered inside these blocks and their interrelations. Depression was revealed to have totally different role among men as it has been clustered in completely separate block. Moreover, high interblock density between block 3 and block 6 reveals an important relation between depression and unemployment in attempting self-poisoning among men. There is evidence from longitudinal study suggesting that unemployment predates depression among men [67]. Depression as one of the main mental diseases can also be referred to a pathway between unemployment and attempting suicide [68]. Since depression has the third highest score of betweenness among men, it should be given the priority in planning prevention strategies for attempting suicide among men. This is in accordance with the fact that major depression provides the background for most of the suicide attempts [69].

Family conflicts and physical illness were found to play similar role in intentional self-poisoning among women. Depression was found to have totally different role from other issues. This may reflect distinct function of different problems among those attempting intentional self-poisoning as well as the function of gender in these differences. Important role of some factors in suicidal behaviors among one gender compared with another has been highlighted in the related literature [65]. As it is evident, factors in block 1 have important relations with the depression among women. This result is consistent with the result of study which reported that family conflicts trigger depression among women [70]. Our findings imply the interrelation between depression and physical illness as well. This is contrary to the result of study in which physical illness was not reported as the trigger for depression [70].

This research may inform public health authorities about the important problems preceding the deliberate self-poisoning and interrelations among those issues in order to establish appropriate prevention strategies. Some consider suicide as a proxy measure for unmet needs among vulnerable individuals [71] and the suicide attempt can be as "a cry for help." Therefore, prevention strategies should be based on providing the vulnerable individuals with the services or skills they need to cope with their problems or to resolve them. The prevention strategies and programs should also be tailored for vulnerable individuals of different genders specifically. Evidence suggests that it is required to put in place a combination of gender-specific preventive approaches in order to address different risk factors and problems preceding suicidal behaviors [72].

Examples of such prevention strategies would be providing free community-based services for family counselling, training living skills, problem solving, effective communication with family members and appropriate parenting mechanism to address family conflicts [73, 74]. It is also required to make available case management services depression in primary care in the population level and to ensure active follow up of depressed patients [75] or to provide suicide screening program for those suffered from mental disorders.

5. Conclusion

Network analysis methods provide useful tools to quantify and better understand a network of interconnections among issues preceding the deliberate self-poisoning. Through information provided from this analysis, the high priority issues contributing to the deliberate self-poisoning can be characterized in order to guide the priorities for intervention programs. Findings from such analyses may also inform the public health authorities for making evidence-based prevention programs in which network of important factors and issues contributing to the deliberate self-poisoning are addressed. A combination of preventive programs can be implemented to influence the network of issues behind the deliberate self-poisoning. Such prevention programs may have much more effective influence than prevention programs that target only one single factor. However, those factors or problems that have high degree and betweenness and have been clustered in separate clusters should be considered in prevention programs.

Additional Points

This research was limited to the data reported by patients or their family on motives behind self-poisoning and recorded in their medical charts. Therefore, there might be a possibility of under reporting some of the issues by them. Data obtained from clinical and psychiatric assessment of patients by clinicians might result in different findings as the statistics on distribution of motives behind deliberate self-poisoning implies. Conducting this analysis on large number of patients was not feasible in this project due to resource limitation. Applying this methodology on large number of data in the future research can shed some light on possibility of sample size effect on the analysis result. Separate network analysis for interrelations of problem among those with mental disorders and without mental disorders can clarify the role of different issues when they are cooccurred with mental disorders.

Competing Interests

The authors declare that there is no conflict of interests.

Acknowledgments

The authors would like to acknowledge Tabriz Health Services Management Research Centre and Tabriz Research

Center of Psychiatry and Behavioral Sciences for supporting this project.

References

[1] C. Rostami, S. Daliri, K. Sayehmiri, A. Delpisheh, and F. Sayehmiri, "The incidence of suicide attempt in Iran (2001–12): meta-analysis," *Journals of Kermanshah University of Medical Sciences*, vol. 19, no. 7, pp. 374–382, 2016.

[2] D. R. Camidge, R. J. Wood, and D. N. Bateman, "The epidemiology of self-poisoning in the UK," *British Journal of Clinical Pharmacology*, vol. 56, no. 6, pp. 613–619, 2003.

[3] M. Eddleston, "Patterns and problems of deliberate self-poisoning in the developing world," *QJM*, vol. 93, no. 11, pp. 715–731, 2000.

[4] C. B. Kelly, J. Weir, T. Rafferty, and R. Galloway, "Deliberate self-poisoning presenting at a rural hospital in Northern Ireland 1976–1996: relationship to prescribing," *European Psychiatry*, vol. 15, no. 6, pp. 348–353, 2000.

[5] M. Shannon, S. Borron, and M. Burns, *Haddad and winchester's clinical management of poisoning and drug overdose*, Elsevier, 2007.

[6] F. Najafi, O. Beiki, T. Ahmadijouybari et al., "An assessment of suicide attempts by self-poisoning in the west of Iran," *Journal of Forensic and Legal Medicine*, vol. 27, pp. 1–5, 2014.

[7] B. Sadock and V. Sadock, Eds., *Kaplan and Sadock's Concise Textbook of Clinical Psychiatry*, LWW, 2008.

[8] L. Rezaie, S. A. Hosseini, M. Rassafiani, F. Najafi, J. Shakeri, and H. R. Khankeh, "Why self-immolation? A qualitative exploration of the motives for attempting suicide by self-immolation," *Burns*, vol. 40, no. 2, pp. 319–327, 2014.

[9] T. M. Kelly, K. G. Lynch, J. E. Donovan, and D. B. Clark, "Alcohol use disorders and risk factor interactions for adolescent suicidal ideation and attempts," *Suicide and Life-Threatening Behavior*, vol. 31, no. 2, pp. 181–193, 2001.

[10] M. Gelder, R. Mayou, and J. Geddes, *Psychiatry: An Oxford Core Text (Oxford Core Texts)*, Oxford University Press, 2005.

[11] K. Hughes, "Suicide screening in the oncology population," *Journal of the Advanced Practitioner in Oncology*, vol. 7, no. 1, pp. 101–104, 2016.

[12] M. Pompili, A. Forte, M. Palermo et al., "Suicide risk in multiple sclerosis: a systematic review of current literature," *Journal of Psychosomatic Research*, vol. 73, no. 6, pp. 411–417, 2012.

[13] D. A. Brent, J. A. Perper, G. Moritz et al., "Familial risk factors for adolescent suicide: a case-control study," *Acta Psychiatrica Scandinavica*, vol. 89, no. 1, pp. 52–58, 1994.

[14] M. J. Marttunen, H. M. Aro, and J. K. Lonnqvist, "Precipitant stressors in adolescent suicide," *Journal of the American Academy of Child & Adolescent Psychiatry*, vol. 32, no. 6, pp. 1178–1183, 1993.

[15] X.-Y. Xing, F.-B. Tao, Y.-H. Wan et al., "Family factors associated with suicide attempts among chinese adolescent students: a national cross-sectional survey," *Journal of Adolescent Health*, vol. 46, no. 6, pp. 592–599, 2010.

[16] M. Nazarzadeh, Z. Bidel, E. Ayubi, K. Asadollahi, K. V. Carson, and K. Sayehmiri, "Determination of the social related factors of suicide in Iran: a systematic review and meta-analysis," *BMC Public Health*, vol. 13, no. 1, article 4, 2013.

[17] R. T. Liu and I. Miller, "Life events and suicidal ideation and behavior: a systematic review," *Clinical Psychology Review*, vol. 34, no. 3, pp. 181–192, 2014.

[18] M. E. Heikkinen and J. K. Lönnqvist, "Recent life events in elderly suicide: a nationwide study in finland," *International Psychogeriatrics*, vol. 7, no. 2, pp. 287–300, 1995.

[19] A. Smith, *Health Related Risk Factors for Elderly Suicide in San Diego County*, University of California, 2004.

[20] J. E. Mitchell, R. Crosby, M. De Zwaan et al., "Possible risk factors for increased suicide following bariatric surgery," *Obesity*, vol. 21, no. 4, pp. 665–672, 2013.

[21] J. A. Bhatti, A. B. Nathens, D. Thiruchelvam, T. Grantcharov, B. I. Goldstein, and D. A. Redelmeier, "Self-harm emergencies after bariatric surgery a population-based cohort study," *JAMA Surgery*, vol. 151, no. 3, pp. 226–232, 2016.

[22] T. T. Jayakrishnan, Y. Sekigami, R. Rajeev, T. C. Gamblin, and K. K. Turaga, "Morbidity of curative cancer surgery and suicide risk," *Psycho-Oncology*, 2016.

[23] I. Mohebi and B. Boushehri, "Influence of stressor factors in attempting suicide with chemical substances: review of 400 cases," *Urmia Medical Journal*, vol. 17, no. 3, pp. 9–15, 2006.

[24] M. Hakim Shooshtari, S. K. Malakouti, L. Panaghi, S. Mohseni, N. Mansouri, and A. R. Movaghar, "Factors associated with suicidal attempts in Iran: a systematic review," *Iranian Journal of Psychiatry and Behavioral Sciences*, vol. 10, no. 1, article e948, 2016.

[25] M. H. Shooshtary, S. K. Malakouti, J. Bolhari et al., "Community study of suicidal behaviors and risk factors among Iranian adults," *Archives of Suicide Research*, vol. 12, no. 2, pp. 141–147, 2008.

[26] A. Fakhari, M. Rostami, T. Hashemi, V. Haji, and B. Agaie Nia, "Relationship of family features, coping styles and stressor life events with suicide attempt," *Journal of Research in Behavioural Sciences*, vol. 12, no. 2, pp. 155–164, 2014.

[27] S. H. Koslow, P. Ruiz, and C. B. Nemeroff, *A Concise Guide to Understanding Suicide Epidemiology Pathophysiology and Prevention*, Cambridge University Press, Cambridge, UK, 2014.

[28] N. Kreitman, *Suicide and Parasuicide*, Churcill Livingstone, Edinburgh, UK, 1982.

[29] Victoria, "Suicide Prevention Taskforce & Kirby, Peter," Sicide Prevention: Victorian Task Force report, Victorian Task Force, Melbourne, Australia, 1997.

[30] T. Wołodźko and A. Kokoszka, "Classification of persons attempting suicide. A review of cluster analysis research," *Psychiatria Polska*, vol. 48, no. 4, pp. 823–834, 2014.

[31] K. L. Gratz, "Risk factors for deliberate self-harm among female college students: the role and interaction of childhood maltreatment, emotional inexpressivity, and affect intensity/reactivity," *American Journal of Orthopsychiatry*, vol. 76, no. 2, pp. 238–250, 2006.

[32] M. Babakhanian, M. Sadeghi, E. Mohamadpur, and H. Rezazadeh, "Deliberate self-harm among patients referring to the emergency room in Damghan, Iran," *Iranian Journal of Psychiatry and Behavioral Sciences*, vol. 8, no. 4, pp. 46–51, 2014.

[33] H. Xu, L. Qin, J. Wang et al., "A cross-sectional study on risk factors and their interactions with suicidal ideation among the elderly in rural communities of Hunan, China," *BMJ Open*, vol. 6, no. 4, Article ID e010914, 2016.

[34] S. L. Brown and A. D. Vinokur, "The interplay among risk factors for suicidal ideation and suicide: the role of depression, poor health, and loved ones' messages of support and criticism," *American Journal of Community Psychology*, vol. 32, no. 1-2, pp. 131–141, 2003.

[35] D. Tidemalm, A. Haglund, A. Karanti, M. Landén, and B. Runeson, "Attempted suicide in bipolar disorder: risk factors in a cohort of 6086 patients," *PLoS ONE*, vol. 9, no. 4, Article ID e94097, 2014.

[36] M. Bazrafshan, F. Sharif, Z. Molazem, and A. Mani, "Exploring the risk factors contributing to suicide attempt among adolescents: A Qualitative Study," *Iranian Journal of Nursing and Midwifery Research*, vol. 21, no. 1, pp. 93–99, 2016.

[37] S. Wasserman and K. Faust, *Social Network Analysis: Methods and Applications*, Cambridge University Press, Cambridge, UK, 1994.

[38] E. I. Fried, S. Epskamp, R. M. Nesse, F. Tuerlinckx, and D. Borsboom, "What are "good" depression symptoms? Comparing the centrality of DSM and non-DSM symptoms of depression in a network analysis," *Journal of Affective Disorders*, vol. 189, pp. 314–320, 2016.

[39] D. Borsboom, A. O. J. Cramer, V. D. Schmittmann, S. Epskamp, and L. J. Waldorp, "The small world of psychopathology," *PLOS ONE*, vol. 6, no. 11, Article ID e27407, 2011.

[40] Y. Shiratori, H. Tachikawa, K. Nemoto et al., "Network analysis for motives in suicide cases: a cross-sectional study," *Psychiatry and Clinical Neurosciences*, vol. 68, no. 4, pp. 299–307, 2014.

[41] M. Bastian, S. Heymann, and M. Jacomy, "Gephi: an open source software for exploring and manipulating networks," in *Proceedings of the 3rd International AAAI Conference on Weblogs and Social Media*, vol. 20, San Jose, Calif, USA, May 2009.

[42] A. Abraham, A. E. Hassanien, and V. Snášel, Eds., *Computational Social Network Analysis: Trends, Tools and Research Advances*, Springer, Berlin, Germany, 2009.

[43] P. Ahookhosh, B. Bahmani, A. Asgari, and H. Hassanian-Moghaddam, "Family relationship and suicide ideation: the mediating roles of anxiety, hopelessness, and depression in adolescents," *International Journal of High Risk Behaviors and Addiction*, 2016.

[44] S. X. Chen, W. C. H. Wu, and M. H. Bond, "Linking family dysfunction to suicidal ideation: mediating roles of self-views and world-views," *Asian Journal of Social Psychology*, vol. 12, no. 2, pp. 133–144, 2009.

[45] D. A. Lamis and P. S. Malone, "Alcohol-related problems and risk of suicide among college students: the mediating roles of belongingness and burdensomeness," *Suicide and Life-Threatening Behavior*, vol. 41, no. 5, pp. 543–553, 2011.

[46] E. A. Thompson, J. J. Mazza, J. R. Herting, B. P. Randell, and L. L. Eggert, "The mediating roles of anxiety depression, and hopelessness on adolescent suicidal behaviors," *Suicide and Life-Threatening Behavior*, vol. 35, no. 1, pp. 14–34, 2005.

[47] P. Arezes and P. Carvalho, *Ergonomics and Human Factors in Safety Management*, CRC Press, Boca Raton, Fla, USA, 2016.

[48] K. Klockner and Y. Toft, "Accident modelling using social network analysis for complex socio-technical systems," in *Proceedings of the Australian System Safety Conference*, T. Cant, Ed., Australian Computer Society, Melbourne, Australia, 2014.

[49] S. Borgatti, M. Everett, and L. Freeman, *Ucinet for Windows: Software for Social Network Analysis*, Analytic Technologies, Harvard, Mass, USA, 2002.

[50] F. Lorrain and H. C. White, "Structural equivalence of individuals in social networks," *The Journal of Mathematical Sociology*, vol. 1, no. 1, pp. 49–80, 1971.

[51] J. Scott, *Social Network Analysis*, SAGE, 3rd edition, 2012.

[52] C. Gramaglia, F. Bert, A. Lombardi et al., "Sex differences in first-admission psychiatric inpatients with and without a comorbid substance use disorder," *Journal of Addiction Medicine*, vol. 8, no. 5, pp. 351–358, 2014.

[53] M. T. Walton and M. T. Hall, "The effects of employment interventions on addiction treatment outcomes: a review of the literature," *Journal of Social Work Practice in the Addictions*, vol. 16, no. 4, pp. 358–384, 2016.

[54] C. Esposito-Smythers and D. B. Goldston, "Challenges and opportunities in the treatment of adolescents with substance use disorder and suicidal behavior," *Substance Abuse*, vol. 29, no. 2, pp. 5–17, 2008.

[55] G. Dedić, S. Djurdjević, and B. Golubović, "Psychological assessment of persons following suicide attempt by self-poisoning," *Vojnosanitetski Pregled*, vol. 67, no. 2, pp. 151–158, 2010.

[56] E. Farzaneh, O. Mehrpour, S. Alfred, H. H. Moghaddam, B. Behnoush, and T. Seghatoleslam, "Self-poisoning suicide attempts among students in Tehran, Iran," *Psychiatria Danubina*, vol. 22, no. 1, pp. 34–38, 2010.

[57] M. Nazarzadeh, Z. Bidel, E. Ayubi, H. Soori, and K. Sayehmiri, "Factors related to suicide attempt in Iran: a systematic review and meta-analysis," *Hakim Research Journal*, vol. 15, no. 4, pp. 352–363, 2013.

[58] A. Ansari-Moghaddam, F. Rakhshani, F. Shahraki-Sanavi, M. Mohammadi, M. Miri-Bonjar, and N.-M. Bakhshani, "Prevalence and patterns of tobacco, alcohol, and drug use among Iranian adolescents: a meta-analysis of 58 studies," *Children and Youth Services Review*, vol. 60, pp. 68–79, 2016.

[59] A. Hajli, M. Zakariyae, and S. Hojjati, "Iranian's values and attitudes to drug abuse in the country," *Iranian Journal of Social Problems*, vol. 10, no. 2, pp. 81–112, 2010.

[60] F. Tatari, S. Mousavi, J. Shakeri, N. Abdoli, V. Mohammadi-Zavaleh, and K. Zarafshani, "Comorbidity of substance dependency in patients with cluster B personality disorders," *Journal of Kermanshah University of Medical Sciences*, vol. 19, no. 6, pp. 365–373, 2016.

[61] K. W. Griffin and G. J. Botvin, "Evidence-based interventions for preventing substance use disorders in adolescents," *Child and Adolescent Psychiatric Clinics of North America*, vol. 19, no. 3, pp. 505–526, 2010.

[62] P. A. Wyman, "Developmental approach to prevent adolescent suicides: research pathways to effective upstream preventive interventions," *American Journal of Preventive Medicine*, vol. 47, no. 3, S2, pp. S251–S256, 2014.

[63] M. Khan and H. Reza, "Attempted suicide in Karachi, Pakistan," *Suicide and Life Threatening Behaviour*, vol. 28, 1998.

[64] M. Navabakhsh and S. Paknia, "Developmental idealism and the proposal of a theoretical model for family change in Iran," *International Journal of Social Sciences*, vol. 5, no. 1, pp. 11–22, 2015.

[65] M. Kim, G. Oh, and Y. Lee, "Gender-specific factors associated with suicide attempts among the community-dwelling general population with suicidal ideation: the 2013 Korean community health survey," *Journal of Korean Medical Science*, vol. 31, no. 12, pp. 2010–2019, 2016.

[66] T. Rajapakse, K. M. Griffiths, H. Christensen, and S. Cotton, "A comparison of non-fatal self-poisoning among males and females, in Sri Lanka," *BMC Psychiatry*, vol. 14, no. 1, article 221, 2014.

[67] S. M. Montgomery, D. G. Cook, M. J. Bartley, and M. E. J. Wadsworth, "Unemployment pre-dates symptoms of depression and anxiety resulting in medical consultation in young men," *International Journal of Epidemiology*, vol. 28, no. 1, pp. 95–100, 1999.

[68] T. A. Blakely, S. C. D. Collings, and J. Atkinson, "Unemployment and suicide. Evidence for a causal association?" *Journal of Epidemiology and Community Health*, vol. 57, no. 8, pp. 594–600, 2003.

[69] K. Tsirigotis, W. Gruszczynski, and M. Tsirigotis, "Gender differentiation in methods of suicide attempts," *Medical Science Monitor*, vol. 17, no. 8, pp. PH65–PH70, 2011.

[70] I. Petersen, J. H. Hancock, A. Bhana, and K. Govender, "Closing the treatment gap for depression co-morbid with HIV in South Africa: voices of afflicted women," *Health*, vol. 5, no. 3, pp. 557–566, 2013.

[71] M. Rezaeian, "Self-immolation as a proxy measure for unmet needs among the vulnerable," *Burns*, vol. 41, no. 2, pp. 417–418, 2015.

[72] World Health Organization, *For Which Strategies of Suicide Prevention is There Evidence of Effectiveness?* WHO Regional Office for Europe, Copenhagen, Denmark, 2012.

[73] S. Sukhawaha, S. Arunpongpaisal, and S. Rungreangkulkij, "Attempted suicide triggers in Thai adolescent perspectives," *Archives of Psychiatric Nursing*, vol. 30, no. 3, pp. 334–341, 2016.

[74] H. Roohafza, S. Mosharraf, G. Mousavi et al., "The prevalence and determinents of suicidal behaviors in the central region of Iran," *International Journal of Body, Mind & Culture*, vol. 1, no. 2, pp. 142–153, 2014.

[75] C. M. van der Feltz-Cornelis, M. Sarchiapone, V. Postuvan et al., "Best practice elements of multilevel suicide prevention strategies: a review of systematic reviews," *Crisis*, vol. 32, no. 6, pp. 319–333, 2015.

14

Prevalence of Depression and Anxiety amongst Cancer Patients in a Hospital Setting

Anish Khalil,[1] Muhammad Faheem,[2] Ammad Fahim,[3] Haran Innocent,[1] Zainab Mansoor,[1] Shehrbano Rizvi,[1] and Hizra Farrukh[4]

[1] *Shifa College of Medicine, Shifa Tameer-e-Millat University, Islamabad, Pakistan*
[2] *Oncology Department, Nuclear Medicine, Oncology and Radiotherapy Institute [NORI], Islamabad, Pakistan*
[3] *Department of Research, Shifa International Hospital, Islamabad, Pakistan*
[4] *Rawalpindi Medical College, Islamabad, Pakistan*

Correspondence should be addressed to Anish Khalil; aanish008@gmail.com

Academic Editor: Takahiro Nemoto

Background. The biomedical care for cancer has not been complemented by psychosocial progressions in cancer care. *Objectives.* To find the prevalence of anxiety and depression amongst cancer patients in a hospital setting. *Design and Setting.* This cross-sectional study was conducted at the tertiary care hospitals Shifa International Hospital Islamabad and Nuclear Medicine, Oncology, and Radiotherapy Institute [NORI]. *Patients and Methods.* 300 patients were interviewed from both the outpatient and inpatient department using The Aga Khan University Anxiety and Depression Scale (AKUADS). *Main Outcome Measures.* Using a score of 20 and above on the AKUADS, 146 (48.7%) patients were suffering from anxiety and depression. *Results.* When cross tabulation was done between different factors and the cancer patients with anxiety and depression, the following factors were found out to be significant with associated p value < 0.05: education of the patient, presence of cancer in the family, the severity of pain, and the patient's awareness of his anxiety and depression. Out of 143 (47.7%) uneducated patients, 85 (59.4%) were depressed, hence making it the highest educational category suffering from depression and anxiety. *Conclusion.* The prevalence of anxiety and depression amongst cancer patients was high showing that importance should be given to screening and counseling cancer patients for anxiety and depression, to help them cope with cancer as a disease and its impact on their mental wellbeing. *Limitations.* The frequency of female patients in our research was higher than those of male patients.

1. Background

Depression, as a disease, is usual in cancer patients. However, only restricted evidence is available for Asian communities [1]. There have been remarkable progressions in biomedical care for cancer which have not been complemented by progressions in providing good quality care for the psychosocial effects of cancer. Various cancer patients report that those in charge did not understand their psychosocial needs, failed to recognize and address depression and anxiety, were unaware of them, and did not refer them to available resources such as counselors or psychiatrists, and overall did not consider psychological support to be an important part of quality medical care [2].

Cancer is a grave illness which has an effect on physical and emotional wellbeing of patients. The recognition of cancer is a tough event causing significant psychological anguish [3–6]. Depression is a difficult task to study in cancer patients as manifestations occur over a range of spectrum being unique in different patients [4, 7]. Anxiety has been shown to mutually exist with depression [7–9]. This is important as it has been shown that patients with coexisting anxiety and depressive disorders tend to have drastic symptoms, extended healing times, worse outcomes, and greater burden on healthcare resources than those with a singular disorder [10].

The objective therefore of this research is to examine the prevalence of anxiety and depression in Pakistani cancer patients and to explore its significance to various influencing demographic factors and social habits.

2. Methods

This cross-sectional study took place from December 2014 till January 2015. Using the WHO sample size calculator, keeping prevalence of depression of 47.2% from a study from Iran, with absolute precision required 6%, the sample size calculated was 300 patients. These patients were selected from the inpatient and outpatient departments of Shifa International Hospital oncology department and Nuclear Medicine Oncology & Radiotherapy Institute (*NORI*). Inclusion criteria were set to those patients seeking treatment and who were 16 years old and older. Through an interview with the patients, the principal investigator and his team asked the patients few questions.

The patients questions were divided into five sections: *Section A: personal information* which consisted of questions including (1) name, (2) age, (3) sex, (4) marital status, that is, married, single, divorced, or widowed, and (5) phone number; *Section B: socioeconomic and educational status* which consisted of questions including (1) occupation, (2) level of education, that is, primary, middle, secondary, higher, bachelors, or masters, (3) level of income and employment status, that is, dependent, independent and unemployed, and independent and employed with either a lower income, middle income, or upper income, (4) source of funding for the treatment, that is, whether he was self-funded or by someone else such as government funds; *Section C: cancer information* which consisted of questions including (1) type of cancer, that is, head and neck, lung cancer, breast cancer, gastrointestinal tract cancer, lymphoma, bone and soft tissue cancer, cervical cancer, and ovarian cancer (for those who did not have the aforementioned cancers, a last category of others was kept), (2) stage of cancer, that is, stage 1, 2, 3, or 4, (3) treatment being sought, that is, radiotherapy, chemotherapy, or cancer related surgery, (4) duration from diagnosis of cancer and from treatment of cancer, and (5) number of cancer patients in the family of the patient other than himself; *Section D: pain scale* which consisted of a pain scale which measured the pain the patient felt at the moment ranging from 0, no pain, to 10, unimaginable unspeakable pain; *Section E: anxiety and depression* which consisted of questions including (1) patient's awareness of whether he or she was anxious and depressed, (2) any treatment sought for his anxiety and depression, (3) whether the caretaker counseled the patient, (4) physical activity, and (5) smoking habits. In the same section, we included the Aga Khan University Anxiety and Depression Scale (AKUADS). The AKUADS is an anxiety and depression scale which was developed in Urdu, the official language of Pakistan. The authors chose AKUADS over other scales available due to various reasons. Only 57.9% of Pakistan's population is literate, that is, aged 15 and over and can read and write [11]; this poses a language barrier as many scales of anxiety and depression are in English. If this factor of language barrier was not kept in mind, the translation of the western scales would vary from investigator to investigator and this would have caused an anomaly in the results. The authors, keeping in mind this language barrier, decided to choose an Urdu scale for their research. Ahmer et al. [12] have already conducted a systemic review on the most extensively evaluated and validated Urdu anxiety and depression scale comparing over 19 questionnaires including questionnaires such as Personal Health Questionnaire (PHQ), General health questionnaire both 12 and 28 version, and Aga Khan University Anxiety and Depression Scale. After analyzing 32 researches which defined these 19 questionnaires, Saeed et al. came to a conclusion in their research that Bradford Somatic Inventory (BSI) [13], Aga Khan University Anxiety and Depression Scale (AKUADS) [14], and self-reporting questionnaire (SRQ) [15] are the most thoroughly judged for an Urdu setting. Out of these three, the AKUADS is indigenously an Urdu scale, the BSI concurrently was developed in English and Urdu, and the SRQ was adapted to Urdu scale. After a contrast of the items in AKUADS, SRQ, and BSI, the authors found out that AKUADS excels in its items as almost all its items are similar to the other two questionnaires. The authors thus decided to choose AKUADS as the scale of choice. The AKUADS consists of 25 questions; each question is answered with a time frame of 2 weeks kept in mind. For example, the first question in the AKUADS is "have you been sleeping less?". This was stated to the patient as "In the past 2 weeks, have you been sleeping less?". The patient then answers this question as never, sometimes, mostly, or always. This scale addresses anxiety and depression of the patient but fails to differentiate between both. Out of these 25 questions, 13 are psychological and 12 are somatic. The questions in AKUADS include those on sleep, interests, anxiety, mood, suicide, gastrointestinal symptoms, pain/burning, breathing, tremulousness, numbness, and voiding. Each of the answers is marked on a 4-point system with never 0, sometimes 1, mostly 2, and always 3. The points of these questions are then summed up. The score of 20 or more on the AKUADS (using a ROC curve analysis) has a sensitivity of 66%, a specificity of 79%, a positive predictive value of 83, and a negative predictive value of 60 [14].

Prior to the research, the ethical approval was granted by Shifa International Hospital's IRB & Ethics Committee and approval from Nuclear Medicine, Oncology, and Radiotherapy Institute [NORI] was taken. Patients were selected at random from the outpatient department (OPD) and the inpatient department (IPD) of the abovementioned hospitals; selection bias was reduced by ensuring that the entire OPD and IPD patients were included in the sample size. Before the patients were interviewed, the principal investigator and his team explained to the patient the research being conducted, the risks and discomforts of the questions, and the benefits the principal investigator and his team hope to be achieved through this research. It was informed to the patients that their data would be kept confidential and any reporting would be done as a group with no identifying information. After being informed, the patients were handed two printed consent forms: one they signed and handed over and the other they kept to themselves as record of voluntarily participating in this research. The patients were also informed that they had every right to refuse to participate without any

Table 1: Frequency of various types of cancers.

Type of cancer	Patients not screened as anxious and depressed AKUADS score < 19	Patients screened as anxious and depressed AKUADS score > 20	Total number of cancer patients in that category
Breast cancer	47	46	93
Gastrointestinal tract	30	23	53
Head and neck	21	21	42
Bone and soft tissue	12	16	28
Lung	8	10	18
Ovarian	3	5	8
Lymphoma	2	2	4
Cervical	0	2	2
Others	31	21	52
Total	154	146	300

penalty. The data collected in the 300 interviews was analyzed using IBM SPSS Statistics version 20 and descriptive statistics were calculated.

3. Results

300 patients were approached to be a part of this research and all 300 patients consented to be a part of the research. The minimum age was 16 and the maximum age was 88 with a mean age of 45.5 years with standard deviation of 15.3. 113 (37.7%) patients were male and the remaining 187 (62.3%) patients were female. 244 (81.3%) patients were married, 41 (13.7%) were single, 3 (1%) were divorced, and 12 (4%) were widowed.

The highest majority of the patients answered occupation as unknown, 123 (41%), followed by housewives, 79 (26.3%), students, 15 (5%), land/cattle farmer, 14 (4.7%), and labour, 14 (4.7%), with the remaining data completely scattered amongst other occupations. 143 (47.7%) patients were uneducated while 33 (11%) had primary, 47 (15.7%) middle, 24 (8%) secondary, 18 (6%) higher, 21 (7%) bachelors, and 13 (4.3%) masters level of education. There was one patient who reported his level of education as unknown and could not be classified in any one of the categories above. When the patients were asked about the employment status, they answered as follows: 210 (70%) dependent on someone, 6 (2%) independent: unemployed, 45 (15%) independent: lower income, 16 (5.3%) independent: middle income, 3 (1%) independent: upper income, and 20 (6.7%) independent: undisclosed. The patients were asked about the source of funds for the treatment they were seeking; 91 (30.3%) said they funded the treatment themselves, 206 (68.7%) said that someone else funded the treatment, and 3 (1%) said that the funding was divided between self-payment and other sources.

The frequencies of various types of cancers are listed in Table 1. Patients were also asked of their stage of cancer with 25 (8.3%) having stage 1 cancer, 33 (11%) having stage 2, 35 (11.7%) having stage 3, 24 (8%) having stage 4, and 183 (61%) not knowing what their cancer stage was. Patients were undergoing various treatments for cancer which included radiotherapy, 29 (9.7%), chemotherapy, 85 (28.3%), cancer related surgery, 28 (9.3%), radiotherapy and chemotherapy, 38 (12.7%), chemotherapy and cancer related surgery, 34 (11.3%), radiotherapy and cancer related surgery, 9 (3%), and all three, 33 (11%). Furthermore, 34 (11.3%) patients did not know what form of treatment they were receiving and 10 (3.3%) answered with a treatment other than the options provided to them. The mean duration from the diagnosis of cancer was 18 months with SD of 17.8 months. The mean duration from initiation of treatment was 12.5 months with SD of 20.5 months. The patients were asked whether someone else had cancer in their family; 21 (7%) answered yes, single person, 11 (3.7%) answered yes, multiple persons, 263 (87.7%) said no one else in their family had cancer, and 5 (17%) said they did not know whether someone else had cancer in their family.

The patients were asked to rate or describe their pain on a pain scale of 0 to 10 using a common hospital pain scale. 79 (26.3%) were in **0**: no pain, 98 (32.7%) were in **1–3**: mild pain, 95 (31.7%) were in **4–6**: moderate pain, and 28 (9.3%) were in **7–10**: severe pain.

Out of 300 patients, 188 (62.7%) patients said they thought they were anxious and depressed and 112 (37.3%) said no they did not think they were anxious and depressed. 44 (14.7%) patients answered that they did seek treatment for their depression and anxiety, 246 (82%) answered no they did not seek treatment for depression and anxiety, and the remaining 10 (3.3%) did not answer this question. The patients were also asked whether their caretaker counseled them or not with 176 (58.7%) answering yes, 122 (40.7%) answering no, and the remaining 2 (0.7%) not answering this question. The patients were asked whether they smoked cigarettes for more than 6 months or not and 39 (13%) were found to be smokers while 238 (79.3%) were nonsmokers. 23 (7.7%) chose not to answer that question. The patients were also asked whether they took time off for physical activities: 146 (48.7%) answered yes, 153 (51%) answered no, and 1 (0.3%) did not answer the question.

Using the score of 20 on the AKUADS as a cut-off value for anxiety and depression, 154 (51.3%) patients were not anxious or depressed (AKUADS score < 19) and 146 (48.7%)

Table 2: Frequency of suicidal thoughts.

Have they thought of taking their life?	Patients not screened as anxious and depressed AKUADS score < 19	Patients screened as anxious and depressed AKUADS score > 20	Total frequency (percentage of total patients)
Never	134	106	240 (80.0%)
Sometimes	18	33	51 (17.0%)
Mostly	2	6	8 (2.7%)
Always	0	1	1 (0.3%)
Total	154	146	300

patients were anxious or depressed (AKUADS score > 20). The AKUADS included a suicidal tendency question stated as whether the patient had thought of taking their life in the previous 2 weeks; the results of this are included in Table 2.

Different factors included in the questionnaire were cross tabulated to the depression of the patient to find out which factor had a significant chi-square p value that is less than 0.05 showing its association with the anxiety and depression of the cancer patient. All these factors, the sex of the patient whether male or female, the occupation, level of income ranging from low income to high income, whether the treatment was self-funded or from other sources such as charity organizations, type of cancer, stage of cancer, treatment being sought for the cancer such as radiotherapy, chemotherapy, or cancer related surgery, duration from diagnosis of cancer, duration from treatment of cancer, whether the caretaker counseled the patient or not, the patient taking time off for physical activities, and the patient being a smoker, showed no significant association with the anxiety and depression of the patient with a p value > 0.05. The significant results of the cross tabulations are shown in Table 3.

It was also found that the type of cancer had no significant link to the number of the people who had cancer in the patient's family, with chi-square test p value of 0.890.

A multiple regression analysis was run to predict AKUADS score from whether the patient was depressed or not (AKUADS > 20), pain scale (0–10), and stage of cancer. These variables statistically significantly predict AKUADS $F(3, 296) = 186$, $p < 0.05$, and R square 0.654. All three variables added statistically significantly to the prediction with $p < 0.05$. The results of these are depicted in Table 4.

4. Discussion

The findings of anxiety and depression amongst cancer patients are comparable and consistent and reinforce the results of a recent study in Pakistan reporting prevalence rates of 52% in cancer patients and a study from Iran showing rates of 47.2% and 57% for depression and anxiety, respectively [16, 17]. Perhaps a better gauge at the level of prevalence we drew from our research would be to compare it to the 66% prevalence of anxiety and depression deduced by a research conducted using the same AKUADS in a different region of Pakistan. These results and their variance from ours draw a hypothesis that maybe regional differences account for variability in the prevalence of anxiety and depression amongst cancer patients [18].

A previously conducted research stated that there was no statistically significant difference between gender, marital status, locality, education, income, occupation, physical activity, smoking, cancer site, illness duration and mode of treatment, surgery related to cancer, and presence of depression and anxiety [18]. Our research enforces majority of these conclusions drawn by that research but at the same time conflicts with only one of the aforementioned factors. In our research, the education of the patient was found to have significance to the presence of depression and anxiety. Bjelland et al. [19] have established that low education levels are linked with anxiety and depression and that a higher level of education plays a preventive role against anxiety and depression. However, they also stated that somatic health is a strong role player for anxiety and depression; further research is needed targeting only level of education, keeping somatic health and other comorbid conditions such as cancer a constant to enhance or reinforce this variable and its significance to depression and anxiety.

Our research showed a higher frequency of breast cancer patients; this may be due to the fact that the frequency of female patients in our research was higher than that of male patients and breast cancer is the commonest cancer amongst female cancer patients [20]. This is indeed a limitation as the female to male ratio of major depressive disorder is 1.64 : 1 with women more likely to report their symptoms then men [21]. As women are more likely to report their symptoms and our research contained 62.3% females, this may have falsely raised our prevalence rates. In retrospect, the authors should have restricted the female and male ratio in order to remove this doubt.

Another interesting finding that the authors would like to draw the reader's attention to is in the second last panel of Table 3. Whether the patient thought they themselves were anxious and depressed or not which can be termed as self-screening did indeed have significant links to the patient being anxious or depressed. 118 out of the 146 anxious and depressed patients had screened themselves; this is an 80.8% self-screening rate. However, attention must be drawn to the fact that 70 had answered that they were anxious and depressed yet they were not. This draws a hypothesis that proper counseling of the patients and relieving of their thoughts that they are anxious and depressed may lower their anxiety and depression. At this point, caution must also be drawn at the 66% sensitivity of the AKUADS scale and to the fact that the abovementioned results may not be a true depiction. This limitation could not be addressed given the

TABLE 3: Cross tabulation of various significant factors to the patients' depression and anxiety with p value < 0.05.

Patient's factors cross tabulated to patient's anxiety and depression	Patients not screened as anxious and depressed AKUADS score < 19	Patients screened as anxious and depressed AKUADS score > 20	Total number of patients in that category	p value
Education				**0.011**
Uneducated	58	85 (85/13 = 59%)	143	
Primary	18	15 (15/33 = 45%)	33	
Middle	28	19 (19/47 = 40%)	47	
Secondary	19	5 (5/24 = 20%)	24	
Higher	10	8 (8/18 = 44%)	18	
Bachelors	11	10 (10/21 = 48%)	21	
Masters	9	4 (4/13 = 31%)	13	
Unknown	1	0 (0/1 = 0%)	1	
Occurrence of cancer in the family				**0.047**
Single person	14	7 (7/21 = 33%)	21	
Multiple persons	4	7 (7/11 = 64%)	11	
None	131	132 (132/263 = 50%)	263	
Unknown	5	0 (0/5 = 0%)	5	
Pain scale				**<0.001**
0, no pain	58	21 (21/79 = 27%)	79	
1–3, mild pain	56	42 (42/98 = 43%)	98	
4–6, moderate pain	30	65 (65/95 = 68%)	95	
7–10, severe pain	10	18 (18/28 = 64%)	28	
Do the patients think they themselves are anxious and depressed?				**<0.001**
Yes	70	118 (118/188 = 63%)	188	
No	84	28 (28/112 = 25%)	112	
Did they seek treatment for their anxiety and depression from any source?				**0.019**
Yes	18	26 (26/44 = 59%)	44	
No	127	119 (119/246 = 48%)	246	
Unanswered	9	1 (1/10 = 10%)	10	

TABLE 4: Multiple linear regression analysis of AKUADS scale as a dependent variable against independent variables.

Model	Unstandardized coefficients		Standardized coefficients	t	Sig.	95.0% confidence interval for B	
	B	Std. error	Beta			Lower bound	Upper bound
(Constant)	−7.766	1.498		−5.185	0.000	−10.714	−4.818
Patient depressed and anxious or not (AKUADS > 20)	15.386	0.789	0.713	19.504	0.000	13.834	16.939
Pain scale	0.777	0.146	0.193	5.328	0.000	0.490	1.065
Stage of cancer	0.590	0.269	0.076	2.192	0.029	0.060	1.119

15

Cognitive Function before and during Treatment with Selective Serotonin Reuptake Inhibitors in Patients with Depression or Obsessive-Compulsive Disorder

Mehdi Sayyah,[1] Kaveh Eslami,[2] Shabnam AlaiShehni,[3] and Leila Kouti[2]

[1]*Education Development Center, Ahvaz Jundishapur University of Medical Sciences, Ahvaz, Iran*
[2]*School of Pharmacy, Ahvaz Jundishapur University of Medical Sciences, Ahvaz 61357-15794, Iran*
[3]*Student Research Committee, Ahvaz Jundishapur University of Medical Sciences, Ahvaz, Iran*

Correspondence should be addressed to Leila Kouti; lkouti.pharmacotherapy@gmail.com

Academic Editor: Lenin Pavón

Objectives. Identification of adverse effects of selective serotonin reuptake inhibitors (SSRIs) is of great importance due to their extensive use in medicine. Some studies have reported the effects of SSRIs on cognitive functions, but the results are conflicting. This study was designed to assess the effect of these drugs on cognition of patients with depression or obsessive-compulsive disorder (OCD). *Methods.* Patients with depression or OCD, naïve to therapy, and candidates of receiving one drug from SSRI class, voluntarily, entered this study. Mini-Mental State Examination (MMSE) test was the tool to assess their cognitive functions. MMSE scores of each patient were recorded prior to taking SSRIs and at weeks 3, 5, and 8 of drug therapy. *Results.* 50 patients met our inclusion criteria, with a baseline mean MMSE score of 23.94. At 3, 5, and 8 weeks of treatment, the mean scores were 22.1, 21.4, and 20.66, respectively. With a p value of <0.0001, the gradual decline was statistically significant. *Conclusion.* The MMSE scores of our patients showed a gradual decline over the consecutive weeks after taking SSRI drugs. It seems that the use of SSRIs in patients with depression or OCD, can cause cognitive dysfunction in the acute phase of treatment.

1. Introduction

Selective serotonin reuptake inhibitors (SSRIs) are the first-line drug treatment of depression and obsessive-compulsive disorder (OCD). Monotherapy with this class is often recommended for patients primarily diagnosed with these conditions [1, 2].

Despite the potential usefulness of SSRIs, they could cause unwanted side effects such as headaches, weight gain, sexual dysfunction, changes in sleep patterns, and gastrointestinal problems [3]. Originally, SSRIs did not appear to cause cognitive impairment, but nowadays there are conflicting evidences regarding this side effect and many patients complain of memory loss during their course of therapy with SSRIs [4, 5].

The aim of this study is to assess the effect of SSRI drugs on cognitive function of patients with depression or OCD, in acute phase of therapy. In this phase, knowledge and management of side effects are very critical for the patient's compliance to therapy, since these patients might not be motivated enough to cope with adverse effects along with their psychiatric symptoms [6]. In many health problems, drug induced memory loss can be an important cause of medication nonadherence [7, 8].

Current study evaluates the patients' cognitive function, prior to taking SSRIs and throughout the acute course of their therapy.

2. Methods

This analytic-descriptive study was conducted in a psychiatric outpatient clinic from April to September 2015. It was permitted by Ahvaz Jundishapur University of Medical Sciences ethics committee. Among patients diagnosed with depression or OCD by a board certified psychiatrist, those who currently were not under any treatment for mental or psychiatric disorders and were candidates of receiving a drug from SSRI class as monotherapy were asked to participate in this study. Inclusion criteria consisted of age between 18 and 60 years, no diagnosed cognitive impairment or mental retardation, no other comorbid disorders in Axis I, the ability to write and read, no visual or auditory impairment, no history of loss of consciousness after head trauma or brain surgery, and no history of using psychoactive drugs such as antidepressants, neuroleptics, benzodiazepines, antiepileptics, or opioids within 14 days prior to the study. Individuals with memory loss complaints in daily functioning would not be included either. If the patient developed any condition in which the use of SSRIs was contraindicated or any disability which interfered with performance of cognitive tests, he/she would be excluded from the study. In addition, patients who stopped their medication for seven consecutive days or did not adhere well with their drug therapy would be excluded. All patients signed a consent form prior to the study.

Several approaches have been developed to help with the diagnosis of cognitive impairment. Some of these tests are Montreal Cognitive Assessment, DemTect, Short Test of Mental Status, Clinical Dementia Rating, and Mini-Mental State Examination (MMSE) [9–12]. Among these, MMSE test is the only valid and reliable test in Farsi; thus, we used this tool for our patients [13, 14]. Aspects of cognitive function assessed by this test include orientation, registration, attention, calculation, recent memory, and language skills. Seyedian et al. translated the Farsi version of MMSE. Its reliability based on Cronbach's Alpha is 81% and a cut-off point of 22 showed a sensitivity of 90% and specificity of 93.5% [13, 14].

The patients' demographic data (age, gender, level of education) were collected in the first visit (week 0 of therapy) and MMSE (a 30-point test) was performed at weeks 0, 3, 5, and 8 of drug therapy. Each patient's drug regimen (type of drug and dosage) remained fixed throughout this 8-week period. If for any reason the patient needed a dose reduction or increase or medication discontinuation, he/she would be excluded from the study. The response to therapy and clinical improvement of OCD/depression signs and symptoms would also be evaluated and recorded.

2.1. Statistical Analysis. The data were analyzed using repeated measures one-way ANOVA. Results with a p value of less than 0.05 were considered significant. Correlations of MMSE scores and age, sex, and level of education were analyzed by Pearson correlation test, one-way ANOVA test, and paired sample t-test, respectively.

3. Results

Fifty patients (28 women and 22 men, ages ranging from 20 to 60 years) participated in this study (50% diagnosed with depression and 50% with OCD). They all completed the study and we had no dropout patients. All of them showed signs of response to treatment of their psychiatric disorder at week 8. In order to analyze the correlation of level of education with MMSE scores, we grouped the patients into six different groups. Nine patients were in the elementary group (under 6 years of education), seven were in the middle school group (7–11 years), and 16 patients had a high school diploma. The number of patients with a bachelor, masters, or Ph.D. degree was 11, 6, and 1, respectively. The prescribed drugs for patients were paroxetine (52%), Zoloft (28%), fluoxetine (12%), and citalopram (8%).

Table 1: Results of patients' cognitive assessment prior to and during treatment with SSRs (number of patients = 50).

Weeks of treatment	Week 0	Week 3	Week 5	Week 8
Mean MMSE score	23.94	22.1	21.4	20.66
p values of comparing MMSE scores of weeks 3, 5, and 8 with baseline score	—	<0.0001	<0.0001	<0.0001
p values of comparing MMSE scores of weeks 5 and 8 with the results of week 3	—	—	<0.0001	0.0709
p values of comparing MMSE scores of week 8 with the results of week 5	—	—	—	<0.0001

The trend of decline shows faster decline by 5 weeks and a more subtle decline until week 8.

Table 1 shows the results of MMSE scores prior to treatment and at weeks 3, 5, and 8. With a p value of less than 0.0001, the patients' MMSE scores lowered significantly from their baseline.

Correlation of age and MMSE scores was also assessed and the results showed no significant relationship between them, neither prior to therapy (p value = 0.4) nor during it (p value = 0.12). MMSE scores among male and female patients had a similar decline trend, when week 8 of treatment was compared with the baseline (95% confidence interval of the difference). Level of education showed no significant correlation with decline of cognitive function (p value = 0.14).

4. Discussion

Cognitive dysfunction subsequent to SSRI therapy remains controversial and different studies have reported inconsistent results [4]. Memory loss as a side effect can be overwhelming for patients and leads to medication nonadherence [7, 8]. We used MMSE test for the evaluation of cognitive function of such patients. It is widely used and easy to perform and takes only few minutes of patient's time but it has its limitations as well. Some of these psychometric limitations of MMSE test include ceiling effect, floor effect, and poor distinguishing between mild cognitive impairment and Alzheimer's disease [15]. This test might not be the preferred tool for cognitive assessment of our patients but so far it is the only test in Farsi language that has approved validity and reliability [13, 14, 16, 17].

Due to these limitations, we evaluated the correlation of age and level of education with MMSE scores to clarify the possible influence of these factors on the subjects' cognitive function. Also, since the cut-off points of MMSE might not accurately correlate to the patient's cognitive state, we compared the mean scores before and after therapy and did not group the patients according to the cut-offs [15]. Future studies with the help of other cognitive assessment tools can help to have a more accurate identification of this problem.

Our findings show that patients taking SSRIs experienced statistically significant memory loss during 8 weeks of treatment; age and gender did not influence this result. In contrast, Levkovitz et al. and Culang-Reinlieb et al. reported that some SSRIs have improved memory function in patients with depression [17, 18]. Herrera-Guzmán and colleagues have investigated the effects of SSRIs on cognitive impairment due to depression, in a series of studies. They performed several cognition tests and evaluated the patients in remission and recovery phase. They reported a positive effect of drug therapy with SSRIs in the long term [19]. Deuschle and colleagues performed California Verbal Learning Test on 24 patients with depression and found a low rate of declarative memory loss after 35 days of treatment with SSRIs (the majority of patients had no change from baseline) but no cognitive impairment at long-term therapy (over 12 months). They concluded that the low-grade impairment is due to depressive symptoms and not a side effect [20]. Nevertheless, some evidences strongly supported our results. The study by Popovic et al. showed that over 20% of patients with depression or anxiety disorders reported memory loss after 6 months of SSRI therapy. This was considered a side effect rather than a symptom of untreated depression/anxiety [21]. Wadsworth et al. and Biringer et al. also reported the probability of memory deficit associated with SSRI use [4, 22]. Two other case reports with memory loss subsequent to fluoxetine use have been published in previous years. In one case report, memory loss was reversed when fluoxetine was changed to another SSRI [23, 24]. Although memory impairments can be due to depression itself, memory loss appears to be more likely due to SSRI therapy rather than depression symptoms. Serretti et al. showed that using SSRIs even in healthy individuals leads to cognitive impairment [25]. The memory loss caused by SSRIs has not yet been convincingly explained; however, serotonin appears to play an important role in learning and memory [26]. Serotonin transporter (SERT) expression has been found to be vital for memory development. Decreased expression of this transporter was found in Alzheimer's disease and other memory impairments and dementia [27]. Benmansour et al. showed a decrease in SERT expression within 21 days (3 weeks) following SSRI use [28]. In order to make a better understanding of this issue, Herzallah et al. studied two groups of patients with major depression (one group naïve to medication (16 patients) and one group under successful treatment with paroxetine (15 patients)) and a control group of 25 healthy volunteers, aged 18–60 years. They performed a task evaluating two different aspects of cognition. The results showed that major depression and SSRIs have different positive and negative effects on cognition. SSRIs may have a positive role in striatal function but can deteriorate hippocampus function, needed for generalization. On the other hand, patients with major depression were normal in the latter function, but slow in learning [29].

Although these findings may partly explain the cause of memory loss due to SSRIs, more studies are needed to discover the exact mechanism responsible for this outcome.

We did not evaluate the effect of disease on cognitive function and only targeted the influence of SSRIs on memory. Although all of the patients had higher baseline MMSE scores compared to short-term treatment with SSRIs, their mean score even prior to therapy was lower than normal population (MMSE = 24–26) [30].

5. Conclusions

Our data show that in patients with OCD or depression and those who are naïve to SSRI therapy, a gradual decline in their memory function can develop within the first 8 weeks of initiation of drug treatment with SSRIs. This decline did not have a relationship with the patient's age or gender, nor his/her level of education. We suggest further follow-up studies of these patients to identify the persistence of memory loss. Our results were obtained via MMSE test and regardless of the specific drug or disorder. We hope that soon other cognitive function tests would be valid and reliable for Iranian population.

Competing Interests

The authors declare no conflict of interests.

Acknowledgments

The authors thank Dr. Ramezani and her kind laboratory staff for their help and support.

References

[1] J. S. Abramowitz, "Treatment of obsessive-compulsive disorder in patients who have comorbid major depression," *Journal of Clinical Psychology*, vol. 60, no. 11, pp. 1133–1141, 2004.

[2] P. A. Marken and J. S. Munro, "Selecting a selective serotonin reuptake inhibitor: clinically important distinguishing features," *The Primary Care Companion for CNS Disorders*, vol. 2, no. 6, pp. 205–210, 2000.

[3] J. Price, V. Cole, and G. M. Goodwin, "Emotional side-effects of selective serotonin reuptake inhibitors: qualitative study," *British Journal of Psychiatry*, vol. 195, no. 3, pp. 211–217, 2009.

[4] E. Biringer, A. Rongve, and A. Lund, "A review of modern antidepressants' effects on neurocognitive function," *Current Psychiatry Reviews*, vol. 5, no. 3, pp. 164–174, 2009.

[5] R. Gallassi, R. Di Sarro, A. Morreale, and M. Amore, "Memory impairment in patients with late-onset major depression: the effect of antidepressant therapy," *Journal of Affective Disorders*, vol. 91, no. 2-3, pp. 243–250, 2006.

[6] M. H. Trivedi, E. H. Lin, and W. J. Katon, "Consensus recommendations for improving adherence, self-management, and outcomes in patients withdepression," *CNS Spectrums*, vol. 12, no. 8, supplement 13, pp. 1–27, 2007.

[7] A. M. Nye, V. B. Clinard, and C. L. Barnes, "Medication nonadherence secondary to drug-induced memory loss," *Consultant Pharmacist*, vol. 25, no. 2, pp. 117–121, 2010.

[8] C.-Y. Cheng, B. Y.-J. Lin, K.-H. Chang, K.-H. Shu, and M.-J. Wu, "Awareness of memory impairment increases the adherence to

immunosuppressants in kidney transplant recipients," *Transplantation Proceedings*, vol. 44, no. 3, pp. 746–748, 2012.

[9] R. Wojtyńska and D. Szcześniak, "DemTect®—effective to asses mci and dementia—validation study of the polish language version," *Aging and Mental Health*, vol. 20, no. 5, pp. 510–516, 2016.

[10] L. A. Cummings-Vaughn, N. N. Chavakula, T. K. Malmstrom, N. Tumosa, J. E. Morley, and D. M. Cruz-Oliver, "Veterans affairs saint louis university mental status examination compared with the montreal cognitive assessment and the short test of mental status," *Journal of the American Geriatrics Society*, vol. 62, no. 7, pp. 1341–1346, 2014.

[11] A. J. Mitchell, "A meta-analysis of the accuracy of the mini-mental state examination in the detection of dementia and mild cognitive impairment," *Journal of Psychiatric Research*, vol. 43, no. 4, pp. 411–431, 2009.

[12] C. Jacova, A. Kertesz, M. Blair, J. D. Fisk, and H. H. Feldman, "Neuropsychological testing and assessment for dementia," *Alzheimer's and Dementia*, vol. 3, no. 4, pp. 299–317, 2007.

[13] M. Seyedian, M. Falah, M. Norouzian, S. Nejat, A. Delavar, and H. Ghasemzadeh, "Validity of the Farsi version of mini-mental state examination," *Journal of Medical Council of Islamic Republic of Iran*, vol. 24, no. 4, pp. 408–414, 2008.

[14] M. Noroozian and L. Kouti, "Severity of Parkinson's disease and memory function: correlation and influencing factors," *The Journal of Nutrition Health and Aging*, vol. 17, supplement 1, pp. S594–S595, 2013.

[15] K. R. Chapman, H. Bing-Canar, M. L. Alosco et al., "Mini mental state examination and logical memory scores for entry into Alzheimer's disease trials," *Alzheimer's Research and Therapy*, vol. 8, article 9, 2016.

[16] M. F. Folstein, S. E. Folstein, and P. R. McHugh, "'Mini-mental state': a practical method for grading the cognitive state of patients for the clinician," *Journal of Psychiatric Research*, vol. 12, no. 3, pp. 189–198, 1975.

[17] Y. Levkovitz, R. Caftori, A. Avital, and G. Richter-Levin, "The SSRIs drug Fluoxetine, but not the noradrenergic tricyclic drug Desipramine, improves memory performance during acute major depression," *Brain Research Bulletin*, vol. 58, no. 4, pp. 345–350, 2002.

[18] M. E. Culang-Reinlieb, J. R. Sneed, J. G. Keilp, and S. P. Roose, "Change in cognitive functioning in depressed older adults following treatment with sertraline or nortriptyline," *International Journal of Geriatric Psychiatry*, vol. 27, no. 8, pp. 777–784, 2012.

[19] I. Herrera-Guzmán, J. E. Herrera-Abarca, E. Gudayol-Ferré et al., "Effects of selective serotonin reuptake and dual serotonergic-noradrenergic reuptake treatments on attention and executive functions in patients with major depressive disorder," *Psychiatry Research*, vol. 177, no. 3, pp. 323–329, 2010.

[20] M. Deuschle, A. Kniest, H. Niemann et al., "Impaired declarative memory in depressed patients is slow to recover: clinical experience," *Pharmacopsychiatry*, vol. 37, no. 4, pp. 147–151, 2004.

[21] D. Popovic, E. Vieta, M. Fornaro, and G. Perugi, "Cognitive tolerability following successful long term treatment of major depression and anxiety disorders with SSRi antidepressants," *Journal of Affective Disorders*, vol. 173, pp. 211–215, 2015.

[22] E. J. K. Wadsworth, S. C. Moss, S. A. Simpson, and A. P. Smith, "SSRIs and cognitive performance in a working sample," *Human Psychopharmacology*, vol. 20, no. 8, pp. 561–572, 2005.

[23] J. D. Joss, R. M. Burton, and C. A. Keller, "Memory loss in a patient treated with fluoxetine," *Annals of Pharmacotherapy*, vol. 37, no. 12, pp. 1800–1803, 2003.

[24] T. Hall, R. D. Barrera, and M. Randon, "Reversible memory loss following treatment with fluoxetine: a case study," *Behavioral Interventions*, vol. 15, no. 3, pp. 217–224, 2000.

[25] A. Serretti, R. Calati, A. Goracci, M. Di Simplicio, P. Castrogiovanni, and D. De Ronchi, "Antidepressants in healthy subjects: what are the psychotropic/psychological effects?" *European Neuropsychopharmacology*, vol. 20, no. 7, pp. 433–453, 2010.

[26] A. Meneses, "5-HT systems: emergent targets for memory formation and memory alterations," *Reviews in the Neurosciences*, vol. 24, no. 6, pp. 629–664, 2013.

[27] A. Meneses, G. Perez-Garcia, T. Ponce-Lopez, R. Tellez, and C. Castillo, "Serotonin transporter and memory," *Neuropharmacology*, vol. 61, no. 3, pp. 355–363, 2011.

[28] S. Benmansour, M. Cecchi, D. A. Morilak et al., "Effects of chronic antidepressant treatments on serotonin transporter function, density, and mRNA level," *The Journal of Neuroscience*, vol. 19, no. 23, pp. 10494–10501, 1999.

[29] M. M. Herzallah, A. A. Moustafa, J. Y. Natsheh et al., "Depression impairs learning, whereas the selective serotonin reuptake inhibitor, paroxetine, impairs generalization in patients with major depressive disorder," *Journal of Affective Disorders*, vol. 151, no. 2, pp. 484–492, 2013.

[30] V. Rashedi, M. Rezaei, and M. Gharib, "Prevalence of cognitive impairment in community-dwelling older adults," *Basic and Clinical Neuroscience*, vol. 5, no. 1, pp. 28–30, 2014.

High Magnitude of Social Anxiety Disorder in School Adolescents

Kindie Mekuria,[1] Haregwoin Mulat,[2] Habtamu Derajew,[3] Tesfa Mekonen,[4] Wubalem Fekadu,[4] Amsalu Belete,[5] Solomon Yimer,[6] Getasew Legas,[5] Melak Menberu,[7] Asmamaw Getnet,[8] and Simegnew Kibret[5]

[1] *Woldia Hospital, Woldia, Ethiopia*
[2] *Psychiatry Department, University of Gondar, Gondar, Ethiopia*
[3] *Amanuel Mental Specialized Hospital, Addis Ababa, Ethiopia*
[4] *Psychiatry Department, Bahir Dar University, Bahir Dar, Ethiopia*
[5] *College of Medicine and Health Sciences, Debre Tabor University, Debre Tabor, Ethiopia*
[6] *Psychiatry Department, Dilla University, Dilla, Ethiopia*
[7] *College of Health Sciences, Mizan-Tepi University, Mizan-Tepi, Ethiopia*
[8] *Finote Selam Hospital, Finote Selam, Ethiopia*

Correspondence should be addressed to Amsalu Belete; amsalu04@gmail.com

Academic Editor: Arif Khan

Introduction. Social phobia is the most prevalent and chronic type of anxiety disorder worldwide and it affects occupational, educational, and social affairs of the individual. Social phobia is also known for its association with depression and substance use disorder. *Objective.* The aim of this study was to assess the prevalence and associated factors of social phobia among high school students in Ethiopia. *Methods.* Cross-sectional study was conducted among 386 randomly selected students. Data were collected using pretested and self-administered questionnaire. Social phobia was assessed by using Social Phobia Inventory (SPIN). Logistic regression was used to analyze the data with 95% confidence interval and variables with p value less than 0.05 were considered as statistically significant. *Results.* From 386 study participants, 106 (27.5%) of them were positive for social phobia. Being female (AOR = 3.1; 95% CI: 1.82–5.27), current alcohol drinking (AOR = 1.75; 95% CI: 1.03–2.98), poor social support (AOR = 2.40; 95% CI: 1.17–4.92), and living with single parent (AOR = 5.72; 95% CI: 2.98–10.99) were significantly associated with social phobia. *Conclusion.* The proportion of social phobia was higher compared to previous evidences. School-based youth-friendly mental health services might be helpful to tackle this problem.

1. Introduction

DSM-V defines social phobia as marked or intense fear or anxiety of social situations in which the individual may be scrutinized by others and this situation interferes significantly with routines, occupational (academic) functioning, social activities, and relationships [1]. Though it is a debilitating psychiatric condition which is treatable, it often remains undetected and untreated. Individuals will have reduced quality of life, disturbed social interactions, poor daily functioning, and poor treatment adherence for other medical or psychiatric conditions [2–4].

The prevalence of social phobia among school adolescents varied from country to country [5]. For instance, in high-income countries, the magnitude ranges from 3.5% to 21% [6–10]. Even though there is scarcity of evidence in developing countries, the available literatures suggested that social phobia is higher, which ranges from 10.3% to 27% [11, 12].

Students with social phobia have difficulty of speaking in front of a group of people and fail or drop out of school due to fear [13]. Students' attention to academic information may be distracted by an excessive focus on their anxiety [14]. The ability to monitor and modify communication with colleagues and teachers may be vague by fear of negative evaluation and when participating in a seminar, socially anxious students judge their competence poorly [15], which leads to academic underachievement [16].

Evidences showed that social phobia was associated with 20% of cases of adult depression [17] and 17% of cases of alcohol and drug dependence [18]. Low socioeconomic status, being unmarried, unemployment, low level of education, and poor social support were identified as a risk factor for social phobia [19]. Society's attitude towards shyness and avoidance as a measure of politeness is also an important factor associated with students' ability to build social interaction [20].

Despite the high worldwide burden of social phobia, limited evidence is available, particularly in developing countries. This study tried to assess factors (social support and wealth index) which were previously not well addressed. The purpose of this study was to assess the prevalence and associated factors of social phobia among school adolescents in Ethiopia.

2. Methods and Materials

School-based cross-sectional study was conducted at Woldia preparatory school. A total of 1516 regular students in 11th and 12th grades in 2015 academic year were enrolled. The school is located in Woldia town, Amhara regional state, 521 kilometers away from Addis Ababa. There is one general hospital and two health centers in the town. All students who were enrolled at Woldia preparatory school in 2014/2015 academic year were included in the study. The sample size for this study was calculated by using single population proportion formula and 424 students were recruited randomly.

Social phobia was the dependent variable and the predictors were sociodemographic variables (sex, age, religion, wealth index, relationship status, current living condition, and origin of residence), clinical factors (past history of psychiatric illness, past history of chronic medical illness, and family history of mental illness), substance use (cigarette, Khat chewing, and alcohol use), and social support. Khat (also called Catha edulis) is a local green leaf plant which had amphetamine-like stimulating effect after chewing due to the active ingredient called cathinone.

Data was collected by pretested self-administered questionnaire and the data collection was facilitated by trained data collectors and supervisors. Social phobia was assessed by using the Social Phobia Inventory (SPIN) which is a 17-item self-rating scale developed by Connor and his colleagues [21]. It shows the symptom domains of social phobia (fear, avoidance, and physiological arousal) and appears to have reliable and valid psychometric properties of screening social phobia in adolescents and other populations [21–24]. It was rated from 0 (not at all) to 4 (extremely) and the sum score ranged from 0 to 68 [21]. A student with a score of 20 and above on SPIN was considered as having social phobia.

Oslo 3-item social support scale was used to determine the level of social support. The total score ranged from 3 to 14 and was categorized into poor support (3–8 scores), moderate support (9–11 scores), and strong support (12–14 scores) [25]. Students' substance use was explained by verbal report of consuming of any alcohol, cigarette, and Khat in the previous three months. Presence and absence of major illness (medical or psychiatric) were also based on report of the participants.

Data were entered by Epi-Info 3.5.3 analyzed by SPSS-21 for Windows version. Factors association was done by running bivariate and multivariable logistic regression. Strength of the association was presented by odds ratio with 95% confidence interval and p value <0.05 was used to identify statistically significant variables.

Ethical clearance was obtained from Institutional Review Board (IRB) of University of Gondar and Amanuel Mental Specialized Hospital. Confidentiality of the participants was maintained by anonymous questionnaire. Participants were fully informed about the purposes of the study prior to the data collection and informed consent (assent) was obtained.

3. Results

3.1. Sociodemographic Characteristics of Respondents. A total of 424 students were included in the study, of which 386 completed the questionnaires with the response rate of 91.03%. 233 (60.4%) of the participants were males and 346 (89.6%) were between the ages of 16 and 19 years. The mean age of the respondents was 18.15 ± 1.24 years (Table 1).

3.2. Clinical and Psychosocial Characteristics of the Respondents. Fourteen (3.6%) students had past psychiatric history and 18 (4.7%) of them had family history of mental illness. About one-third of the participants reported that they did not use any mass media (Table 2).

3.3. Prevalence and Associated Factors of Social Phobia. The overall prevalence of social phobia was 27.5%. In multivariable logistic regression analysis, sex, current use of alcohol, social support, and students raised by single parent were significantly associated with social phobia (Table 3).

4. Discussion

The overall prevalence of social phobia was 27.5% and it was consistent with the study done elsewhere which was 26.5% [26]. However, the present study was higher than the study conducted in Nigeria, 9.4% [27], Swedish high school students, 21% [9], Iran, 6.2% [6], Delhi, 10.3% [11], and china, 14.1% [12], as well as the national comorbidity survey in USA, 9% [8]. It was also higher compared to a comparative study among high school students in Egypt, Saudi Arabia, and United Arab Emirates where the percentages were 13%, 9.8%, and 7.8%, respectively [28]. This discrepancy might be due to sociocultural differences between those countries and Ethiopia. For instance, in Ethiopia, shyness as a measure of politeness has been emphasized as a dominant cultural norm [23]. The other possible reason for this difference might be the tool used in the current study, which is nondiagnostic self-administered tool, and this might overestimate the prevalence of social phobia among students [21, 22, 24].

In this study, social phobia had significant association with sex, current alcohol drinking, social support, and students' living status. In female students, the odds of having social phobia were 3 times more than those of male students

Table 1: Sociodemographic distribution of the respondents (n = 386).

Sociodemographic variables	Frequency	Percent
Sex		
Male	233	60.4
Female	153	39.6
Age		
16–19	346	89.6
>19	40	10.4
Relationship status		
Single	350	90.4
Married	36	9.6
Ethnicity		
Amhara	377	97.7
Others	9	2.3
Religion		
Orthodox	304	78.8
Muslim	71	18.4
Protestant	11	2.8
Place of upbringing		
Urban	236	61.1
Rural	150	38.9
Lived with		
Both parents	267	69.2
Single parent	61	15.8
Relative/alone	58	15
Semester result (performance)		
Low	236	61.2
Medium	119	30.8
High	31	8.0
Wealth index		
Lowest (poor)	35	9.1
Second	151	39.1
Medium	46	11.9
Fourth	109	28.2
Highest (rich)	45	11.7

Note. Ethnicity (others) = Tigre, 6, and Afar, 3; performance (average academic score): low ≤ 70, medium = 70–84.99, and high ≥ 85.

Table 2: Clinical conditions of respondents (n = 386).

Variables	Frequency (n)	Percent (%)
Past psychiatric history		
Yes	14	3.6
No	372	96.4
Family psychiatric history		
Yes	18	4.7
No	368	95.3
Previous medical illness		
Yes	37	9.6
No	349	90.4
Social support		
Poor	65	16.8
Moderate	159	41.2
Strong	162	42.0
Using mass media		
Yes	274	71.0
No	112	29.0
Using social media		
Yes	220	57.0
No	166	43.0
Alcohol		
Yes	135	34.9
No	251	65.1

and this was supported by the study done in Poland [26] and Baghdad [29]. The community's perception towards shyness and politeness as a measure of predominant cultural norm might have high influence on female students' social phobia status [23]. Students who were current alcohol users were about 2 times more likely to have social phobia as compared with their counterparts. Students with social phobia tend to engage themselves into heavy drinking and alcohol use problems [30]. This finding was consistent with previous studies conducted in Nigeria [27] and USA [10]. The students probably use alcohol as self-medication for their fear and for their concerns of negative evaluation by others [18].

Social support was another important factor associated with social phobia. Students with poor and moderate social support had about two times more odds to have social phobia as compared with students who had strong social support and the finding was in line with the study done in Iran [7]. Social connectedness is important for the development of confidence and positive social skills. In addition to poor social support, students who lived with single parent were more than 5 times more likely to have social phobia as compared with students who lived or were raised by both parents. This finding was supported by study done in Saudi Arabia [31]. However, students' media usage, wealth index, past psychiatric history, and family history of mental illness did not show any association with social phobia in this study.

5. Limitations of the Study

The first limitation of the study may be the fact that we used nondiagnostic self-rating screening tool; the prevalence of social phobia might be overestimated. The other limitation is that we did not measure substance use by a standard tool and consuming a substance for one day and daily use of a substance were reported as substance use, and the association may not be real if standard tool has been used. The last limitation is our design which cannot show the direction of association.

TABLE 3: Factors associated with social phobia.

Variables	Social phobia Yes	Social phobia No	COR (95% CI)	AOR (95% CI)
Sex				
Male	41	192	1.00	1.00
Female	65	88	3.44 (2.17, 5.51)	**3.10 (1.82, 5.27)***
Age (years)				
16–19	102	244	3.76 (1.31, 10.84)	2.02 (.66, 6.26)
>19	4	36	1.00	1.00
Alcohol (current use)				
Yes	47	88	1.74 (1.10, 2.75)	**1.75 (1.03, 2.98)****
No	59	192	1.00	1.00
Psychiatric history				
Yes	7	7	2.76 (.94, 8.06)	3.15 (.97, 10.29)
No	99	273	1.00	1.00
Social support				
Poor	25	40	2.75 (1.45, 5.20)	**2.40 (1.17, 4.92)****
Moderate	51	108	2.08 (1.24, 3.49)	**2.14 (1.20, 3.80)****
Strong	30	132	1.00	1.00
Living status (students were raised by or lived with)				
Both parents	53	214	1.00	1.00
Single parent	38	23	6.67 (3.67, 12.14)	**5.72 (2.98, 10.99)***
Alone/others	15	43	1.41 (.73, 2.73)	1.86 (.91, 3.82)

Note: $^{*}p < 0.001$ and $^{**}p < 0.05$.

6. Conclusion

The proportion of social phobia was higher which was predicted by female gender, current alcohol use, living with single parent, and having poor social support. School and community intervention on students' alcohol use is important. Moreover, school-based youth-friendly mental health service might be very helpful to tackle this problem and to help students with this problem. Further longitudinal and interventional studies are needed to describe the longitudinal nature of the illness and to identify risk factors.

Competing Interests

All authors declared that they have no competing interests regarding the publication of this paper.

Authors' Contributions

Kindie Mekuria conceived the original idea and participated in proposal development, data collection, analysis of the data, and preparation of the manuscript and in all stages of the project. Haregwoin Mulat, Habtamu Derajew, Tesfa Mekonen, Wubalem Fekadu, Amsalu Belete, Solomon Yimer, Getasew Legas, Melak Menberu, Asmamaw Getnet, and Simegnew Kibret participated in proposal development, design, analysis, interpretation of data, and preparation of the manuscript and in all stages of the research.

Acknowledgments

The authors would like to thank the study participants for their unlimited cooperation and Amanuel Mental Specialized Hospital for the financial support. They also would like to thank Woldia preparatory school staff members for their support during the data collection.

References

[1] American Psychiatric Association, "Anxiety disorders," in *Diagnostic and Statistical Manual of Mental Disorders*, American Psychiatric Association, Washington, DC, USA, 5th edition, 2013.

[2] S. M. Valente, "Social phobia," *Journal of the American Psychiatric Nurses Association*, vol. 8, no. 3, pp. 67–75, 2002.

[3] D. Villiers, *Perfectionism and social anxiety among college students [Counseling psychology Disssertations]*, Northeastern University, Boston, Mass, USA, 2009.

[4] M. H. Pollack, "Social anxiety disorder (social phobia): effective treatment," *Journal of Clinical Psychiatry*, vol. 62, no. 12, pp. 24–29, 2006.

[5] H. Wittchen, "Social phobia: new perspectives on neglected mental disorder," *Psychiatric Networks*, vol. 3, no. 1, pp. 5–8, 2007.

[6] N. Dodangi, N. Habibi Ashtiani, and B. Valadbeigi, "Prevalence of DSM-IV TR psychiatric disorders in children and adolescents of Paveh, a Western City of Iran," *Iranian Red Crescent Medical Journal*, vol. 16, no. 7, Article ID e16743, 2014.

[7] S. Talepasand and M. Nokani, "Social phobia symptoms: prevalence and sociodemographic correlates," *Archives of Iranian Medicine*, vol. 13, no. 6, pp. 522–527, 2010.

[8] M. Burstein, J.-P. He, G. Kattan, A. M. Albano, S. Avenevoli, and K. R. Merikangas, "Social phobia and subtypes in the National Comorbidity Survey-Adolescent Supplement: prevalence, correlates, and comorbidity," *Journal of the American Academy of Child and Adolescent Psychiatry*, vol. 50, no. 9, pp. 870–880, 2011.

[9] L. Wetterberg, "Social anxiety in 17-year-olds in Stockholm, Sweden—a questionnaire survey," *South African Psychiatry Review*, vol. 7, no. 2, pp. 30–32, 2004.

[10] F. R. Schneier, T. E. Foose, D. S. Hasin et al., "Social anxiety disorder and alcohol use disorder co-morbidity in the national epidemiologic survey on alcohol and related conditions," *Psychological Medicine*, vol. 40, no. 6, pp. 977–988, 2010.

[11] V. Chhabra, M. Bhatia, S. Gupta, P. Kumar, and S. Srivastava, "Prevalence of Social Phobia in school-going adolescents in an urban area," *Delhi Psychiatry Journal*, vol. 12, no. 1, pp. 18–25, 2009.

[12] Y. Jin, L. He, Y. Kang et al., "Prevalence and risk factors of anxiety status among students aged 13–26 years," *International Journal of Clinical and Experimental Medicine*, vol. 7, no. 11, pp. 4420–4426, 2014.

[13] M. Van Ameringen, C. Mancini, and P. Farvolden, "The impact of anxiety disorders on educational achievement," *Journal of Anxiety Disorders*, vol. 17, no. 5, pp. 561–571, 2003.

[14] Z. Acarturk, *Epidemiology and Psychological Treatment of Social Phobia*, Department of Clinical Psychology of The Vrije University in Amsterdam, Amsterdam, The Netherlands, 2009.

[15] M. M. Ohayon and A. F. Schatzberg, "Social phobia and depression: prevalence and comorbidity," *Journal of Psychosomatic Research*, vol. 68, no. 3, pp. 235–243, 2010.

[16] B. K. Gültekin and I. F. Dereboy, "The prevalence of social phobia, and its impact on quality of life, academic achievement, and identity formation in university students," *Turkish Journal Of Psychiatry*, vol. 22, no. 3, pp. 150–158, 2011.

[17] J. D. Buckner, N. B. Schmidt, A. R. Lang, J. W. Small, R. C. Schlauch, and P. M. Lewinsohn, "Specificity of social anxiety disorder as a risk factor for alcohol and cannabis dependence," *Journal of Psychiatric Research*, vol. 42, no. 3, pp. 230–239, 2008.

[18] B. O. Olatunji, J. M. Cisler, and D. F. Tolin, "Quality of life in the anxiety disorders: a meta-analytic review," *Clinical Psychology Review*, vol. 27, no. 5, pp. 572–581, 2007.

[19] H.-U. Wittchen and L. Fehm, "Epidemiology, patterns of comorbidity, and associated disabilities of social phobia," *Psychiatric Clinics of North America*, vol. 24, no. 4, pp. 617–641, 2001.

[20] K.-I. Okano, "Shame and social phobia: a transcultural viewpoint," *Bulletin of the Menninger Clinic*, vol. 58, no. 3, pp. 323–338, 1994.

[21] K. M. Connor, J. R. T. Davidson, L. Erik Churchill, A. Sherwood, E. Foa, and R. H. Weisler, "Psychometric properties of the social phobia inventory (SPIN). New self- rating scale," *British Journal of Psychiatry*, vol. 176, no. 4, pp. 379–386, 2000.

[22] M. M. Antony, M. J. Coons, R. E. McCabe, A. Ashbaugh, and R. P. Swinson, "Psychometric properties of the social phobia inventory: further evaluation," *Behaviour Research and Therapy*, vol. 44, no. 8, pp. 1177–1185, 2006.

[23] S. D. Messing and J. S. Prince, "Health practices in Ethiopian pre-urban communities," *Journal of Health and Human Behavior*, vol. 7, no. 4, pp. 272–276, 1966.

[24] K. Ranta, R. Kaltiala-Heino, P. Rantanen, M. T. Tuomisto, and M. Marttunen, "Screening social phobia in adolescents from general population: the validity of the Social Phobia Inventory (SPIN) against a clinical interview," *European Psychiatry*, vol. 22, no. 4, pp. 244–251, 2007.

[25] H. Bøen, "Characteristics of senior centre users—and the impact of a group programme on social support and late-life depression," *Norsk Epidemiologi*, vol. 22, no. 2, pp. 261–269, 2012.

[26] J. Bracik, K. Krysta, and A. Zaczek, "Impact of family and school environment on the development of social anxiety disorder: a questionnaire study," *Psychiatria Danubina*, vol. 24, no. 1, pp. 125–127, 2012.

[27] F. R. Schneier, T. E. Foose, D. S. Hasin et al., "Social anxiety disorder and alcohol use disorder co-morbidity in the National Epidemiologic Survey on Alcohol and Related Conditions," *Psychological Medicine*, vol. 40, no. 6, pp. 977–988, 2010.

[28] H. M. Azab, U. A. Mussttafa, and M. A. El-Khouli, "Social phobia among secondary school students: a comparative study between Egypt, Saudi Arabia and the United Arab Emirates," *The Egyptian Journal of Psychiatry*, vol. 26, no. 1, 2007.

[29] B. F. Hummadi and A. K. AlObaidi, "Social phobia among secondary school students in Baghdad/Iraq," *Journal of the Canadian Academy of Child and Adolescent Psychiatry*, vol. 23, no. 1, pp. 70–71, 2014.

[30] R. M. Crum and L. A. Pratt, "Risk of heavy drinking and alcohol use disorders in social phobia: a prospective analysis," *American Journal of Psychiatry*, vol. 158, no. 10, pp. 1693–1700, 2001.

[31] M. Ali and S. A. Al-Qahtani, "Prevalence and risk factors of social phobia among secondary school male students in Khamis Mushayt," *Medical Journal Cairo University*, vol. 80, no. 1, pp. 871–876, 2012.

17

Comparison of Sexual Experience and Behavior between Bipolar Outpatients and Outpatients without Mood Disorders

Jennifer Downey,[1] Richard C. Friedman,[2] Elizabeth Haase,[3] David Goldenberg,[4] Robinette Bell,[5] and Sidney Edsall[6]

[1] *Department of Psychiatry, New York State Psychiatric Institute and Columbia University College of Physicians and Surgeons, New York, NY 10032, USA*
[2] *Department of Psychiatry, Weill Cornell Medical School, New York, NY 10021, USA*
[3] *Department of Psychiatry, Carson Tahoe Health System, Carson City, NV 89701, USA*
[4] *Department of Psychiatry, Weill Cornell Medical College, New York, NY 10021, USA*
[5] *Department of Psychiatry, University of Colorado School of Medicine, Aurora, CO 80045, USA*
[6] *Behavioral Health and Recovery Services, San Mateo County Psychiatric Department, San Mateo, CA 94403, USA*

Correspondence should be addressed to Jennifer Downey; jidl@cumc.columbia.edu

Academic Editor: Umberto Albert

Sexual behavior over the past year of 32 outpatients with Bipolar disorder is compared to that of 44 Comparison patients that had never had an episode of affective illness. Subjects were outpatients treated with drugs and psychotherapy in routine office practice. Differences in sexual behavior between the two groups as a whole were minimal, but meaningful differences emerged when subgroups were compared. Compared to control men, Bipolar men had had more partners in the last year and were more likely to have had sex without condoms. Compared to Bipolar females, Bipolar males had more sex partners, had more sex with strangers, and were more likely to have engaged in homosexual behavior. Even so, some patients in the Comparison group also had engaged in risky sexual behavior. They had failed to use condoms and had had sex with strangers and prostitutes during the previous year.

1. Introduction

This paper discusses a study of sexuality in Bipolar outpatients treated in private practice in comparison to outpatients without affective disorder or schizophrenia.

The evidence that sexuality is often increased in adults with Bipolar disorder during hypomanic or manic episodes includes controlled and uncontrolled studies and clinical case reports [1]. The DSM-IV-TR description of mania listed hypersexuality in criteria B #6 and #7 as "increased goal driven behavior…sexually" and/or "excess involvement in pleasurable activities that have a high potential for painful consequences: for example, sexual indiscretions" [2]. The DSM-5 [3] had not been published at the time this study was carried out but continues to list hypersexuality as a frequently occurring feature of bipolar mania and hypomania.

The study we discuss below was designed to assess a dimension of sexuality not included in most research to date. We were interested in sexuality as part of the person's temperamental trait behavior, rather than simply being influenced by affective state. We sought to assess whether sexuality was different among individuals with Bipolar disorder even when they are well treated and stable compared with those without affective disorder. As part of the preparation for the study, our group reviewed the literature on sexuality in Bipolar disorder, which we now discuss.

Controlled Studies of Sexuality in Patients with Bipolar Disorder. We found 10 English-language controlled studies of sexuality in patients with Bipolar disorder. These were conducted in different subcultures over a time-span of over 45 years during which diagnostic criteria and clinical treatment changed dramatically. Most studies asked only a few questions about sex, and there was no uniformity across studies of the questions asked or instruments used to acquire information. Medication status of patients was sometimes not reported and the phase of illness studied ranged from mania to depression. Some studies found aspects of sexuality to be increased in Bipolar patients but some were negative.

Positive Studies. Clayton et al. [4] found increased sexuality in manic compared to depressed patients. Jamison et al. [5] found increased sexuality in manic or hypomanic patients compared to major depressive controls. Additionally, 40 percent of the Bipolar I and II patients in this study reported elevated sexuality as an enduring interepisodic trait. Raja and Azzoni [6] found that Bipolar patients were more likely to be having stable sexual relations, to be married, and to have more frequent intercourse than schizophrenic patients at hospital admission. Dell'Osso et al. [7] reported that increased interest in sex and frequent change of sexual partners were more common among patients with Bipolar disorder compared with patients with unipolar depression and normal controls. Mazza et al. [8] found that Bipolar I patients placed more value on sex, had more interest in sex, and desired and engaged in intercourse more frequently than Bipolar II or Comparison patients.

Negative Studies. Beigel et al. [9] reported higher lifetime incidence of periods of celibacy in Bipolar than unipolar patients. Spalt [10] reported that Bipolar patients were less sexually active than unipolar patients, or patients with affective disorders secondary to primary psychiatric or medical illness or nonaffective disorder patients. Casper et al. [11] studied depressed Bipolar patients and reported more loss of interest in sex among them compared to normal controls. Raboch [12] found that Bipolar inpatients in states of both mania and depression did not differ from gynecology patient controls in sexual knowledge and attitude, function, or developmental history. Additionally, Frank et al. [13] compared couples in which one partner was Bipolar to nonpsychiatrically disordered control couples and found no difference in satisfaction between them.

Uncontrolled Studies of Sexuality in Patients with Bipolar Disorder. The uncontrolled studies include Allison and Wilson [14] who studied sexual behavior in manic or hypomanic patients. In their group, of 13 women, seven had markedly increased sexual display and provocative or seductive behavior. The investigators did not comment on provocative or seductive behavior in the 12 men in the study. However, 7/12 men and 10/12 women experienced a marked increase in libido in an elevated mood state. Similarly, Winokur et al. [15] found that 65 percent of manic episodes were characterized by increased sexuality, evenly divided between those in committed and noncommitted relationships. Carlson and Goodwin [16] studied 20 unmedicated manic patients admitted for four months for an observational study of a complete episode and found hypersexuality in 80 percent, although no specific sexual behavior is described. Loudon et al. [17], however, found sexual preoccupation in only 25 percent of 16 manic inpatients who started medication by the third day of admission.

In a retrospective chart review study of 1,000 Bipolar II patients, Akiskal [18] found that 40 percent of cyclothymic patients had "episodic or unexplained promiscuity or extramarital affairs" and that Bipolar II patients manifested diverse types of sexual excess including sexual infidelity, overt bisexuality, and sexual activity many times per day.

Of the uncontrolled studies, Jamison et al.'s study [5] uniquely addressed aspects of sexuality in Bipolar individuals who were in the euthymic state, conceptualized sexuality in terms of the whole person, highlighted sex differences between men and women in sexual experience, and directed attention to state versus trait sexual phenomena.

Recognizing the value of this approach, we were prompted to investigate diverse aspects of sexuality in relatively stable Bipolar individuals. We also wished to study a group of Bipolar patients underreported in the literature—those treated in routine office practice.

We compared a Bipolar patient group to other psychiatric patients with no affective disorder seen in a private practice setting, with the goal of increasing knowledge about their sexual behavior. We expected Bipolar patients to have more sexual thoughts and behaviors than other patients treated by private practitioners, even when Bipolar patients were euthymic and on medication.

2. Study Methods

2.1. Method of Recruiting Subjects. One purpose in carrying out this investigation was to utilize a patient population different from that usually reported in scientific studies. Psychiatrists in private practice often obtain valuable information that is not routinely published. We collected such information by systematically querying each psychiatrist in our group about the characteristics of patients that he/she knew well, having treated them for months and even years. The data collected would therefore supplement that usually reported in studies of more conventional design. Participating psychiatrists were all psychodynamically trained and provided both psychotherapy and psychotropic medication to the patients studied. They knew the patients in depth. This was an advantage since subjects may be reticent to report sexual information in questionnaire studies or to impart such information to researchers with whom they have no relationship. Since data were coded and only reported in aggregate, no individual patient could be identified. All study procedures were approved by the New York State Psychiatric Institute Institutional Review Board. Participants gave written informed consent.

Patients ($N = 76$) were psychiatric outpatients of the study psychiatrists, all members of the Human Sexuality Committee of the Group for the Advancement of Psychiatry

(GAP), an affiliate organization of the American Psychiatric Association (APA). These patients had presented for treatment with diverse symptoms and complaints. No patient was aware that his or her psychiatrist was a member of a study group on sexual behavior or Bipolar disorder. The patients that each psychiatrist reported on therefore were those that happened to be part of his or her routine office practice (total number of psychiatrists = 7: M = 3 and F = 4).

Psychiatrists had practices in the Far West (1), Rocky Mountain states (1), and Northeastern United States (5). All Bipolar patients and 59 percent of Comparison patients were taking at least one psychotropic medication (see below for details).

2.2. Inclusion Criteria. In order to be reported on, patients had to be 18 years of age or older, to have attended at least four appointments in the 12 months before the study, and to have been seen during the last five business days before the study data collection period. Each psychiatrist reported on *every* patient that met inclusion criteria for Bipolar disorder or Comparison group as described below. This means that subject recruitment was *consecutive* for the period of time studied. Patients whose symptoms were in remission were included so long as they were still in treatment.

Psychiatrists filled out a questionnaire for each patient, based on what they knew about him or her (see below). Although they did not further query any patient in order to answer the questions, they consulted patients' charts as needed. We felt it would be intrusive for psychiatrists to suddenly inquire about specific aspects of their sexual behavior.

2.3. Method of Information Collection. The study questionnaire, titled *Sexual History Form*, was created by the GAP Committee on Human Sexuality and may be obtained from the senior author (Jennifer Downey at jidl@cumc.columbia.edu). The questionnaire consisted of demographic (Q1–10), psychiatric (Q11–31), and sexual history questions (Q32–72) and took 30–45 minutes to fill out for each patient. Sexual history questions fell into the following categories, all for the last year: Current Sexual History (Q32–35), Nature of Partners (Q36–42), Frequency of Sexual Behaviors (Q43–54), Sexual Risk-taking (Q55–58), STD status (Q59-60), Sexual Orientation Identity and Gender Identity (Q61–64), Hormonal Status for Female Patients (Q65), and Special Circumstances Affecting Sexuality (Q66–69). The last section asked about presence of probable Bipolar disorder in the patient's sexual partner and family of origin (Q70-71) and clarification of any answer (Q73). These last 3 questions did not specify a period of time.

All DSM IV-TR diagnoses were listed for each patient [2]. The Global Assessment of Functioning Scale (GAF) [19] was used to assess average overall psychological function for the past year. A second GAF score was assigned to assess the lowest level of functioning during a one-week period in the last year. Episodes of affective illness in the last year were assessed as were psychotropic medications. Questions concerning lifetime psychiatric illness included age of onset at first illness and number of psychiatric hospitalizations. Diagnosis of Bipolar disorder in the patient's family was also assessed. The remainder of the psychiatric items concerned the nature and severity of the worst episode of mania or hypomania the patient had ever had.

2.4. Method of Data Management and Analysis. IBM SPSS was used for data analysis. In preliminary analyses we examined the distribution, means, and standard deviations of the demographic and other continuous measures, as well as the distributions of categorical measures. All but three continuous measures were found to be normally distributed (see below). There was a series of questions regarding specific sexual practices (Q43–51) for which "Don't know" was the most common response. These data are not presented.

Seven questions (Q36–42) address the "Nature of Partners In The Past Year," ranging from primary partners to strangers to paid phone/internet sex. The affirmative answers to these questions were summed and considered a partner risk measure. Items Q55, 57, and 58 (substance use, sex with strangers, and anal/vaginal intercourse without condoms with nonmonogamous partners) were also summed as a risk-taking measure.

Continuous measures were compared across the two patients groups using the t-test statistic. If Levene's test indicated unequal variances (Age in years @ onset 1st Psychiatric Illness, Duration of Current Treatment (months), and Hypomanic/Manic Symptoms), we report the separate variance estimates for the t-test and significance level. For the categorical measures, many of which exhibited small cell frequencies, we used Fisher's Exact Test (FET) throughout. All tests were two-tailed and the alpha for significance was set at $p < 0.050$.

3. Results

3.1. Subject Characteristics. Psychiatric diagnoses are presented first since diagnosis (plus the treatment characteristics noted above) was the criterion by which patients were selected.

3.2. Psychiatric Diagnosis of the Subjects. The Bipolar group consisted of individuals diagnosed with a primary diagnosis of one of the Bipolar disorders according to DSM-IV-R criteria. Total N was 32. Of these individuals $N = 10$ were receiving treatment for Bipolar I disorder, $N = 20$ were receiving treatment for Bipolar II disorder, and $N = 2$ bore the diagnosis Bipolar disorder NOS.

The Comparison group of psychiatric outpatients consisted of individuals who never had an episode of affective illness, either Bipolar disorder or unipolar depression. Total N was 44. Of these, the majority were receiving treatment for the primary diagnosis of an Anxiety Disorder ($N = 24$) or Adjustment Disorder with Anxiety ($N = 7$). Other primary diagnoses were lightly represented: Attention Deficit Disorder $N = 1$, Substance Abuse Disorder $N = 1$, Posttraumatic Stress Disorder $N = 1$, Pain Disorder $N = 1$, and Delusional Disorder $N = 1$. Only one patient had no Axis I diagnosis; that person was being treated for Personality Disorder NOS.

A number of patients in each study group had more than one Axis I disorder. The Bipolar group of $N = 32$ had nine patients with a second Axis I disorder and three patients with a third Axis I disorder. Of the 44 patients in the Comparison group, nine had a second Axis I diagnosis, four had a third Axis I disorder, and two had a fourth Axis I disorder.

Some patients also had Axis II disorders. Of the Bipolar group, 8 patients had received diagnosis of diverse Axis II conditions.

Of the Comparison group, 16 patients had received Axis II diagnoses.

Subject demographics are listed in Table 1. All subjects were at least 18 years of age and were English-speaking. The Bipolar group consisted of 16 males and 16 females. The Comparison group consisted of 26 males and 18 females. Average age for both groups was early 40s. Slightly over than 50% of each subject group had a live-in partner.

Educational level for the patients in both groups was high. The majority of patients were college graduates or had a graduate degree. The Comparison group had a higher occupational status according to the Hollingshead Scale [20] and also a higher calculated Hollingshead Socio-Economic Status, which uses both educational and occupational levels.

Additional Psychiatric Information about the Subjects. As noted above, the Global Assessment of Functioning (GAF) scale was used to measure overall psychological functioning. This psychometrically valid and reliable instrument yields scores varying from 1 to 90 with 90 being good functioning in all areas and 1 being functioning so severely impaired that the patient's life is threatened. Although the average GAF for the last year did not differ significantly for the Bipolar and Comparison groups, the Bipolar group differed from the Comparison patient group on a variety of other parameters, demonstrating more impairment in the Bipolar individuals. For instance, GAF score for the lowest-functioning week over the last year was significantly lower for the Bipolar group. Statistical tests and significance levels for all parameters discussed in this section may be found in Table 2.

Other measures of psychopathology also showed the Bipolar group to be generally more severely affected. Thus, mean age of onset of psychiatric symptoms in the Bipolar group was 15.7 years while the Comparison group had onset at 21.3 years. Duration of present treatment differed by more than 30 months on average with Bipolar individuals having been in treatment longer. This was not a significant difference due to large standard deviations. More patients with Bipolar disorder were reported to be taking psychiatric medications than Comparison patients (100% versus 59%; Yates $\chi^2 = 14.92$, $p < 0.001$) and to have experienced psychiatric hospitalization (FET: $p < 0.0001$).

Patients with Bipolar disorder were more likely to be taking antipsychotics and mood stabilizers. There were no differences between the patient groups in percentages taking SSRI antidepressants, other antidepressants, anxiolytics, stimulants, sleep medications, and phosphodiesterase inhibitors.

Psychiatrists were asked whether the patient's parents, siblings, or children had definite or probable Bipolar disorder. Over 50% of B patients but only 4.5% of C patients had at least one Bipolar relative related by blood, a highly significant difference.

3.3. Sexual History: Whole-Group Comparison. The Bipolar patients were more likely to report sexual experiences that may be described as nontraditional than were the Comparison subjects. Although this might not have been revealed in comparisons of individual items because of relatively small numbers of subjects, the *sum* of affirmative items (Q36–42) regarding nature of sexual partners was statistically significant ($p = 0.05$ by t-test).

In other ways the groups were similar in sexual behavior over the previous year. For instance, patients in both groups reported an average of "moderate enjoyment" of their sex lives (Q32). Mean frequency of sexual activity with another person over the last year was "sometimes" defined as two to eight times/month (Q34).

Questions 43–51 and 53-54 concerned the frequency of certain sexual behaviors/experiences—masturbation, orgasm, sexual desire, and novelty-seeking sexual behavior—for the year and for the most intense week of the year. For these items there were too much missing data for analyses to be meaningful, and the results are not presented here. This was a result of research design. The practicing clinicians did not always have readily available details about the patients' most intense week in the last year. If the questionnaire had been administered to patients directly, this information would have been straightforward to elicit.

Another type of question assessed diagnosis of a DSM-IV Sexual Dysfunction or Paraphilia (Q52). Very few patients in either group had received one of these diagnoses (Bipolar $N = 4$ versus Comparison $N = 3$), and there was no difference between the groups.

Sexual risk-taking was assessed with six questions (Q55–60). We found no significant differences between Bipolar and Comparison groups for any of the items. The first four were frequency with which they engaged in recreational substance use with sex (Q55), substances they used if any (Q56), sex with strangers (Q57), and receptive anal or vaginal intercourse without a condom with partners of unknown HIV status (Q58). One person in each group was known to have positive HIV status, not a significant difference. There was also no difference in how many patients had been diagnosed with any other STD in the last year.

Sexual orientation identity and gender identity were assessed with four questions (Q61–64). Sexual *activity* in the last year was rated by Kinsey scale where 0 is exclusively heterosexual activity and 6 is exclusively homosexual activity [21]. The two groups did not differ in sexual behavior Kinsey scores. The majority were reported to have engaged exclusively in heterosexual activity in the last year.

A separate question asked was for the psychiatrists to rate patients' sexual *fantasy* over the last year using the same Kinsey scale. Again, the two patient groups did not differ. Thirty-four percent of Bipolar patients and 45.5 percent of Comparison patients were reported to have had only heterosexual fantasies. Thirteen percent of Bipolar and 16 percent of Comparison patients ($N = 7$) had had only

Table 1: Demographics: statistics are the t-test for continuous measures and the Fisher's Exact Test for categorical measures.

Demographic measures	Bipolar disorders $N = 32$		Comparison $N = 44$		Group effect		
	Mean	sd	Mean	sd	t	df	p
Age	41.6	(13.2)	42.2	(14.3)	0.17	74	0.869
Hollingshead occupation code	7.4	(1.5)	8.1	(1.2)	2.10	67	0.040*
Hollingshead SES	55.6	(8.6)	60.1	(6.7)	2.43	67	0.018*
	%	N	%	N	Fisher's Exact p		
Gender (female % and N)	50	(16)	41	(18)	0.488		
Education level							
High school/GED	3	(1)	0	(0)			
Some college	9	(3)	7	(3)			
B.A./B.S. degree	47	(15)	36	(16)			
Graduate school	41	(13)	57	(25)	0.364		
Current employment status							
Retired	9	(3)	5	(2)	0.644		
Homemaker	16	(5)	2	(1)	0.077[t]		
Unemployed	16	(5)	9	(4)	0.480		
Student	9	(3)	14	(6)	0.726		
Race							
White	88	(28)	96	(42)			
Black	3	(1)	0	(0)			
Asian/PAC. ISL	3	(5)	5	(2)			
Other	6	(2)	0	(0)	0.215		
Hispanic	13	(4)	2	(1)	0.233		
Marital status							
Married	38	(12)	48	(21)			
Single	53	(17)	46	(20)			
Widowed/divorced	9	(3)	7	(3)	0.678		
Live-in partner	56	(18)	57	(25)	1.0		
Religion							
Protestant	28	(9)	30	(13)			
Catholic	19	(6)	14	(6)			
Jewish	28	(9)	43	(19)			
Other	6	(2)	7	(3)			
None	19	(6)	7	(3)	0.460		

*indicates significance and [t]trend.

homosexual fantasies. A fairly substantial number of patients experienced both heterosexual and homosexual fantasies at times—Bipolar 22 percent versus Comparison 9 percent. Psychiatrists reported not enough information to rate Kinsey fantasy level for about 30 percent of the patients.

Sexual orientation self-identity in the last year (Q63) was assessed separately from the Kinsey scale questions and was found not to differ significantly between groups. Most patients were reported by their psychiatrists as having a "straight" identity. The percentages with a self-identity as gay or lesbian were about the same for both groups—16 percent versus 18 percent (Bipolar versus Comparison). One Bipolar person was reported to have a bisexual identity and one to have "other." Gender identity in the last year was exclusively male or female in all cases except for the one Bipolar patient reported as transgender, male to female.

Special circumstances which might affect sexual functioning were assessed with five questions (65–69). Hormonal

Table 2: Psychiatric history and clinical characteristics.

Clinical measures	Bipolar disorders $N = 32$		Comparison $N = 44$		Group effect		
	Mean	sd	Mean	sd	t	df	p
Age in years @ onset 1st Psychiatric Illness	15.7	(5.8)	21.3	(11.7)	2.72	$67^{\dagger}$	0.008^{*}
Global assessment of function							
Average over the past year	68.7	(8.7)	72.6	(9.6)	1.80	74	0.076^{t}
Lowest week during last year	54.8	(13.7)	64.9	(12.1)	3.41	74	0.001^{*}
Duration of current treatment (months)	77.3	(107.1)	46.6	(67.4)	1.43	$74^{\dagger}$	0.158
Hypomanic and manic symptoms	5.7	(1.5)	0.14	(.50)	18.16	$46^{\dagger}$	$<0.001^{*}$
	%	N	%	N		Fisher's Exact p	
Episodes during the past year							
Manic episodes	6	(2)	0	(0)		0.174	
Depressive episodes	31	(10)	0	(0)		0.000^{*}	
Mixed episodes	50	(16)	0	(0)		0.000^{*}	
Hospitalizations (lifetime)							
0	63	(20)	98	(41)			
1	19	(6)	2	(1)			
2 or more	19	(6)	0	(0)		$<0.0001^{*}$	
Current psychotropic medications							
Antipsychotics	44	(14)	7	(3)		$<0.001^{*}$	
SSRI	47	(14)	32	(14)		0.228	
Antidepressants	23	(7)	14	(6)		0.363	
Mood stabilizers	72	(23)	0	(0)		$<0.001^{*}$	
Anxiolytics	48	(15)	41	(18)		0.638	
Stimulants	13	(4)	9	(4)		0.711	
Sleep	19	(6)	18	(8)		1.00	
Phosphodiesterase	10	(3)	2	(1)		0.300	
Other	16	(5)	5	(2)		0.129	
Number of medications prescribed Mean (sd) t-test	2.8	(1.3)	1.3	(1.3)	5.20	74	$<0.001^{*}$
Bipolar family history First degree relatives	53	(16)	5	(2)		$<0.001^{*}$	
Significant medical illness (during the last year)	34	(11)	30	(13)		0.803	

*indicates significance, †separate variance est., and ^{t}trend.

status was assessed for women in both groups and did not differ. Most women were premenopausal.

When the entire Bipolar and Comparison groups, both males and females, were compared, there were no special circumstances over the last year reported that might affect sexual functioning (falling in love, pregnancy, ill health, and sexual abuse) that differed between groups.

A question (70) assessed bipolarity in the patients' relationships. One patient in each group was reported to definitely or probably have a Bipolar partner.

3.4. Sexual History: Analysis of Subgroups. Additional information sometimes emerges when statistical tests are performed on subgroups of interest. We looked at two additional comparisons for sexual history items. We compared patients by gender so that Bipolar males were compared to Comparison males, and Bipolar females were compared to Comparison females. We also compared Bipolar males with Bipolar females and Comparison males with Comparison females.

For the comparison between men, more Bipolar patients were reported to have had additional lovers ($p = 0.047$

by Fisher's Exact Test, question 37). There was a trend for Bipolar men to have engaged in receptive intercourse without condoms in the last year relative to the Comparison group ($p = 0.061$ by Fisher's Exact Test; question 58). Comparisons of Bipolar with Comparison female patients showed no differences.

Finally, meaningful differences in the sexual behavior of the men versus women in each group were examined. Bipolar males differed from Bipolar females on two items only. More Bipolar males than females had had two or more sexual partners *n* the last year—males 67% versus females 19% ($p = 0.034$ by Fisher's Exact Test, question 33). More Bipolar males than females had engaged in homosexual activity in the last year ($p = 0.018$ by Fisher's Exact Test, question 61). The easiest way to understand this since the Kinsey score was on a spectrum, not binary, is to consider that 67% of Bipolar males but 94% of Bipolar females had engaged only in heterosexual activity in the last year. There was also a trend for Bipolar males to be more likely than females to have a homosexual identity ($p = 0.083$ by Fisher's Exact Test, question 63).

Comparisons of Comparison males to females showed that Comparison males had engaged in more frequent sexual activity during the most intense week over the last year ($p = 0.049$ by Fisher's Exact Test, question 35). More males than females were reported to have engaged in the last year in homosexual activity ($p = 0.012$ by Fisher's Exact Test, question 61) and in homosexual fantasy ($p = 0.037$ by Fisher's Exact Test, question 62). When sexual orientation self-identity was reported, eight Comparison men but no women reported a gay/lesbian identity ($p = 0.014$ by Fisher's Exact Test, question 63).

3.5. Sexual History: Risk-Taking among All Patients. Another way to look at the sexual risk-taking among this outpatient sample is to note how many people had engaged in these behaviors *ever* in the last year. Despite the fact that these patients had an average age in their 40s, were married, were highly educated, and were in an ongoing therapy with a psychiatrist, a surprising number of patients in both groups had engaged in risky sexual behavior over the last year. For instance, the number of patients who engaged in recreational drug use and sex at the same time (Q55) was over 40 percent for each group—Bipolar = 46.9 percent ($N = 15$) versus Comparison = 43.2 percent ($N = 19$). The percentage of patients who had engaged in sex with a stranger over the last year (Q57) was over 20 percent—Bipolar = 26 percent ($N = 8$) versus Comparison = 21 percent ($N = 8$). The number of patients who had engaged in receptive anal and/or vaginal intercourse without condoms with partners not known to be monogamous was 19% ($N = 6$) for the Bipolar individuals and 8% ($N = 3$) for the Comparison patients.

4. Discussion

This naturalistic comparison study of the sexual experience and activity of Bipolar patients had unique design features. We hoped that our research approach might demonstrate the usefulness of systematic investigation of patients not usually studied and of harvesting data that is often not shared in the professional community. In our view the method we devised could be adapted for the investigation of diverse types of patients other than those with Bipolar disorders and of diverse forms of behavior other than sexuality.

To the best of our knowledge there has been no previous controlled study of sexuality in Bipolar outpatients carried out in such depth and detail. Indeed studies of sexuality in psychiatric patients have been scant. In the case of our own study, the patients received both psychotherapy and medication from their doctors and had largely durable and positive working alliances with them. This is clear from the mean duration of treatment with the psychiatrists—almost four years for the Comparison group and over six years for the Bipolar group. To learn about sexuality, the topic of the questionnaire discussed in this report, the trusting therapeutic relationships that our respondents had with these patients proved crucial.

4.1. The Questionnaire. The psychiatrists who provided study data were all members of the Human Sexuality Committee of Group for the Advancement of Psychiatry. Based on an inclusive review of the literature in Bipolar disorder, the group had constructed a questionnaire, which they subsequently filled out about the patients. Respondents had no hypothesis about which specific aspects of sexual experience and activity would be increased.

4.2. Validity of Diagnosis of Bipolar Disorder. A crucial question about the sample reported on in this study is whether their psychiatric disorders were accurately diagnosed. The usual indices of diagnostic accuracy are reliability and validity. No effort was made to establish diagnostic reliability in our study using commonly accepted methods. Psychiatrist respondents were experienced in using the DSM-IV-TR and carefully reviewed diagnostic criteria for each subject selected.

A number of measures indicate that the diagnosis of the Bipolar patients was *valid*. For example, among Bipolar patients, more than half had first-degree relatives with definite or probable Bipolar disorder. Only two of the Comparison individuals had a first-degree relative with Bipolar disorder. The difference between the groups was highly significant. This is meaningful because of Bipolar disorder clusters among family members [1].

Given that individuals with schizophrenia and mood disorders were excluded from the Comparison group, it is not surprising that the Bipolar group had had more episodes of severe illness during the course of their lives than the Comparison group. Over one third of Bipolar patients ($N = 12$) had been psychiatrically hospitalized in contrast to only one Comparison patient.

Although the current GAF score between the two groups was similar, those in the Bipolar group were likely to have been more impaired during the worst week of the past year (mean score of 54.7 or "serious impairment"), while mean score for Comparison patients during the worst week was 64.8 or "moderate symptoms."

Mean age of onset of psychiatric symptoms in the Bipolar group was significantly younger than in the Comparison group (15.6 versus 21.2 years), compatible with the overall trend of psychopathology in the sample.

In keeping with what has been reported elsewhere [22], Bipolar patients in this study took more than twice as many psychiatric medications as Comparison patients and were much more likely to be prescribed antipsychotic medicines. Perhaps more importantly as another indicator of validity, 71.9 percent of Bipolar patients were prescribed thymoleptic mood stabilizers, in contrast with no Comparison patients. This finding is both statistically and clinically significant.

The fact that the Bipolar patients and Comparison patients were well-balanced with respect to use of SSRI medications is particularly important given the well-known sexual inhibitory effects of these drugs [23]. Of course, the SSRI drugs might also induce hypomanic or manic states in predisposed patients, but that did not appear to occur in the population we report.

It is important for diagnostic accuracy that no patient with unipolar depression was included in the Comparison group. In two surveys of members of the National Depressive and Mani-Depressive Association (DMDA), most Bipolar patients were initially misdiagnosed [24, 25]. The most common incorrect diagnosis was unipolar depression. This may have been because the first affective episode of Bipolar disorder is often depression.

4.3. Comorbidity. Of the Bipolar patients in our study, nine (28 percent) had more than one Axis I disorder and eight (25 percent) had Axis II disorders. The Comparison patients were similar in this regard, with nine (20 percent) having more than one Axis I disorder and 16 (36 percent) having an Axis II disorder.

These findings are consistent with what might be expected from published studies showing significant comorbidity in Bipolar individuals [26, 27]. Comorbidity prevalence with Bipolar disorder varies substantially across studies and may be as high as 75 percent [1].

4.4. Sexuality Findings. Our group of psychiatrists had discussed the literature on Bipolar disorder and sexuality among ourselves and expected our Bipolar patients to be more sexual in some sense than controls. This expectation was only modestly supported by the pooled data, however.

The group of Bipolar patients had more sexual partners than did Comparison patients and increased frequency of risky sexual behavior.

In addition, Bipolar males had more sexual partners during the past year than Bipolar females and more Bipolar males had engaged in homosexual activity. Bipolar males were also somewhat more likely than Comparison males to have engaged in receptive intercourse without condoms during the past year.

4.5. Similarity in Sexual Behavior between Bipolar and Comparison Patients. We note that risky sexual behavior has been reported to be increased in psychiatric patients generally [28, 29]. Some studies have reported risky behavior among psychiatric patients to be increased in females compared to males [30]. A recent study reported high-risk behavior to be increased during hypomanic states, generally [31].

Our investigation did find certain risky behaviors to be increased particularly in the males who were Bipolar, but these findings were modest. One reason for this may well have been that every patient with Bipolar disorder in this investigation was medicated. Although the patients were treated with psychotherapy as well, we conjecture that the dimensions of sexual motivation that were embedded in hypomanic or manic affective tendencies were diminished by pharmacological agents. It might also be that the particular patients reported on in this sample, although clearly Bipolar, were not drawn from the most extreme segment of the illness spectrum, particularly at the time of data collection.

An astonishing and clinically important finding of this investigation was the frequency of unconventional and risky sexual behavior among the Comparison patients. This included sex with strangers, failure to use condoms with partners not known to be monogamous, and sex with prostitutes. This indicates the importance of the sexual history in the general assessment of psychiatric patients, not just Bipolar individuals.

Additional Points

Our study had a number of limitations. The convenience group of patients that the therapists reported on was not representative of Bipolar patients generally. The fact that the patients were largely Caucasian and well-educated and able to pay for private treatment limited generalizability of our findings. The greatest strengths of our design were also its greatest weaknesses. Therapists with preconceived beliefs about the questions being studied provided data about their patients. Obviously this might have biased responses. Interestingly, however, the therapists' expectations were frequently not confirmed. The advantage of using the therapeutic alliance to study sexuality seemed apparent to our group. In order to protect the alliance, closed ended questions about sexuality were not part of our design. Therapists provided only historical data that they had acquired from their psychotherapeutic work with patients. We judged that the truthfulness of patient responses, however, outweighed the limitations of this approach. Due to practical limitations we focused only on the past year. The sexual history of patients prior to that was not explored. The longer arc of sexuality in Bipolar individuals over the life cycle remains for others to explore. Another limitation is that we did not use independent standardized measures to document possible temperamental differences between the two groups and to provide additional mood data. This would be straightforward to do in a future study. Similarly, it would be straightforward to administer the questionnaire directly to Bipolar and control individuals in a research clinic, thus obtaining much more information about the fine details of sexual variations (e.g., during the most sexual week) over the time period studied. In conclusion we stress that our study might be thought of at two levels: as research about sexuality in Bipolar patients and as a feasibility study of carrying out research in a private practice setting.

Disclosure

All authors were members of the Human Sexuality Committee of the Group for the Advancement of Psychiatry (GAP). Jennifer Downey and Richard C. Friedman were Chairpersons of the committee.

Competing Interests

The authors declare that they have no competing interests.

Acknowledgments

The authors acknowledge the insight, advice, and steadfast help of Drs. Jean Endicott, Ph.D., and Ray Goetz, Ph.D., of the Clinical Phenomenology Division, New York State Psychiatric Institute/Department of Psychiatry of Columbia University College of Physician & Surgeons, and of Dr. Stewart Adelson, M.D., of the Departments of Psychiatry, Columbia University and Weill-Cornell School of Medicine. The authors appreciate the careful reading of an earlier version of the paper by the Publications Committee of the Group for the Advancement of Psychiatry.

References

[1] F. K. Goodwin and K. R. Jamieson, "Sexual Behavior in Manic Depressive Illness. Chapter 2: clinical description and diagnosis, Chapter 10: personality, personality disorders, and interpersonal functioning," in *Manic Depressive Illness*, Oxford University Press, New York, NY, USA, 2007.

[2] American Psychiatric Association, *Diagnostic and Statistical Manual of Mental Disorders (DSM-4 TR)*, American Psychiatric Association, Washington, DC, USA, 4th edition, 2000.

[3] American Psychiatric Association, *Diagnostic and Statistical Manual of Mental Disorders (DSM-5)*, American Psychiatric Association, Washington, DC, USA, 2013.

[4] P. J. Clayton, F. N. Pitts Jr., and G. Winokur, "Affective disorder. IV: Mania," *Comprehensive Psychiatry*, vol. 6, no. 5, pp. 313–322, 1965.

[5] K. R. Jamison, R. H. Gerner, C. Hammen, and C. Padesky, "Clouds and silver linings: positive experiences associated with primary affective disorders," *American Journal of Psychiatry*, vol. 137, no. 2, pp. 198–202, 1980.

[6] M. Raja and A. Azzoni, "Sexual behavior and sexual problems among patients with severe chronic psychoses," *European Psychiatry*, vol. 18, no. 2, pp. 70–76, 2003.

[7] L. Dell'Osso, C. Carmassi, M. Carlini et al., "Sexual dysfunctions and suicidality in patients with bipolar disorder and unipolar depression," *Journal of Sexual Medicine*, vol. 6, no. 11, pp. 3063–3070, 2009.

[8] M. Mazza, D. Harnic, V. Catalano et al., "Sexual behavior in women with bipolar disorder," *Journal of Affective Disorders*, vol. 131, no. 1–3, pp. 364–367, 2011.

[9] A. Beigel, D. L. Murphy, and W. E. Bunney, "The manic-state rating scale: scale concentration, reliability and validity," *Archives of General Psychiatry*, vol. 25, no. 3, pp. 256–262, 1971.

[10] L. Spalt, "Sexual behavior and affective disorders," *Disease of the Nervous System*, vol. 36, no. 12, pp. 644–647, 1975.

[11] R. C. Casper, D. E. Redmond Jr., M. M. Katz, C. B. Schaffer, J. M. Davis, and S. H. Koslow, "Somatic symptoms in primary affective disorder," *Archives of General Psychiatry*, vol. 42, no. 11, pp. 1098–1104, 1985.

[12] J. Raboch, "Sexual development and life of psychiatric female patients," *Archives of Sexual Behavior*, vol. 15, no. 4, pp. 341–353, 1986.

[13] E. Frank, S. D. Targum, E. S. Gershon et al., "A comparison of nonpatient and bipolar patient-well spouse couples," *American Journal of Psychiatry*, vol. 138, no. 6, pp. 764–768, 1981.

[14] J. B. Allison and W. P. Wilson, "Sexual behavior of manic patients: a preliminary report," *Southern Medical Journal*, vol. 53, no. 7, pp. 870–874, 1960.

[15] G. Winokur, P. J. Clayton, and T. Reich, *Manic Depressive Illness*, C. V. Mosby, St. Louis, Mo, USA, 1969.

[16] G. A. Carlson and F. K. Goodwin, "The stages of mania: a longitudinal analysis of the manic episode," *Archives of General Psychiatry*, vol. 28, no. 2, pp. 221–228, 1973.

[17] J. B. Loudon, I. M. Blackburn, and C. M. Ashworth, "A study of the symptomatology and course of manic illness using a new scale," *Psychological Medicine*, vol. 7, no. 4, pp. 723–729, 1977.

[18] H. S. Akiskal, "Searching for behavioral indicators of bipolar II in patients presenting with major depressive episodes: the 'red sign,' the 'rule of three' and other biographic signs of temperamental extravagance, activation and hypomania," *Journal of Affective Disorders*, vol. 84, no. 2-3, pp. 279–290, 2005.

[19] J. Endicott, R. L. Spitzer, J. L. Fleiss, and J. Cohen, "The global assessment scale. A procedure for measuring overall severity of psychiatric disturbance," *Archives of General Psychiatry*, vol. 33, no. 6, pp. 766–771, 1976.

[20] A. B. Hollingshead, *Four Factor Index of Social Status*, Unpublished Manuscript, Yale University, New Haven, Conn, USA, 1975.

[21] A. C. Kinsey, W. Pomoroy, and C. Martin, *Sexual Behavior in the Human Female*, WB Saunders, Philadelphia, Pa, USA, 1953.

[22] R. J. Baldessarini, L. Leahy, S. Arcona, D. Gause, W. Zhang, and J. Hennen, "Patterns of psychotropic drug prescription for U.S. patients with diagnoses of bipolar disorders," *Psychiatric Services*, vol. 58, no. 1, pp. 85–91, 2007.

[23] G. Corona, V. Ricca, E. Bandini et al., "Selective serotonin reuptake inhibitor-induced sexual dysfunction," *Journal of Sexual Medicine*, vol. 6, no. 5, pp. 1259–1269, 2009.

[24] J. D. Lish, S. Dime-Meenan, P. C. Whybrow, R. A. Price, and R. M. A. Hirschfeld, "The National Depressive and Manic-depressive Association (DMDA) survey of bipolar members," *Journal of Affective Disorders*, vol. 31, no. 4, pp. 281–294, 1994.

[25] R. M. A. Hirschfeld, L. Lewis, and L. A. Vornik, "Perceptions and impact of bipolar disorder: how far have we really come? Results of the National Depressive and Manic-Depressive Association 2000 Survey of individuals with bipolar disorder," *Journal of Clinical Psychiatry*, vol. 64, no. 2, pp. 161–174, 2003.

[26] E. L. George, D. J. Miklowitz, J. A. Richards, T. L. Simoneau, and D. O. Taylor, "The comorbidity of bipolar disorder and axis II personality disorders: prevalence and clinical correlates," *Bipolar Disorders*, vol. 5, no. 2, pp. 115–122, 2003.

[27] A. Altindag, M. Yanik, and M. Nebioglu, "The comorbidity of anxiety disorders in bipolar I patients: prevalence and clinical correlates," *Israel Journal of Psychiatry and Related Sciences*, vol. 43, no. 1, pp. 10–15, 2006.

[28] M. P. Carey, K. B. Carey, S. A. Maisto, K. E. E. Schroder, P. A. Vanable, and C. M. Gordon, "HIV risk behavior among

psychiatric outpatients: association with psychiatric disorder, substance use disorder, and gender," *Journal of Nervous and Mental Disease*, vol. 192, no. 4, pp. 289–296, 2004.

[29] L. L. Otto-Salaj and L. Y. Stevenson, "Influence of psychiatric diagnoses and symptoms on HIV risk behavior in adults with serious mental illness," *The AIDS Reader*, vol. 11, no. 4, pp. 197–204, 2001.

[30] K. McKinnon, F. Cournos, and R. Herman, "A lifetime alcohol or other drug use disorder and specific psychiatric symptoms predict sexual risk for HIV infection among people with severe mental illness," *AIDS and Behavior*, vol. 5, no. 3, pp. 233–240, 2001.

[31] K. Fletcher, G. Parker, A. Paterson, and H. Synnott, "High-risk behaviour in hypomanic states," *Journal of Affective Disorders*, vol. 150, no. 1, pp. 50–56, 2013.

Prevalence of Antipsychotic Polypharmacy and Associated Factors among Outpatients with Schizophrenia Attending Amanuel Mental Specialized Hospital, Addis Ababa, Ethiopia

Siranesh Tesfaye,[1] Nigussie Debencho,[2] Teresa Kisi,[3] and Minale Tareke[4]

[1]*Department of Psychiatry, Felege Hiwot Referral Hospital, Bahir Dar, Ethiopia*
[2]*Department of Pharmacology, Amanuel Mental Specialized Hospital, Addis Ababa, Ethiopia*
[3]*Department of Epidemiology and Biostatistics, Institute of Public Health, College of Medicine and Health Science, University of Gondar, Gondar, Ethiopia*
[4]*Bahir Dar University, College of Medicine and Health Science, Bahir Dar, Ethiopia*

Correspondence should be addressed to Siranesh Tesfaye; siratesfaye@yahoo.com

Academic Editor: Umberto Albert

Background. Despite recommendations by guidelines to avoid combinations of antipsychotics unless after multiple trials of antipsychotic monotherapy, it is quite a common practice to use combinations. This practice leads to unnecessary expenses and exposes the patient to severe drug adverse effects. *Methods.* An institution based cross-sectional study was conducted from April to May 2014. Systematic random sampling technique was used to select 423 study subjects. Logistic regression analysis was conducted to identify associated factors of antipsychotic polypharmacy among schizophrenia outpatients. *Result.* The overall prevalence of antipsychotic polypharmacy was found to be 28.2%. Extra pyramidal side effects (AOR = 2.80; 95% CI: 1.38, 5.71), repeated psychiatric hospitalization (AOR = 2.83; 95% CI: 1.45, 5.50), history of substance use (AOR = 2.82; 95% CI: 1.36, 5.88), longer duration of treatment (AOR = 2.10; 95% CI: 1.14, 3.87), and drug nonadherence (AOR = 1.84; 95% CI: 1.14, 2.98) were found to be significantly associated with antipsychotic polypharmacy. *Conclusion.* Prevalence of antipsychotic polypharmacy was found to be high among the current study participants. Individuals who had extra pyramidal side effects, admission, substance use, duration of treatment, and drug nonadherence were associated with antipsychotic polypharmacy.

1. Introduction

Schizophrenia is a severe mental illness with a serious impact on the lives of patients and their families. Treatment with antipsychotic drugs has been the main part of treatment and management of psychotic patients globally [1]. These patients exhibit marked interindividual variability in their response to antipsychotics and some of them have poor response to several antipsychotics or even no response at all. Therefore, common strategy in management of these difficult to treat patients is combination of antipsychotic agents [2].

Antipsychotic polypharmacy (APP) is the use of two or more antipsychotic drugs at a time for a given patient. Study in USA reported a prevalence of 27.5% antipsychotic combination which is similar to that in South Africa (28.6%) and the study done in six East Asian countries and territories (China, Hong Kong, Japan, Korea, Singapore, and Taiwan) revealed that the prevalence of antipsychotic polypharmacy was 45.7% [3, 4], while a Nigerian study reported a 92% prevalence polypharmacy [5]. These discrepancies in prevalence of antipsychotic combination across studies may be accounted for by differences in the definition of antipsychotic combination and also availability and type of medical insurance for schizophrenia patients as well as clinical experience and knowledge of psychopharmacology by medical practitioners [6].

Despite recommendations by guidelines to avoid combinations of antipsychotics unless after multiple trials of antipsychotic monotherapy, it is quite a common practice to use combinations [7]. In addition to this, patients who need antipsychotic doses more than the maximum recommended are often prescribed two antipsychotics [3].

When more than one antipsychotic drug is prescribed at a time, it is difficult to identify the antipsychotic agent which reduced the psychotic symptoms and the other which is responsible for the adverse effects. The frequently reported reason for antipsychotic polypharmacy is that if one agent does not achieve the desired therapeutic outcome for controlling positive and/or negative symptoms, another medication within the same class can be added to address the uncontrolled symptoms. But this practice on the contrary leads to unnecessary expenses and exposes the patient to severe drug adverse effects.

Therefore, long term use of antipsychotic polypharmacy is recommended only as a last resort after having exhausted monotherapy alternatives [2, 8]. In this study, frequency of antipsychotic combinations in Amanuel Mental Specialized Hospital was examined. Furthermore, factors associated with antipsychotic combination were investigated.

2. Methods

A cross-sectional study design was conducted at Amanuel Mental Specialized Hospital (AMSH) in Addis Ababa from April to May, 2014. AMSH is one of the oldest hospitals established in 1937 and located in western part of Addis Ababa, the capital city of Ethiopia. The hospital is playing its pivotal role as a training institute for psychiatric professionals so as to expand psychiatry service to the primary health care system of the country. There were about 51,204 schizophrenia patients who had regular follow-up in a year period at outpatient department; and on average 4,267 schizophrenia patients had monthly follow-up. The study population was schizophrenia outpatients who were on regular treatment and who had follow-up during the study period at AMSH. Patients aged 18 years and above and who had one or more previous visits were involved in the study. Patients with medical or neurological illnesses, who had no insight, and who were unable to communicate were excluded from the study.

2.1. Sample Size and Sampling Procedures. The sample size was calculated using the formula [$n = ((z\alpha/2)2p(1 - p))/d2$] for estimating a single population proportion at 95% confidence interval (CI) ($Z\alpha/2 = 1.96$) and 5% margin of error. Due to absence of data in the country, proportion of population who took polypharmacy antipsychotic among schizophrenia patients was assumed to be 50%, and by adding 10% contingency for nonresponse rate, a total of 423 study populations were involved.

The total number of schizophrenia patients who visit the hospital over the previous 6 months was taken from records and the average number per month calculated and it was found to be 4267. Systematic random sampling technique was used to select the study subjects. The sampling fraction is 4267/423 = 10. Hence, patient was selected every ten intervals. The first individual was selected by lottery method among the first ten patients who visited the hospital.

2.2. Data Collection and Quality Control. The data was collected using a pretested structured questionnaire developed in English and translated to Amharic and then to English by expertise and senior psychiatrist to ensure its consistency. The questionnaire was pretested on 5% of the sample size at St. Paul's Hospital one week before data collections. Both chart review and interview aided questionnaire were used to collect information from the study participants. Data was collected by three trained diploma psychiatry nurses and one supervisor (B.S. nurse) for a period of one month. Face-to-face interview was employed using local Amharic language.

Data regarding type of antipsychotics, duration of treatment, admission frequency, and duration of illness was filled from patient record. Drug nonadherence was assessed using the eight-item version of self-reporting questionnaire of Morisky medication adherence rating scale (MMARS); it is validated and is used as a tool in certain African countries including South Africa, Nigeria, and Kenya. The cut point of 3 and above is used to define nonadherence [9, 10] and the extra pyramidal side effects (EPS) were assessed using Simpson-Angus Scale (SAS); it is a 10-item rating scale that has been used widely for assessment of Neuroleptic Induced Parkinsonism (NIP) in both clinical practice and research settings. It consists of one item measuring gait (hypokinesia), six items measuring rigidity, and three items measuring glabella tap, tremor, and salivation, respectively. The cut-off value for screening NIP is 0.65 or more [11]. The use of two or more antipsychotic drugs at a time/simultaneously for a given patient for at least 30 days was taken as antipsychotic polypharmacy.

Two-day training was given to orient data collectors and supervisor on the questionnaire to be used, the purpose of the study, and how to approach respondents and obtain consent. The data collectors were supervised daily and the filled questionnaires were checked for completeness and consistency by supervisor and principal investigator.

2.3. Data Management and Analysis. Data was cleaned, edited, and entered using Epi info version 3.5 statistical software and then exported to SPSS version 20 for further analysis. Description of the collected data was done using frequency, percentages, means, and standard deviations. Logistic regression was performed to assess the association between binary outcomes and different explanatory variables. Bivariate analysis was first conducted for each potentially explanatory risk factor. Variables that satisfied p value <0.2 were selected for further analysis using multivariate logistic regression analysis in order to control confounding effects. The strength of association was interpreted using odds ratio (OR) and confidence interval (CI). p value <0.05 was considered statistically significant in this study.

2.4. Ethical Consideration. Ethical clearance was obtained from University of Gondar and AMSH. Informed consent was obtained from each respondent. They were given the right to refuse to take part in the study as well as to withdraw at any time during the interview process. Confidentiality was maintained throughout the study.

Table 1: Distribution of sociodemographic characteristics of schizophrenia outpatients attending AMSH, June 2014.

Variable		Frequency	Percentage (%)
Sex	Male	287	69.7
	Female	125	30.3
Age	≤25	71	17.2
	26–35	163	39.6
	≥36	178	43.2
Marital status	Single	270	65.5
	Married	80	19.4
	Divorced	32	7.8
	Widowed	6	1.5
Residence	Urban	280	68.0
	Rural	132	32.0
Religion	Orthodox	231	65.5
	Muslim	80	19.4
	Protestant	51	12.4
	Others	4	2.7
Ethnicity	Amhara	148	35.9
	Oromo	112	27.2
	Gurage	93	22.4
	Tigre	21	5.1
	Others	38	9.2
Educational status	Uneducated	49	11.9
	1–8 grades	126	30.6
	9–12 grades	157	38.1
	Diploma and above	80	19.4
Occupation	Employed	68	16.5
	Private business	70	17.0
	Daily laborer	37	9.0
	Jobless	196	47.6
	Student	20	4.9
	Housewife	21	5.1
Monthly income (ETB)	<750 birr	302	73.3
	750–1199 birr	47	11.4
	≥1200 birr	63	15.3

3. Results

3.1. Sociodemographic Characteristics and Other Related Factors. A total of 412 patients of schizophrenia were included in the study with a response rate of 97.4%. The mean age of the participants was 35.28 (±10.35 years), with age range of 18–85. The majority (69.7%) of participants were males, Orthodox Christians (65.5%), never married (65.5%), and from urban area (68.0%) and earn less than 750 birr monthly income (73.3%) (Table 1).

3.2. Clinical and Patient Related Factors. Among the participants, the duration of illness and duration of treatment above ten years were 38.6% and 28.9%, respectively. On the other hand, 13.6% of the participants had two or more previous psychiatric admissions, had good adherence (59.0%) to their antipsychotic treatment, and had extra pyramidal side effect (10.4%) (Table 2).

Table 2: Distribution of clinical and patient related factors among schizophrenia patients at AMSH, Addis Ababa, Ethiopia, June 2014 ($n = 412$).

Variable name		Frequency	Percent
Duration of illness	<5 years	143	34.7
	5–10 years	110	26.7
	>10 years	159	38.6
Antipsychotic polytherapy	Yes	116	28.2
	No	296	71.8
Duration of treatment	<5 years	198	48.1
	5–10 years	95	23.1
	>10 years	119	28.9
Type of antipsychotics	*FGA	250	60.7
	*SGA	46	11.2
	FGA + FGA	96	23.3
	FGA + SGA	19	4.6
	FGA + FGA + SGA	1	0.2
Number of admissions	None	290	70.4
	One	66	16.0
	≥two	56	13.6
EPS	Yes	43	10.4
	No	369	89.6
Drug adherence	Yes	243	59.0
	No	169	41.0
Substance use (alcohol, Khat, and tobacco)	No	250	60.7
	Yes	162	39.3

*FGA: first generation antipsychotics. *SGA: second generation antipsychotics.

3.3. Factors Associated with Antipsychotic Polypharmacy. The overall prevalence of any antipsychotic polypharmacy was 28.2%; of these 27.9% were on two antipsychotics; that is, 23.3% were on FGA + FGA and 4.6% were on FGA + SGA (Table 2).

Bivariate logistic regression analyses were done for the relationship of sociodemographic variables, patient related variables, and treatment or medication related variables with antipsychotic polypharmacy. The result of bivariate analysis revealed that sex, ethnicity, place of residence, marital status, occupational status, duration of illness, duration of treatment, number of psychiatric hospitalization days, history of active substance use, extra pyramidal side effect, and drug adherence were found to be significantly associated with antipsychotic polypharmacy. However, by multivariate logistic regression only duration of treatment, number of hospitalization days, history of active substance use, extra pyramidal side effect, and drug nonadherence were found to be statistically significant. Accordingly, patients who were on treatment for more than ten years were found to be about two times

TABLE 3: Factors associated with antipsychotic polypharmacy among schizophrenia outpatients under follow-up at AMSH Addis Ababa, Ethiopia, June 2014 ($n = 412$).

Variables		Polypharmacy (%) Yes	No	COR, 95% CI	AOR, 95% CI
Sex	Male	92	195	**1.99 (1.19, 3.30)**	1.16 (0.58, 2.31)
	Female	24	101	1.00	1.00
Ethnicity	Amhara	37	75	1.07 (0.48, 2.35)	1.17 (0.46, 2.94)
	Oromo	32	116	0.60 (0.27, 1.31)	0.74 (0.29, 1.85)
	Tigre	10	11	1.97 (0.65, 5.89)	1.54 (0.43, 5.52)
	Gurage	25	68	0.80 (0.35, 1.81)	0.87 (0.82, 2.74)
	Others	12	26	1.00	1.00
Residence	Urban	88	192	**1.70 (1.04, 2.77)**	1.50 (0.82, 2.74)
	Rural	28	104	1.00	1.00
Marital status	Married	15	65	1.00	1.00
	Single	81	189	**1.86 (1.00, 3.45)**	0.73 (0.37, 1.43)
	Separated	11	13	**3.67 (1.37, 9.76)**	2.11 (0.83, 5.35)
	Divorced	8	24	1.44 (0.54, 3.84)	0.80 (0.32, 2.02)
	Widowed	1	5	0.86 (0.09, 7.97)	0.64 (0.06, 5.97)
Occupational status	Employed	17	51	3.17 (0.66, 15.02)	2.60 (0.45, 14.93)
	Private business	18	52	3.29 (0.69, 15.53)	1.79 (0.30, 10.66)
	Daily laborer	11	26	4.02 (0.79, 20.28)	2.26 (0.35, 14.56)
	Jobless	66	130	**4.82 (1.09, 21.33)**	2.99 (0.52, 16.91)
	Student	2	18	1.06 (0.13, 8.31)	1.16 (0.11, 12.13)
	Housewife	2	19	1.00	1.00
Duration of illness	<5 years	28	115	1.00	1.00
	5–10 years	34	76	**1.83 (1.03, 3.27)**	0.72 (0.29, 1.75)
	>10 years	54	105	**2.11 (1.24, 3.58)**	0.43 (0.13,1.46)
Duration of treatment	<5 years	37	161	1.00	1.00
	5–10 years	35	60	2.53 (1.46, 4.39)	**1.93 (1.07, 3.49)***
	>10 years	44	75	**2.55 (1.52, 4.27)**	**2.24 (1.29, 3.89)***
Number of admissions	None	65	225	1.00	1.00
	One	20	46	1.51 (0.83, 2.72)	1.50 (0.80, 2.80)
	Two or more	31	25	**4.29 (2.36, 7.78)**	**3.16 (1.68, 5.94)***
Substance use (Khat, alcohol, and tobacco)	No	54	196	1.00	1.00
	Yes	62	100	**2.25 (1.45, 3.48)**	**1.69 (1.06, 2.71)***
Extra pyramidal side effect	No	94	275	1.00	1.00
	Yes	22	21	**3.07 (1.61, 5.82)**	**2.76 (1.38, 5.53)***
Drug adherence	Yes	52	191	1.00	1.00
	No	64	105	**2.24 (1.44, 3.46)**	**1.96 (1.22, 3.15)***

*p value is significant at $p < 0.05$.

more likely to be on antipsychotic polypharmacy as compared to those who are on treatment for less than five years (AOR = 2.24; 95% CI: 1.29, 3.89). Concerning hospitalization status of study participants, patients who had two or more previous admissions were found to be three times more likely to be on antipsychotic polypharmacy as compared to those who had no previous admission (AOR = 3.16, 95% CI: 1.68, 5.94).

Regarding substance use, patients who were using psychoactive substances after initiation of treatment were found to be three times more likely to be on APP than patients who had no history of substance use (AOR = 1.69, 95% CI: 1.06, 2.71). Patients who had extra pyramidal side effect (EPS) were about three times more likely to be on APP when compared to those who had no EPS during the study period (AOR = 2.76, 95% CI: 1.38, 5.53). Patients who were nonadherent to their treatment were found to be two times more likely to be on APP as compared to those who had good adherence to antipsychotic treatment (AOR = 1.96, 95% CI: 1.22, 3.15) (Table 3).

4. Discussion

This study has attempted to identify the prevalence of antipsychotic polypharmacy (APP) and associated factors among schizophrenia outpatients attending AMSH. The overall prevalence of APP was found to be 28.2%.

The prevalence of antipsychotic polypharmacy in the current study area was found to be similar with the studies in USA, South Africa, and Jordan which were 27.5%, 28.6%, and 24.7%, respectively [3, 4, 12], but lower than the findings in Singapore, France, and Egypt which were 71.7%, 37.7%, and 37.6%, respectively [1, 12, 13]. On the contrary the finding of APP in this study is relatively higher than reports in Bahrain which is 10.8% [14]. The possible reason for discrepancies in prevalence rates of antipsychotic polypharmacy among studies could be explained by differences in sociodemographic characteristics, population difference, and instrument used which involves clinical judgments. Besides these, certain studies had used different inclusion criteria; for instance, in USA participants were those who were on treatment for 60 days [15].

Among participants who were on antipsychotic polypharmacy in the current study, almost all (99.1%) were taking two antipsychotics; of those 82.7% were taking combination of typical antipsychotics which is in line with findings in France [13]. This might be because of availability and cost of typical (first generation) antipsychotic drugs. Regarding the associated factors, participants who had history of substance use since the initiation of treatment were three times more likely to be on APP. The possible reason could be that psychoactive substances decrease the effect of antipsychotic drugs and the patient may have poor adherence; these in turn lead the patient to be on APP.

There was a strong association between extra pyramidal side effect (EPS) and APP in this study; individuals who had EPS were about three times more likely to be on APP as compared to those who had no EPS. This is in line with the findings in USA which reports a high prevalence of antipsychotic polypharmacy cases among patients who had EPS [16]. The possible reason could be that patients treated for schizophrenia receive antipsychotic drugs more than the necessary total daily doses and also limited access of antipsychotic drugs (atypical antipsychotic drugs) with less extra pyramidal side effects.

Those who had history of repeated admission were about three times more likely to be on APP as compared to those who do not have admission. This is similar with findings in USA schizophrenia outpatients which report an increased likelihood of hospital admission among polypharmacy cases [17]. The possible reason might be use of psychoactive substances, having poor compliance to their treatment, or increased medication side effects and finally these all worsen the positive symptom of schizophrenia and increase the relapse rate so patient might be admitted repeatedly.

Participants who had poor adherence to their treatment were two times more likely to be on APP. These patients could have a higher likelihood of acute psychiatric hospitalization because of forgetting or being unable to take medications and increasing side effects of medications and finally this would suggest interventions on multiple antipsychotics when compared to those who had good adherence.

A statistically significant association was also found between long treatment duration and APP. The possible reason could be that these patients might be lost to follow-up after initiation of treatment, might have poor prognosis, and experience increased adverse effects as a result of excess antipsychotic exposure to control the aggravated psychotic symptoms.

The strength of this study is the first of its kind in Ethiopia that determined the prevalence and associated factors for antipsychotic polypharmacy among schizophrenia patients. However, our limitations include clinical data pertaining to illness severity which were difficult to assess using cross-sectional studies.

5. Conclusion

Prevalence of APP was found to be high among the current study participants. Individuals who had extra pyramidal side effects, repeated psychiatric admission, history of active substance use, longer duration of treatment, and drug nonadherence were found to have significant association with antipsychotic polypharmacy. Clinicians have to monitor patients for treatment adherence and development of side effects before proceeding to APP. Further cohort study is needed to test the potential benefits and risks of specific antipsychotic combination therapies.

Conflict of Interests

The authors declare that they have no competing interests.

Authors' Contribution

Siranesh Tesfaye, Nigussie Debencho, Teresa Kisi, and Minale Tareke conceived and designed the study; Siranesh Tesfaye collected, analyzed, and interpreted data; Siranesh Tesfaye and Minale Tareke drafted the paper for important intellectual content. All authors read the draft paper and approved the final copy for submission.

Acknowledgments

This study received financial support from University of Gondar and AMSH. The authors would like to thank the staffs of AMSH for their cooperation during the study. They are also grateful to the study participants without whom the current study would not have been realized.

References

[1] K. Sim, A. Su, Y. H. Chan, N. Shinfuku, E. H. Kua, and C. H. Tan, "Clinical correlates of antipsychotic polytherapy in patients with schizophrenia in Singapore," *Psychiatry and Clinical Neurosciences*, vol. 58, no. 3, pp. 324–329, 2004.

[2] M. Šagud, B. Vuksan-Čusa, M. Živković et al., "Antipsychotics: to combine or not to combine?" *Psychiatria Danubina*, vol. 25, no. 3, pp. 306–310, 2013.

[3] L. Koen, P. Magni, D. J. H. Niehaus, and A. Le Roux, "Antipsychotic prescription patterns in Xhosa patients with schizophrenia or schizoaffective disorder," *African Journal of Psychiatry*, vol. 11, no. 4, pp. 287–290, 2008.

[4] K. Sim, A. Su, S. Fujii et al., "Antipsychotic polypharmacy in patients with schizophrenia: a multicentre comparative study in East Asia," *British Journal of Clinical Pharmacology*, vol. 58, no. 2, pp. 178–183, 2004.

[5] R. M. Procyshyn, N. B. Kennedy, G. Tse, and B. Thompson, "Antipsychotic polypharmacy: a survey of discharge prescriptions from a tertiary care psychiatric institution," *Canadian Journal of Psychiatry*, vol. 46, no. 4, pp. 334–339, 2001.

[6] A. B. Adeponle, A. O. Obembe, S. O. Adeyemi, and G. T. Suleiman, "Polypharmacy in psychiatric outpatient practice in northern Nigeria: original article," *African Journal of Psychiatry*, vol. 10, no. 4, pp. 215–218, 2007.

[7] B. L. Crabtree, V. G. Dostrow, C. J. Evans, B. J. Cuffel, J. M. J. Alvir, and K. N. Sanders, "Outcome assessment of an antipsychotic drug algorithm: effects of the Mississippi State Hospital algorithm project," *Psychiatric Services*, vol. 62, no. 8, pp. 963–965, 2011.

[8] J. A. Kreyenbuhl, M. Valenstein, J. F. McCarthy, D. Ganoczy, and F. C. Blow, "Long-term antipsychotic polypharmacy in the VA health system: patient characteristics and treatment patterns," *Psychiatric Services*, vol. 58, no. 4, pp. 489–495, 2007.

[9] D. E. Morisky, A. Ang, M. Krousel-Wood, and H. J. Ward, "Predictive validity of a medication adherence measure in an outpatient setting," *The Journal of Clinical Hypertension*, vol. 10, no. 5, pp. 348–354, 2008.

[10] S. Mahaye, T. Mayime, S. Nkosi et al., "Medication adherence of psychiatric patients in an outpatient setting," *African Journal of Pharmacy and Pharmacology*, vol. 6, no. 9, pp. 608–612, 2012.

[11] S. Janno, M. M. Holi, K. Tuisku, and K. Wahlbeck, "Validity of Simpson-Angus Scale (SAS) in a naturalistic schizophrenia population," *BMC Neurology*, vol. 5, no. 1, article 5, 2005.

[12] M. Amr, T. T. Amin, D. Al-Raddad, A. El-Mogy, and G. Trifirò, "Antipsychotic polypharmacy among Arab patients with schizophrenia," *The Arab Journal of Psychiatry*, vol. 23, no. 2, pp. 115–121, 2012.

[13] A. Millier, E. Sarlon, J.-M. Azorin et al., "Relapse according to antipsychotic treatment in schizophrenic patients: a propensity-adjusted analysis," *BMC Psychiatry*, vol. 11, no. 1, article 24, 2011.

[14] K. A. Al Khaja, M. K. Al-Haddad, R. P. Sequeira, and A. R. Al-Offi, "Antipsychotic and anticholinergic drug prescribing pattern in psychiatry: extent of evidence-based practice in bahrain," *Pharmacology & Pharmacy*, vol. 3, no. 4, pp. 409–416, 2012.

[15] D. E. Faries, H. Ascher-Svanum, B. Zhu, C. U. Correll, and J. Kane, "Antipsychotic monotherapy and polypharmacy in the naturalistic treatment of schizophrenia with atypical antipsychotics," *BMC Psychiatry*, vol. 5, no. 1, article 26, 2005.

[16] F. Centorrino, J. L. Goren, J. Hennen, P. Salvatore, J. P. Kelleher, and R. J. Baldessarini, "Multiple versus single antipsychotic agents for hospitalized psychiatric patients: case-control study of risks versus benefit," *American Journal of Psychiatry*, vol. 161, no. 4, pp. 700–706, 2004.

[17] F. Sun, E. M. Stock, L. A. Copeland, J. E. Zeber, B. K. Ahmedani, and S. B. Morissette, "Polypharmacy with antipsychotic drugs in patients with schizophrenia: trends in multiple health care systems," *American Journal of Health-System Pharmacy*, vol. 71, no. 9, pp. 728–738, 2014.

19

Community Perception towards Mental Illness among Residents of Gimbi Town, Western Ethiopia

Misael Benti,[1] Jemal Ebrahim,[2] Tadesse Awoke,[3] Zegeye Yohannis,[4] and Asres Bedaso[2]

[1]*Psychiatry Department, Gimbi General Hospital, Oromia, Ethiopia*
[2]*School of Nursing and Midwifery, College of Medicine and Health Sciences, Hawassa University, Hawassa, Ethiopia*
[3]*Department of Biostatistics and Epidemiology, College of Medicine and Health Sciences, University of Gondar, Gondar, Ethiopia*
[4]*Research and Training Directorate, Amanuel Specialized Mental Hospital, Addis Ababa, Ethiopia*

Correspondence should be addressed to Jemal Ebrahim; jemebrie@gmail.com

Academic Editor: Yvonne Forsell

Background. Despite the increased burden of mental health problem, little is known about knowledge and perception of the public towards mental health problems in Ethiopia. *Methods.* Community based cross-sectional study was conducted among selected 845 Gimbi town residents from May 28 to June 28, 2014. *Results.* Out of the total study participants, 304 (37.3%) were found to have poor perception (a score below mean five semantic differential scales for positive questions and above mean for negative questions) of mental illness. Being above 28 years of age (AOR = 0.48 CI (0.23, 0.78)), private workers (AOR = 0.41 CI (0.19, 0.87)), and lack of mental health information were found to be associated with poor perception of mental illness (AOR = 0.133 CI (0.09, 0.20)). Absence of family history of mental illness was also found to be associated with poor perception of mental illness (AOR = 0.37 CI (0.21, 0.66)). *Conclusions.* Significant proportions of the community in Gimbi town were found to have poor perception of mental illness. Poor perception is common among old aged, less educated, private workers, those unable to access mental health information, and those with no family history of mental illness. Mental health education on possible causes, treatment options, and possible outcome of treatment to the community is required.

1. Background

Mental and behavioral problem exist in all countries, in women and men at all stages of life, among the poor and rich and among rural and urban people. As many as 450 million people worldwide are estimated to be suffering at any given time from some kind of mental or brain disorder, including behavioral and substance related disorders [1]. Worldwide it is estimated that life time prevalence ranges from 12.2% to 48.6% and 12-month prevalence between 8.25% and 29.1% [2].

Community's perception of mental health varies across the culture, and there are various myths and beliefs regarding mental health [3]. The conceptualization and perceived cause of mental illness vary from community to community. Accordingly, people with mental health problem get different names in different societies [4–6].

People tend to have strong beliefs about the mental illness, and many of these concepts are based on prevailing local systems of belief. Most of the society's perception and attitude towards mental illness are far from the scientific view and this may negatively affect treatment seeking and adherence [7, 8].

Several studies show that people's belief regarding mental illness is also the main factor which leads to stigmatization and labeling. Stigma against people with mental illness remains a significant barrier to positive outcomes across cultures and nations, related to the threat value of mental symptoms, intolerance for diversity, and inaccurate conceptions of mental disorder [9, 10].

Community's perception is dynamic and tends to change as the awareness and education changes. Education and social media are the major factors which move the perception of the community to the scientific perspectives [11].

Globally, including developed and developing countries, people held different explanation regarding mental illness, especially its causal and treatment option. A report of the behavioral risk factor surveillance system shows that in USA

80% of the adult population in the state surveyed agree that mental illness treatment is effective. The rest either disagree or have no idea about that and only 35%–67% of the population agreed that people are caring and sympathetic to people with mental illness [12].

Mental health, neglected for far too long, is crucial to the overall well-being of individuals, societies, and countries and must be universally regarded in a new light. Unfortunately, in most parts of the world, mental health and mental disorders are not regarded with anything like the same importance as physical health [13].

Poor perception of mental illness in different community contributed to low treatment seeking and stigmatization of people with mental illness. They often go to hospitals after they have tried all options and after the symptom has got worse and this in turn negatively affects the prognoses of treatment [14].

Hence, assessing community's perception is important to have appropriate plan of health promotion and scaling up publics' utilization of mental health services, particularly in multiethnic and multicultural Ethiopia as the community's view of mental illness varies with culture.

Studies done in different areas have shown that poor perception towards the mentally ill is mainly deep rooted with various sociodemographic and other factors [7, 8, 10, 13–18].

In Ethiopia there are few published studies [18] assessing community perception towards people with mental illness and no studies were done in Gimbi town concerning this topic. Therefore, this study has great value on assessing the perception of the community towards mental illness. Also the result of this study is very important to the mental health strategy developed so far and to other stakeholders as describing the community's deep rooted belief and perception regarding mental illness in West Wellega, particularly Gimbi town.

2. Method and Materials

2.1. Study Design and Period. Community based cross-sectional study design was conducted from May 28 to June 28, 2014, at Gimbi town, West Wellega Zone of Oromia region, Ethiopia. The town is located at a distance of 441 Km from the capital city, Addis Ababa to the west. Gimbi town has got two hospitals and one health center. The town has 4 kebeles and according to the 2007 National Housing and Population Census, the projected population of Gimbi town for the year 2014/15 was about 42,286 and the estimated number of households was 8629 [19].

2.2. Sampling Techniques. Single population proportion with the assumptions of 95% level of confidence, 5% error, and 50% proportion was used to estimate the minimum sample size for the study. Considering the design effect of two (multiplied by 2) and 10% nonresponse rate, the final sample size became 845.

Following purposive selection of the administrative town (Gimbi town), the two kebeles out of four (the smallest administrative level) were selected randomly. Households in the selected kebeles were approached by systematic sampling method with the first household selected randomly. From each selected household, one individual, 18 years of age and older (based on information from household head), was included for the interview. A lottery method was used to select one individual in a house hold where more than one individual, 18 years of age and older, was found.

2.3. Data Collection and Measurements. Data were collected through face to face interview by trained data collectors. A case vignette based standardized questionnaire which explains cases like schizophrenia, major depressive disorder, epilepsy, and generalized anxiety disorder [18] as well as questionnaires adopted from previous studies to assess sociodemographic characteristics and other associated factors was used. Standard 9 items of five semantic deferential scales were also used to assess community perception about mental illness. A score above mean score of five semantic differential scales for positive questions and below mean score for negative questions was considered as having good perception of mental illness. Four trained diploma nurses interviewed the community and were supervised in the field during data collection. Eligible participants not available at home during the first visit of data collection were revisited once on the next day and then registered as nonresponse if not found.

2.4. Data Quality Control. The tool was first developed in English language and translated to Amharic language with back translation to English for consistency. Amharic version questionnaire was used to collect data as Amharic is the national official language that majority of Ethiopians speak.

To assure the quality of data the questionnaire was pretested 1 week before the actual data collection time among 40 people not included in the actual sample and appropriate modification was made. The reliability of the tool was found to be $\alpha = 0.73$.

Training on objectives of the study, over all data collection procedure and ethics of the study, was given to data collectors and supervised by principal investigators on the actual data collection site. To ensure confidentiality, interview was conducted in private setting. Throughout the course of the data collection, interviewers were supervised at each site; regular meetings were held between the data collectors and the principal investigator. Two more additional visits were made for eligible respondent not accessed in the first visit. The collected data was reviewed and checked for completeness before data entry.

2.5. Data Processing and Analysis. Data clean-up and cross checking were done before analysis. Checked, cleaned, and coded data was entered into EPI info version 7 and exported to SPSS version 20.0 for analysis. Descriptive statistics like frequencies, percentages, mean, and standard deviation were used to present data. Tables and figures were also used to present data. Binary logistic regression was used to see associated factors with the dependent variable. Those variable with p value less than 0.02 were entered to multivariate analysis to identify the independent associated factors after confounders are controlled. Finally the variables which had independent association with community perception were identified on the basis of OR, with 95% CI and p value less than 0.05.

2.6. Ethical Considerations. Ethical clearance was obtained from the Institutional Review Board of University of Gondar and Amanuel mental specialized hospital. Permission letter was obtained from Oromia regional health bureau, West Wellega Zonal health department, and Gimbi town health office hierarchically.

Written informed consent was obtained from each study participant. After reading the consent statement by the data collectors, finger prints were obtained from those participants who could not read and write. The respondents were informed that their inclusion in the study is voluntary and they are free to withdraw from the study if they are not willing to participate.

Also all respondents are informed that they did not have direct payment for their participation in the study. Anonymity was maintained to ensure confidentiality of respondents.

3. Results

A total of 845 selected peoples in Gimbi town were interviewed, out of which 29 responses were excluded for gross incompleteness and considered as nonresponse. Therefore, analysis was made based on 816 questionnaires, yielding a response rate of 96.5%.

3.1. Sociodemographic Characteristics of Respondents. Among the total respondents, 414 (50.73%) were females and the mean age of participants was 33.0 ± 10 SD. The majority, 706 (86.5%), of study participants were Oromo in ethnicity and four hundred and sixty-seven (57.2%) were Orthodox followers by religion. 577 (70.7%) were married, 285 (34.9%) have elementary level education, and 31.4% of the respondents were merchant. Six hundred and fifteen (75.4%) of the respondents had an average family monthly income less than or equal to 651 Ethiopian birr (Table 1).

Table 1: Sociodemographic characteristics of respondents (n = 816) in Gimbi town, West Wellega Zone, Oromia region, Ethiopia, 2014.

Variables	Category	Frequency	Percentage
Age	18–28	313	38.4
	29–38	301	36.9
	≥39	202	24.8
Sex	Male	402	49.3
	Female	414	50.7
Religion	Orthodox	467	57.2
	Protestant	266	32.6
	Muslim	83	10.2
Ethnicity	Oromo	704	86.3
	Amhara	84	10.1
	Gurage	18	2.2
	Tigre	8	1.2
	Others	2	0.2
Educational status	Degree and above	38	4.7
	Diploma	119	14.6
	High school	280	34.3
	Elementary	285	34.9
	Uneducated	94	11.5
Marital status	Single	221	27.1
	Married	577	70.7
	Divorced	18	2.2
Occupational status	Government	113	13.8
	Private	270	33.1
	Merchant	256	31.4
	Student	66	8.1
	Housewife	111	13.6
Family monthly income in Ethiopian birr	≤450	27	25.4
	451–650	215	26.3
	651–1300	193	23.7
	≥1301	201	24.6

3.2. Mental Health Information. Mental health information refers to information on the types of mental illness, causes, possibility of treatment, treatment options, and magnitude of mental illness. Accordingly, among all study participants, 564 (69.1%) were reported as having mental health information in the past 12 months while the remaining 252 did not receive any information related to mental health illness. Among 564 respondents having information regarding mental illness 21.3%, 12.4%, and 11% believe that mental illnesses are caused by excessive worry, substance use, and evil spirit, respectively. Mental illness are serious problem (18.5%) and stress can cause mental illness (11.3%), which were among the statements frequently mentioned.

3.3. Family History of Mental Illness. Presence of family member/s with any type of mental health problem was considered here. Among the total participants, 100 (12.3%) were reported to have family history of mental illness (Figure 1).

3.4. Respondents' Perception of Mental Illness. A score below 27 for 9 items of five semantic deferential scales was considered having poor perception towards mental illness in this study. Accordingly (37.3%) respondents were found having poor perception towards mental illness (Table 2).

3.5. Respondents' Perceived Cause of Mental Illness. Majority of the respondents attributed the cause of mental illness in the case vignette to supernatural causes like evil spirit, God's punishment, and witchcraft. Table 3 shows the distribution of perceived cause of mental illness in the case vignettes (Table 3).

3.6. Respondents' Recognition of the Case Vignette as Mental Illness. Schizophrenia was the case identified as mental illness by the majority of respondents. Seven hundred and seventy-four (94.9%) of the respondents identified schizophrenia as mental illness. General Anxiety Disorder

TABLE 2: Distribution of community's perception of mental illness among the residents of Gimbi town, Oromia region, Ethiopia ($n = 816$), 2014.

S. number	Questions	1		2		3		4		5	
		N	%	N	%	N	%	N	%	N	%
1	Do you agree that substance misuse like alcohol or drug could result in mental illness?	12	1.5	50	6.5	106	13.0	444	55.4	204	25.0
2	Do you agree that genetic inheritance could be the cause of mental illness?	220	27.0	130	15.9	150	18.4	222	27.2	94	11.5
3	Do you agree that head injury can be the cause of mental illness?	52	6.4	130	15.9	111	13.6	308	37.7	215	26.3
4	Do you agree that physical illness (like diabetes, HIV/AIDS) can be the cause of mental illness	54	6.6	221	27.1	49	6.0	273	33.5	219	26.8
5	Do you agree that mental illness is treatable?	12	1.5	220	27.0	60	7.4	304	37.3	220	27.0
6	Do you agree that stress in daily life can cause mental Illness?	19	2.3	107	24.1	65	8.0	270	33.1	265	32.5
7	Do you agree that mental illness is contagious?	435	53.3	152	18.6	171	21	40	4.9	18	2.2
8	Do you agree that mental illness is punishment from God?	38	4.7	88	10.8	400	49.0	226	27.7	64	7.8
9	Do you agree that evil sprite can be the cause of mental illness?	32	3.9	35	4.3	221	27.0	413	50.6	115	14.0

1: strongly disagree; 2: disagree; 3: not sure; 4: agree; 5: strongly agree.

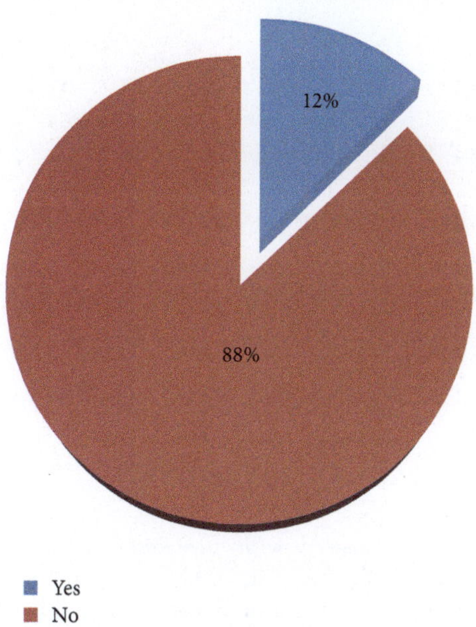

FIGURE 1: Distribution of family history of mental illness among residents of Gimbi town, 2014.

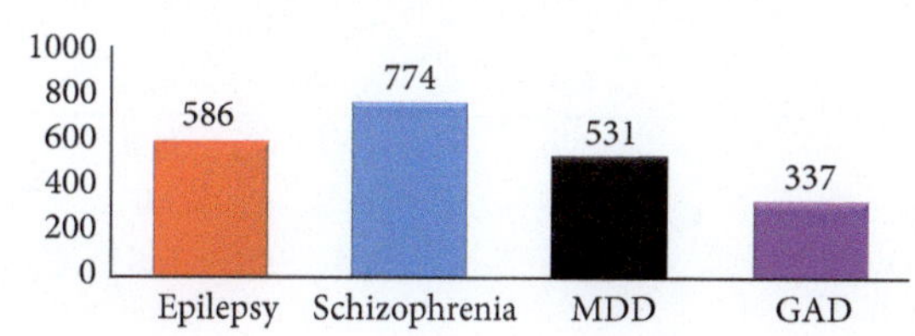

FIGURE 2: Distribution of respondents' recognition of mental illness among residents of Gimbi town, 2014.

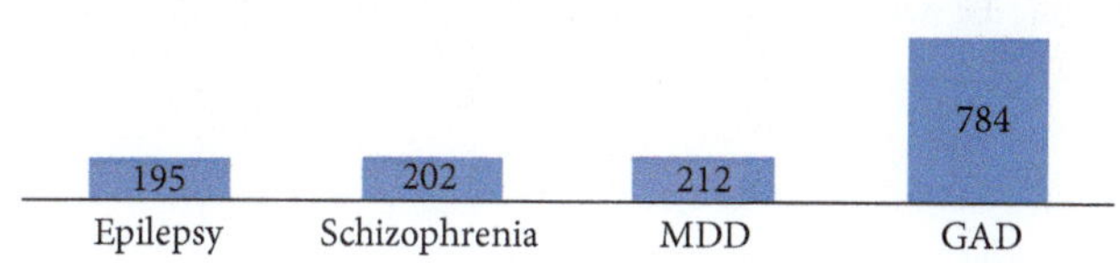

FIGURE 3: Distribution of respondents' perception regarding possibility of treatment of mental illness ($n = 816$), Gimbi town, 2014.

(GAD) was the least case identified as mental illness by the respondents (Figure 2).

3.7. Perception regarding Possibility of Treatment of Mental Illness on the Case Vignette. Great discrepancy was observed among case vignettes regarding the respondents' view of whether or not they can be treated. Majority of the respondents (784) (96.1%), reported that GAD can be treated while 202 (24.8%) of the respondents reported that schizophrenia is treatable (Figure 3).

3.8. Respondents Preferred Place of Treatment for the Case Vignettes. Regarding preferred place of treatment: 538 (65.9%), 470 (57.6%), 454 (55.6%), and 254 (31.1%) of respondents prefer health institution for epilepsy, schizophrenia, MDD, and GAD, respectively. See Table 4 for the distribution of the respondents' preferred place of treatment.

3.9. Respondents Perceived Severity of Mental Illness. Respondents were asked to rank the case vignette from the most serious to the least. Schizophrenia was seen as the most severe by majority of the respondents. Following schizophrenia,

TABLE 3: Distribution of respondents' perceived cause of mental illness among residents of Gimbi town, West Wellega Zone, Oromia region, Ethiopia (multiple responses), 2014.

Causes		Mental illness							
		Epilepsy		Schizophrenia		MDD		GAD	
		N	%	*N*	%	*N*	%	*N*	%
Evil spirit	No	262	32.1	232	28.4	280	34.3	334	40.9
	Yes	554	67.9	584	71.6	536	65.7	482	59.1
God's punishment	No	644	78.9	646	79.2	706	86.5	732	89.7
	Yes	172	21.1	170	20.8	110	13.5	84	10.3
Witchcraft	No	648	79.4	640	78.4	668	81.9	684	83.8
	Yes	168	20.6	176	21.6	148	18.1	132	16.2
Daily stress	No	596	73.0	254	31.1	774	94.9	202	24.8
	Yes	220	27.0	562	68.9	42	5.1	614	75.2
Biological	No	736	90.2	710	87.0	204	25.0	185	22.7
	Yes	80	9.8	106	13.0	612	75.0	631	77.3
Substance use	No	630	77.2	394	48.3	632	77.5	696	85.3
	Yes	186	22.8	422	51.7	184	22.5	120	14.7
Physical illness	No	488	59.8	664	81.4	632	77.5	756	92.6
	Yes	328	40.2	152	18.6	184	22.5	60	7.4

TABLE 4: Distribution of respondents preferred place of treatment mental illness among residents of Gimbi town, West Wellega Zone, Ethiopia, 2014.

Treatment option		Mental illness							
		Epilepsy		Schizophrenia		MDD		GAD	
		N	%	*N*	%	*N*	%	*N*	%
Family	No	808	99.0	810	99.3	784	96.1	612	75.0
	Yes	8	1.0	6	.7	32	3.9	204	25.0
Hospital/HC	No	278	34.1	346	42.4	362	44.4	562	68.9
	Yes	538	65.9	470	57.6	454	55.6	254	31.1
Holly water	No	658	80.6	656	80.4	658	80.6	728	89.2
	Yes	158	19.4	160	19.6	158	19.4	88	10.8
Traditional healer	No	772	94.6	770	94.4	758	92.9	796	97.5
	Yes	44	5.4	46	5.6	58	7.1	20	2.5
Prayer	No	572	70.1	538	65.9	380	46.6	334	40.9
	Yes	244	29.9	278	34.1	436	53.4	482	59.1
Witchcraft	No	782	95.8	790	96.8	790	96.8	804	98.5
	Yes	34	4.2	26	3.2	26	3.2	12	1.5

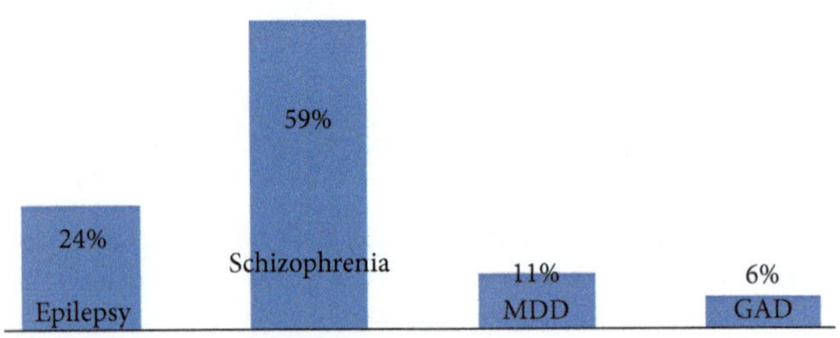

FIGURE 4: Distribution of respondents' perceived severity of mental illness among residents of Gimbi town, West Wellega Zone, Oromia region, Ethiopia, 2014 ($n = 816$).

epilepsy, major depressive disorder, and generalized anxiety disorder were seen from the most severe to the least, respectively (Figure 4).

3.10. Factors Associated with the Respondents' Perception of Mental Illness. In bivariate analyses age of respondents, educational status, occupational status, mental health information, and family history of mental illness were found to be significantly associated with perception of mental illness.

Respondent age, educational level, occupation, mental health information, and family history of mental illness were found to be independently associated after multivariate analysis.

The likelihood of having poor perception of mental illness among those above age 39 is higher than those below 28 years old (AOR = 0.5 (0.30, 0.80)). The proportion of poor perception is observed among those who have no formal education (AOR = 0.09 CI (0.02, 0.46)), elementary education (AOR = 0.07 CI (0.02, 0.33)), and high school level (AOR = 0.13 CI (0.03, 0.61)), when compared with those with

TABLE 5: Distribution of factors associated with community's perception of mental illness among residents of Gimbi town, West Wellega Zone, Oromia region, Ethiopia, 2014.

Variable	Perception		Crud OR 95% CI	Adjusted OR
	Good (%)	Poor (%)		
Age				
18–28	215 (68.7)	98 (31.3)	1.00	1.00
29–38	210 (69.8)	91 (30.2)	1.05 (0.7, 1.5)	1.2 (0.8, 1.9)
≥39	87 (43.1)	115 (56.9)	0.35 (0.24, 0.50)	**0.5 (0.30, 0.80)***
Education				
Illiterate	40 (42.6)	54 (57.4)	0.41 (0.01, 0.18)	**0.09 (0.02, 0.46)***
Elementary	138 (48.4)	147 (51.6)	0.05 (0.01, 0.22)	**0.07 (0.02, 0.33)***
High school	187 (66.8)	93 (33.2)	0.11 (0.03, 0.47)	**0.13 (0.03, 0.61)***
Diploma	118 (93.3)	8 (6.7)	0.77 (0.16, 3.80)	1.35 (0.25, 7.24)
Degree & above	36 (94.7)	2 (5.3)	1.00	1.00
Occupation				
Government	100 (88.5)	13 (11.5)	1.00	RC
Private	121 (44.8)	149 (55.2)	0.11 (0.06, 0.20)	**0.41 (0.19, 0.87)***
Merchant	188 (73.4)	68 (26.6)	0.36 (0.19, 0.68)	1.25 (0.60, 2.69)
Student	42 (63.6)	24 (36.4)	0.23 (0.11, 0.49)	0.62 (0.25, 1.56)
Housewife	61 (55.0)	50 (45.0)	0.16 (0.08, 0.32)	0.84 (.36, 1.96)
Mental health information	Yes 423 (75.0)	141 (25.0)	1.00	RC
	No 89 (35.3)	161 (64.7)	0.18 (0.13, 0.25)	**0.133 (0.09, 0.2)***
Family history of mental illness	Yes 74 (74.0)	26 (26.0)	1.00	RC
	No 438 (61.2)	278 (38.8)	0.14 (0.35, 0.89)	**0.37 (0.21, 0.66)***

* p value < 0.05; RC: reference category.

degree and above. This shows that perception towards mental illness is higher among educated people.

Community's perceptions of mental illness were also found associated with occupational status. Private workers will have poor perception when compared with government employees (AOR = 0.41 CI (0.09, 0.87)). Mental health information is also associated with perception of mental illness. Having mental health information from any sources is more likely associated with good perception of mental illness (AOR = 0.133 CI (0.09, 0.2)).

The likelihood of having good perception among individual with no family history of mental illness is 63% less when compared with those having family history of mental illness (AOR = 0.37 CI (0.21, 0.66)) (Table 5).

4. Discussion

This community based cross-sectional study identified important information on community perception towards mental illness. Significant number of the respondents from Gimbi community had poor perception of mental illness. This study is in line with the study conducted in India where 39.4% of the respondents were found to have poor perception about mental illness [14]. But it is not consistent with study done in Iraq where 30% of the respondents were with poor perception of mental illness [13]. The variation might be due to socioeconomic and cultural difference among respondents.

This study demonstrated that there was higher proportion of poor perception of mental illness among those above 39 years of age compared to the youth. The finding is not consistent with a study done in North Western Ethiopia, Agaro town, where younger respondents were more likely to hold socioenvironmental deprivation responsible for mental and physical illnesses than older respondents [18]. This could be due to the difference in educational level between these two groups or may be due to the fact that the younger respondents may have access to information. Also in study done in Iraq and India no significant association was found with age regarding the community's view of mental illness. This could be due to the tool used or sample characteristics as rural and urban community are involved in both studies [13, 14].

Educational level was found to be one of the sociodemographic characteristics significantly affecting perception of mental illness in this study. Respondents who have no formal education are by 90% more likely to have poor perception when compared with degree holders and above. This finding is in agreement with the study done in Agaro town [18]. Study done in Nigeria also found out that perception of mental illness correlates with educational level [20]. Less educated respondents were more likely to attribute mental illnesses to supernatural retribution. This could be due to poor understanding of scientific explanation regarding causation of mental illness.

Occupational status was significantly associated with perception of mental illness. Government employees will have good perception of mental illness compared to private workers, which implies those in government organization may have more access to current policies, directions, and strategies relatively than those in private organizations. However this finding is not clearly observed in other studies. This may be due to the difference of tool used.

In addition, respondents having information about mental illness from any source were of good perception of mental illness compared to those having no information. This finding is in line with the study done in Karfi region of Nigeria [15]. Theory of psychology also supports this fact. According to psychologists' point of view, perception can be deductive or inductive. If perception is deductive, no probabilistic association needs to be added and no cognition is required. Information is sufficient and deductive perception is possible. If however perception is inductive some premises come from cognition and memory [21].

Family history of mental illness is also another factor found associated with perception of mental illness among Gimbi community. Those who do not have family history of mental illness are found more likely to have poor perception of mental illness than those having family history of mental illness. This may be due to the fact that those having family history of mental illness may share experience. This experience may help them to develop good perception. This factor is also supported by psychologists' explanation. According to Bill, perceptual experiences are experiences of mind-independent things and are themselves an account of the way in which they provide peculiarly basic reasons for beliefs about the world around the perceiver [22].

4.1. Conclusion and Recommendation. Significant proportions of community in Gimbi town have poor perception of mental illness. Poor perception of mental illness was common among old age people, those with low educational level, private workers, those who do not have mental health information, and those who do not have family history of mental illness. High level of educational status and access to mental health information strengthen the community's perception of mental illness.

It is important to address the poor perception towards the mentally ill in order to make community based mental health care a reality. The community health professionals should work on awareness creation on mental ill issues at the community level providing relevant information. There is the need to provide more knowledge and increased awareness on the causes of mental illness and also dispel the myths around the causes of the disorders and treatment options.

Competing Interests

The authors declare they have no conflict of interests.

Authors' Contributions

Jemal Ebrahim, Misael Benti, Tadesse Awoke, and Zegeye Yohannis designed the study, collected data, and participated in data analysis and interpretation. Jemal Ebrahim and Asres Bedaso prepared the manuscript. All the authors saw and approved the final version of the manuscript.

Acknowledgments

The authors would like to thank Amanuel Mental Specialized Hospital for financial support and providing necessary materials in support of undertaking this research. They would also like to appreciate Gimbi Town Health Office, supervisors, and data collectors who showed the greatest effort in acquiring appropriate information. Finally, they would like to acknowledge the study subjects who have kindly cooperated in providing the required information.

References

[1] WHO, *Stigmatization and Human Rights Violations Mental Health a Call for Action by World Health Ministers*, 2001.

[2] WHO, *Scaling Up Care for Mental, Neurological and Substance Use Problem*, Mental Health Gap Action Program, 2008.

[3] D. Saint Arnault, "Cultural determinants of help seeking: a model for research and practice," *Research and Theory for Nursing Practice*, vol. 23, no. 4, pp. 259–278, 2009.

[4] S. Teferra and T. Shibre, "Perceived causes of severe mental disturbance and preferred interventions by the Borana semi-nomadic population in southern Ethiopia: a qualitative study," *BMC Psychiatry*, vol. 12, article 79, 2012.

[5] T. Stolovy, Y. M. Levy, A. Doron, and Y. Melamed, "Culturally sensitive mental health care: a study of contemporary psychiatric treatment for ultra-orthodox Jews in Israel," *International Journal of Social Psychiatry*, vol. 59, no. 8, pp. 819–823, 2013.

[6] J. S. Payne, "Influence of race and symptom expression on clinicians' depressive disorder identification in African American men," *Journal of the Society for Social Work and Research*, vol. 3, no. 3, pp. 162–177, 2012.

[7] J. R. Nsereko, D. Kizza, F. Kigozi et al., "Stakeholder's perceptions of help-seeking behaviour among people with mental health problems in Uganda," *International Journal of Mental Health Systems*, vol. 5, article 5, 2011.

[8] P. Ventevogel, M. Jordans, R. Reis, and J. De Jong, "Madness or sadness? Local concepts of mental illness in four conflict-affected African communities," *Conflict and Health*, vol. 7, article 3, 2013.

[9] A. Stier and S. P. Hinshaw, "Explicit and implicit stigma against individuals with mental illness," *Australian Psychologist*, vol. 42, no. 2, pp. 106–117, 2007.

[10] O. Gureje, V. O. Lasebikan, O. Ephraim-Oluwanuga, B. O. Olley, and L. Kola, "Community study of knowledge of and attitude to mental illness in Nigeria," *British Journal of Psychiatry*, vol. 186, pp. 436–441, 2005.

[11] B. A. Pescosolido, J. K. Martin, B. G. Link et al., "Americans' views of mental health and illness at century's end: continuity and change," Public Report on the MacArthur Mental Health Module, General social survey. Indian Consortium for Mental Health Services Research, 1996.

[12] BRFSS, "Attitude toward mental illness," BRFSS Mental Illness Stigma Report, Behavioral Risk Factor Surveillance System, Atlanta, Ga, USA, 2012.

[13] S. Sadik, M. Bradley, S. Al-Hasoon, and R. Jenkins, "Public perception of mental health in Iraq," *International Journal of Mental Health Systems*, vol. 4, article 26, 2010.

[14] H. Salve, K. Goswami, R. Sagar, B. Nongkynrih, and V. Sreenivas, "Perception and attitude towards mental illness in an urban community in South Delhi—a community based study," *Indian*

Journal of Psychological Medicine, vol. 35, no. 2, pp. 154–158, 2013.

[15] M. Kabir, Z. Iliyasu, I. S. Abubakar, and M. H. Aliyu, "Perception and beliefs about mental illness among adults in Karfi village, northern Nigeria," *BMC International Health and Human Rights*, vol. 4, article 3, 2004.

[16] J. Crabb, R. C. Stewart, D. Kokota, N. Masson, S. Chabunya, and R. Krishnadas, "Attitudes towards mental illness in Malawi: a cross-sectional survey," *BMC Public Health*, vol. 12, no. 1, article 541, 2012.

[17] E. Girma, M. Tesfaye, G. Froeschl, A. M. Möller-Leimkühler, N. Müller, and S. Dehning, "Public stigma against people with mental illness in the Gilgel Gibe Field Research Center (GGFRC) in Southwest Ethiopia," *PLoS ONE*, vol. 8, no. 12, Article ID e82116, 2013.

[18] Y. S. T. Deribew, "How are mental health problems perceived by a community in Agaro town?" *Ethiopian Journal of Health Development*, vol. 9, no. 2, pp. 153–159, 2005.

[19] CSA (Central Statistical Agency), *The 2007 Population and Housing Census of Ethiopia. Statistical Report*, CSA, Addis Ababa, Ethiopia, 2008.

[20] A. O. Adewuya and R. O. A. Makanjuola, "Lay beliefs regarding causes of mental illness in Nigeria: pattern and correlates," *Social Psychiatry and Psychiatric Epidemiology*, vol. 43, no. 4, pp. 336–341, 2008.

[21] J. E. Cutting, "Perception and information," *Annual Review of Psychology*, pp. 3–30, 1987.

[22] B. Bill, "Experience and reason in perception," http://www2.warwick.ac.uk/fac/soc/philosophy/people/brewer/erp.pdf.

20

Forethought in Youth with Attention Deficit/Hyperactivity Disorder: An fMRI Study of Sex-Specific Differences

H. Poissant,[1] L. Rapin,[2] S. Chenail,[3] and A. Mendrek[3]

[1]*Department of Education and Pedagogy, UQAM, Montreal, QC, Canada H2L 2C4*
[2]*Department of Linguistics, UQAM, Montreal, QC, Canada H2L 2C4*
[3]*Department of Psychology, Bishop's University, Sherbrooke, QC, Canada J1M 1Z7*

Correspondence should be addressed to H. Poissant; poissant.helene@uqam.ca

Academic Editor: Umberto Albert

Objective. The majority of studies investigating neurocognitive processing in attention deficit/hyperactivity disorder (ADHD) have been conducted on male participants. Few studies evaluated females or examined sex differences. Among various cognitive anomalies in ADHD, deficit in forethought seems particularly important as children with ADHD often fail to adequately use previous information in order to prepare for responses. The main goal of this study was to assess sex-specific differences in behavioral and neural correlates of forethought in youth with ADHD. *Methods.* 21 typically developing (TD) youth and 23 youth with ADHD were asked to judge whether two pictures told a congruent or incongruent story. Reaction time, performance accuracy, and cerebral activations were recorded during functional magnetic resonance imaging (fMRI). *Results.* Significant sex-specific differences in cerebral activations appeared, despite equivalent performance. Relative to the boys TD participants, boys with ADHD had extensive bilateral frontal and parietal hypoactivations, while girls with ADHD demonstrated more scattered hypoactivations in the right cerebral regions. *Conclusion.* Present results revealed that youth with ADHD exhibit reduced cerebral activations during forethought. Nevertheless, the pattern of deficits differed between boys and girls, suggesting the use of a different neurocognitive strategy. This emphasizes the importance of including both genders in the investigations of ADHD.

1. Introduction

Attention deficit/hyperactive disorder (ADHD) is a neurodevelopmental disorder defined by persistent inattention and/or hyperactivity/impulsivity [1]. The disorder negatively impacts social, academic, or occupational functioning. Most of the studies have been conducted on male participants resulting in a limited knowledge regarding sex and gender differences in ADHD [2]. The higher prevalence of ADHD in boys could partly explain this gap in the literature [3], but we need more information regarding ADHD females, especially in the realm of neurocognitive dysfunction. Thus, the present study was designed to examine neural sex differences in ADHD.

The expression of ADHD appears to be sexually dimorphic. Boys seem to exhibit more hyperactivity, inattention, impulsivity, and externalizing problems. Girls generally show more internalizing problems (depression, anxiety) and intellectual impairment [4, 5]. Larger deficits in inhibition have also been reported in males [6]. Differences in age of onset and differences in symptoms could be due to neurochemical and hormonal factors. For example, boys show a significant increase in dopamine (DA) receptor density before and during puberty, which could contribute to more hyperactivity symptoms at an earlier stage [7]. In comparison, girls demonstrate a later increase in DA receptors related to an increase in estrogen during puberty [7].

Several executive dysfunctions have been found in children with ADHD, including difficulties with prioritizing, time management, and initiating and completing tasks as well as difficulty in shifting cognitive sets and poor working memory (WM) [8]. Working memory, defined as the ability to retain information for prospective execution of an action [9], seems specifically affected in ADHD [3]. A meta-analysis indicated that children with ADHD scored lower than control children on verbal storage, verbal central executive, visual-spatial storage, and visual-spatial central executive [10].

Another meta-analysis [11] found significant patterns of hypoactivity in ADHD, which affected the anterior cingulate cortex (ACC), dorsolateral and inferior prefrontal cortex (PFC), basal ganglia, thalamus, and portions of the parietal cortex. Other findings also point to deficits in the neural activity of the frontostriatal and frontoparietal pathways [12]. Studies on inhibition alone indicate hypoactivation, especially pronounced in the PFC, and greater activity in the medial frontal gyrus and the parietal paracentral lobule in individuals with ADHD [11].

Only a few neuroimaging studies on ADHD have included females. The percentage of females across all studies has been estimated to be less than 20% [2] while the male to female ratio among ADHD is estimated to be 2.28 : 1 [13]. Valera and colleagues (2010) [14] found that while performing a verbal WM task, males with ADHD showed significantly less activation in the right frontal, right temporal, left occipital, cerebellar, and some subcortical regions. However, no differences in activation were found between females with and without ADHD. Similar results were obtained in a subsequent fMRI study [15], while the electroencephalography (EEG) investigation revealed markedly different EEG profiles in boys and girls with ADHD [16].

Forethought is a prospective function of WM related to the ability to conjecture possible future related events [17]. Children with ADHD often fail to adequately use previous information in order to prepare for upcoming responses. One study found that children with ADHD showed diminished activation in the ventral PFC and ACC when having to react to a stimulus that was not expected from a past stimulus [18]. More recently, Poissant et al. (2012) [19] also found hypoactivation of the PFC in youth with ADHD and higher reaction times during a task requiring forethought.

In the present study we examined neural sex differences in ADHD during a forethought task. Based on previous findings, it was expected that boys with ADHD would demonstrate poorer performance and greater cerebral hypoactivation during the task relative to girls with ADHD.

2. Method

2.1. Participants. Forty-four children (21 control (12 girls) and 23 with ADHD (7 girls); age range: 7–15 years old) composed the two groups of this cross-sectional study. Control participants (TD) were recruited through schools in the Montreal area. Participants with ADHD were recruited through a specialized clinic for ADHD in Montreal. All participants with ADHD had received a diagnosis by a specialized medical team based on DSM-IV-TR criteria (APA, 2000). In the following weeks, all parents filled out the Risk Factor Questionnaire (RFQ) [20] to confirm diagnosis in participants with ADHD as well as to exclude signs of the disorder in TD. Recruitment of patients was done over two and a half years, from 2009 to 2012. In addition, both sustained and selective attention were measured with the Continuous Performance Task (CPT) [21]. The ability to shift sets was measured by the Wisconsin Card Sorting Test (WCST) [22] and working memory with the Auditory Consonant Trigrams (ACT) test for children [23]. Mean composite IQ scores (K-BIT) [24] were also assessed in both groups. All adolescents were assessed in two sessions: neuropsychological and cerebral imagery while they were deprived of methylphenidate (MPH) for at least 24 hr. Children with motor, auditory or vision deficits, central nervous system abnormalities, and major health problems were excluded.

2.2. Functional Magnetic Resonance Imaging (fMRI). The neural activation was assessed with fMRI. While in the scanner, participants were asked to judge whether two consecutive pictures told a congruent or incongruent story. There were 56 stories: 28 congruent (e.g., a picture of a girl grabbing a pint of milk followed by a picture of the same girl pouring milk in cereal: COherent condition) and 28 noncongruent (e.g., a picture of a girl grabbing a pint of milk followed by a picture of the same girl pouring water into a flower vase: INCOherent condition). The number of correct responses for each condition and the reaction time for each item were recorded. An fMRI blood oxygenation level dependent (BOLD) signal was recorded during performance of the task. A single-shot, gradient-recalled echo-planar imaging sequence (repetition time = 2000 ms, echo time = 30 ms, flip angle = 90 degrees, and matrix 64 × 64 voxels) was used on a MRI Siemens TRIO system at 3.0 Tesla at Institut Universitaire Gériatrique de Montréal (IUGM). The images consisted of 32 continuous axial slices, with a 3 mm × 3 mm in-plane resolution. The slice thickness was 3 mm. During the run, 270 volumes were continuously acquired over a total duration of 540 seconds. A high-resolution T1-weighted scan (1 mm^3 voxel size) was provided for each subject for anatomical coregistration. Prospective acquisition correction was applied to the images for better correction of head movement.

2.3. Data Analysis. Analyses of standardized neurological tests were done on the *T*-scores of all CPT and WCST measures and on raw scores for ACT. A 2 ∗ 2 ANOVA with the diagnosis and sex as between-subjects factors was performed on each measure. Interaction effects and pairwise comparisons were explored using the Bonferroni correction with the alpha level set to 0.05. A log10 transformation was necessary to normalize the forethought data distribution and a 2 ∗ 2 ANCOVA with age as a covariate was performed for the number of correct responses (Hits), number of missed responses (Misses), reaction time (RT), and reaction time per correct responses (RT/Hit) for both the CO and INCO conditions. Previous to performing ANOVAs and ANCOVAs, assumptions of normality, homogeneity of variance, and presence of outliers were checked for each test and none were violated.

The fMRI data were processed using statistical parametric mapping (SPM8, Wellcome Department of Cognitive Neurology, London, UK). Individual cerebral activation of INCO > CO contrast served as the measure of forethought. A 2 × 2 ANCOVA was conducted in SPM8, with diagnosis and sex as independent factors and age as the covariate, to assess level of neural activation related to forethought. Because the literature is quite dispersed regarding the neural deficits in

TABLE 1: Age and IQ of participants with ADHD and typically developing youth (TD).

ADHD	Boys				Girls			
	Mean	SD	Min	Max	Mean	SD	Min	Max
Age	10	2.3	7	15	11	1.51	7	14
K-Bit_Voc	103	13.3	75	130	99	11.6	85	120
K-Bit_mat.	110	16.3	91	150	107	12.8	93	127
K-Bit_total	107	15.3	83	134	103	8	94	115
TD	Boys				Girls			
	Mean	SD	Min	Max	Mean	SD	Min	Max
Age	11	1.2	9	12	11	1.9	7	14
K-Bit_Voc	98	14.3	78	113	107	14.1	72	119
K-Bit_mat.	108	16.3	69	136	118	12.2	96	136
K-Bit_total	103	17.6	74	128	114	13.7	82	129
ANOVA	*F*: Diagnosis	*p*		*F*: Sex	*p*	*F*: Group × Sex		*p*
Age	0.70	0.408		0.72	0.402	0.96		0.332
K-Bit_Voc	0.21	0.651		0.31	0.541	2.40		0.129
K-Bit_mat.	0.69	0.410		0.54	0.465	1.69		0.200
K-Bit_total	0.54	0.466		0.61	0.439	2.60		0.114

Note. K-Bit_Voc, Kaufman brief intelligence test_Vocabulary; K-Bit_mat., Kaufman brief intelligence test_Matrices; TD, typically developing youth; ADHD, youth with attention deficit and hyperactivity disorders.
All *ps* are two-tailed.

ADHD (except for the frontostriatal network hypothesis), a whole brain analysis was conducted. The effects of diagnosis and sex were investigated in the contrasts [TD > ADHD] and [ADHD > TD],and interaction effects in the following simple contrasts: [TD boys > ADHD boys], [TD girls > ADHD girls], [ADHD boys > TD boys], and [ADHD girls > TD girls]. Statistical tests were performed for group comparisons at a threshold level of $p = 0.001$ uncorrected for multiple comparisons with a cluster threshold of 10 voxels. This more liberal threshold was used because the expected effects are broad but weak [25].

3. Results

3.1. Neuropsychological Profiles. Mean composite IQ scores (K-BIT) [24] varied between 103 and 114 and no IQ differences were found between diagnostic groups, sex or group-by-sex interaction (Table 1). Most neuropsychological measures indicated that boys with ADHD were in the mildly atypical clinical range pointing mostly to inattentive symptoms (CPT: omission, Hit RT, Hit RT SE). Their larger T-scores (> 60) on WCST also suggested lower mental flexibility (Table 2). Analysis of CPT indicated several main effects and sex-by-diagnostic interactions. A significant difference of omission was found between boys with ADHD and TD boys ($p = 0.017$) but not between TD girls and girls with ADHD. Regarding Hit RT, higher scores for boys with ADHD compared to girls with ADHD were observed ($p = 0.01$). For the Hit RT SE, the ADHD groups obtained higher scores and, specifically, boys with ADHD obtained significantly higher scores compared to TD boys ($p = 0.016$) and to TD girls ($p = 0.037$). The analysis of Hit RT Block change revealed that boys with ADHD obtained a higher score compared to girls with ADHD ($p = 0.024$) but no difference appeared between girls and boys in the TD group. The same pattern of results occurred with Standard Errors for reaction time over Blocks (Hit SE Block change). Boys with ADHD displayed larger scores compared to girls with ADHD ($p = 0.004$) and to TD girls ($p = 0.003$). A main effect of diagnostic was found for the Standard Error of reaction time slope over different interstimulus intervals (HIT SE ISI change); youth with ADHD demonstrated less consistency compared to TD groups ($p = 0.006$), a tendency more acute in boys with ADHD. The ACT analysis revealed a lesser performance for the groups with ADHD ($p = 0.013$) but no sex difference nor interaction between sex*diagnostic group was observed. No subtest of WCST was statistically significant in terms of group differences (for brevity, we did not include these data in Table 2).

3.2. Forethought Performance. Behavioral performance results are presented in Table 3. No significant difference was found in the number of correct answers. However, reaction times (RT) analyses revealed group differences. For the CO condition, the TD group provided systematically faster responses (RT) ($p = 0.003$) and faster RT per hit ($p = 0.008$) compared to the group with ADHD. For the INCO condition, the TD group demonstrated marginally faster RT Inco/Hits compared to the ADHD group ($p = 0.073$). Although neither sex nor interaction effects were found, boys with ADHD showed systematically longer reaction times compared to girls with ADHD.

3.3. Neural Correlates of Forethought. Cerebral activation findings are presented in Table 4. The diagnostic group contrast (TD > ADHD) showed significantly more activation

TABLE 2: Neuropsychological profile of participants with ADHD and typically developing youth (TD).

	ADHD boys		ADHD girls		TD boys		TD girls		F-value		
ACT	Mean	SD	Mean	SD	Mean	SD	Mean	SD	*F*: group	*F*: sex	*F*: (G) × (S)
Total	32.13	11.2	44.50	8.4	48.44	8.3	48.50	15.9	5.35**	2.00	1.86
CPT											
Omission	58.11	9.8	47.18	3.7	45.68	7.3	49.07	11.3	3.05	1.56	5.63*
Commission	53.54	5.4	56.78	6.3	46.58	21	59.96	18.5	0.16	3.10	1.16
Hit RT	58.42	12.3	40.42	5.2	48.89	6.9	48.21	13.5	0.06	6.65*	5.73*
Hit RT SE	61.46	10.5	49.42	11.1	47.10	7.8	49.56	12.1	4.21*	1.91	4.37*
Hit RT ISI	62.83	16.1	51.24	9.5	53.18	12.6	52.05	12.7	0.97	2.01	1.36
Hit SE ISI	59.48	11.7	55.24	11.5	45.09	9.5	49.67	8.8	8.51**	0.00	1.69
Hit RT Block	60.45	11.3	48.2	13.4	50.07	13.6	48.77	11.9	0.47	5.96*	4.38*
Hit SE Block	59.08	7.9	40.95	11.3	48.88	11.7	49.11	7.53	0.12	9.46*	9.96*

Note. ACT, Auditory Consonant Trigrams test; CPT, Continuous Performance Task; omission, number of times the subject fails to respond when target was presented; commission, number of response in absence of target; Hit RT, overall reaction time; Hit RT Block, slope of change in RTs over the six time blocks; Hit SE Block, slope of change in RTs standard errors over the six time blocks; Hit RT ISI, slope of change in RTs over the three interstimulus intervals; Hit SE ISI, slope of change in RTs SE over the three ISI; *F*: group corresponds to the Fisher test comparing youth with ADHD to youth without; *F*: sex corresponds to the Fisher test comparing boys to girls and *F*(G × S) corresponds to the Fisher measure observed for the interaction between the group and the sex.
*$p < 0.05$; **$p < 0.01$; all *p*s are two-tailed.

TABLE 3: Forethought performance in participants with ADHD and typically developing (TD) youth.

Measures	ADHD boys		ADHD girls		TD boys		TD girls		2 × 2 ANCOVA		
	Mean	SD	Mean	SD	Mean	SD	Mean	SD	*F*: (G)	*F*: (S)	*F*: (G) × (S)
Co_hit	24.19	6.0	26.14	1.95	27.33	0.71	27	1.04	0.87	0.03	0.49
Co_miss	2.63	5.9	1.14	1.22	0.44	0.53	0.5	0.91	3.29	0.08	0.21
RT_Co	1412	256	1407	555	931.5	180	1150	270	10.02**	2.49	0.97
RT Co/hit	74.94	69.8	55.15	26.7	34.07	6.48	42.73	10.3	7.93**	0.87	1.39
Inco_hit	23.38	6.5	26	1.9	27.22	0.8	26.75	1.2	0.74	0.07	0.53
Inco_miss	2.81	6.5	1.14	1.5	0.33	0.5	0.92	1.1	0.98	0.12	0.57
RT_Inco	1474	605	1341	551	996.6	228	1255	310	2.93	1.86	1.36
RT Inco/hit	95.9	134	52.49	24.6	36.59	8.14	47.22	12.9	3.38†	0.40	1.88

Note. Co_hit, good answer in authorized delay for coherent condition; Inco_hit, good answer in authorized delay for incoherent condition; Co_miss, error in authorized delay for coherent condition; Inco_miss, error in authorized delay for incoherent condition; RT_Co, mean reaction time (ms.) for coherent condition; RT Co/hit, mean reaction time (ms.) per hit for coherent condition; RT_Inco, mean reaction time (ms) for incoherent condition; RT Inco/hit, mean reaction (ms.) per hit for incoherent condition; *F*: group corresponds to the Fisher test comparing youth with ADHD to youth without; *F*: sex corresponds to the Fisher test comparing boys to girls and *F*(G × S) corresponds to the Fisher measure observed for the interaction between the group and the sex.
**$p < 0.01$; † = 0.07; all *p*s are two-tailed.

in the right parietal postcentral gyrus (BA 1), left cingulate gyrus (BA 24), right middle frontal gyrus (MFG, BA 6), and the right culmen (cerebellum). No significant activation was observed in the opposite contrast (ADHD > TD). Relative to TD boys, boys with ADHD had extensive bilateral frontal and parietal hypoactivation, including bilateral superior frontal gyrus (BA 6), left inferior parietal lobule (IPL; BA 40), and right superior parietal lobule (SPL; BA 7). Boys with ADHD were also found to activate significantly more the right amygdala and left superior temporal gyrus than TD boys. Girls with ADHD demonstrated more scattered neural hypoactivation in comparison to TD girls including the right culmen, the right postcentral gyrus (BA 2), right middle temporal gyrus (MTG; BA 21), left claustrum (basal ganglia), and right inferior frontal gyrus (BA 47-10). There was no significant activation for the opposite contrast (ADHD girls > TD girls).

4. Discussion

Our expectations that ADHD boys would demonstrate more deficits than ADHD girls in sustained and selective attention and in cerebral activation during forethought were partially supported by the present study. Indeed, ADHD boys expressed greater inattentiveness, greater impulsivity, and lesser vigilance than TD boys, while ADHD girls did not differ from TD girls. Boys with ADHD also showed greater variability. Overall, WM capacities were lower in ADHD relative to TD group, confirming previous reports [3, 10]. Moreover, diagnosis by sex interactions observed on several occasions were compatible with studies reporting that boys with ADHD usually show more severe inattention symptoms [4] and greater executive deficits than girls with ADHD [15].

Table 4: Brain activations during forethought: contrast INCO-CO in participants with ADHD and typically developing (TD) youth.

Comparison/region	K (voxel)	Z value	MNI x	MNI y	MNI z	p value
TD-ADHD						
Right parietal postcentral gyrus, BA 1	124	4.42	66	−22	40	0.000
Left cingulate gyrus, BA 24	126	3.69	−3	−4	46	0.000
Right middle frontal gyrus, BA 6	92	4.10	27	−7	67	0.000
Right anterior lobe, culmen	64	3.62	30	−52	−32	0.000
ADHD-TD						
No voxel activated						
TD boys-ADHD boys						
Bilateral superior frontal gyrus, BA 6	3300	4.36	−18	−4	58	0.000
Left inferior parietal lobule, BA 40	158	3.81	−66	−34	31	0.000
Right superior parietal lobule, BA 7	110	3.22	12	−64	61	0.001
ADHD boys-TD boys						
Right amygdala	578	3.18	39	−4	−20	0.001
Left superior temporal gyrus	114	3.15	−39	8	−23	0.001
TD girls-ADHD girls						
Right cerebellum, culmen	549	3.61	69	−22	34	0.000
Right, postcentral gyrus, BA 2	180	3.25	30	−55	−29	0.001
Right middle temporal gyrus, BA 21	137	3.70	57	−55	−1	0.000
Left claustrum	38	3.25	−24	26	−8	0.001
Right frontal gyrus, BA 10	32	3.15	45	53	1	0.001
Right, inferior frontal gyrus, BA 47	21	3.03	33	20	−20	0.001
ADHD girls-TD girls						
No voxel activated						

Note. Minimum cluster threshold = 10 voxels; TD, typically developing youth; ADHD, youth with attention deficit and hyperactivity disorders; INCO-CO, contrast between incoherent and coherent conditions; MNI, Montreal Neurological Institute; BA, Brodmann Area; K (voxel) gives the number of voxels in each cluster; the Z value is the Z-score given for that specific cluster with its p value associated; x, y, z corresponds to the x, y, z MNI coordinates of the most central voxel of the cluster.

4.1. Forethought. The ADHD participants showed a tendency to be slower, but as accurate as the TD group on the forethought task. The forethought slowness was apparent especially in boys and was coherent with the CPT findings. As expected, extensive brain activation was observed in the TD group, including parietal and prefrontal regions as well as part of the cingulate gyrus and the cerebellum, during the forethought task performance. In contrast, the ADHD group showed no neural activation during forethought. This finding is consistent with reports of attenuated cerebral activation in ADHD tapping cognitive control [26, 27], working memory [2], and inhibition and vigilance/attention [28]. Overall, our study confirms the hypothesis of impairment in the frontal-parietal pathway in ADHD [11, 12, 28]. Lateral portions of the PFC are part of the attentional network [29] and thus it is plausible that its malfunction is responsible for the encountered forethought slowness. Moreover, cerebral hypoactivation in ADHD youth is in accordance with their greater inattention and lack of vigilance, as well as weaker working memory.

4.2. Boys with ADHD. TD boys showed more extensive bilateral frontal activation relative to boys with ADHD, including the premotor cortex and the supplementary motor area (SMA). Our results are compatible with findings observed in TD adolescent groups [11, 19, 28] although no sex differentiation was made in these studies. Premotor cortex and SMA are involved in motor sequencing and planning [30], working memory [31], and visuospatial attention [32]. All these functions are essential for optimal performance of forethought. Moreover, hypoactivation of the SMA and the superior frontal gyrus has been accounted for motoric hyperactivity in ADHD [28].

TD boys also exhibited greater activation in the bilateral parietal cortex, left IPL and right SPL, relative to ADHD boys. The SPL is involved in visual representation of movements [33] and in WM related to motor sequence performance [34]. Thus, hypoactivation of SPL in boys with ADHD could have contributed to their impairment of forethought due to its link with WM. Similar results were observed by Dickstein et al. (2006) [11] where controls demonstrated significantly greater activation relative to ADHD in the left prefrontal and bilateral parietal lobes (IPL and SPL). The inferior part of SPL is related to inhibition, WM, and attention processes [28], all components of forethought. This region is part of the ventral attention network (VAN) that supports reorientation to behaviorally relevant external stimuli [35]. Thus, a deficient engagement of the VAN in ADHD may account for difficulties in adequately shifting attention to salient external stimuli [36]. Moreover, hypoactivation in VAN underpins ADHD-related deficits in detecting irregularities in the environment [28]. These considerations are relevant considering the present impairment in forethought, which involves a reflection on an incongruent succession of events.

Furthermore, boys with ADHD were found to hyperactivate a region adjacent to the medial temporal lobe, which is a part of the default mode network (DMN). This region was previously found to be hyperactivated in children with ADHD [28]. Fluctuations in activation of the DMN tend to correlate negatively with fluctuations in networks activated during task performance, typically the frontoparietal attention network [37]. The current findings in ADHD boys corroborate this pattern of activation. Indeed, their lesser functioning of the frontoparietal network might have impacted the DMN, resulting in disruption of the ongoing forethought performance. Together with the CPT results, this finding supports the recent perspective suggesting a link between variability and intrusion of "task-negative brain network" [38]. According to this perspective, RT variability is related to increased activity in DMN. The present study also supports the increasing recognition of motivational and emotional dysfunction in models of ADHD [39]. Boys with ADHD possibly perceived the task as more difficult or unpleasant, as it required a certain amount of time staying still and attentive, so that they had to rely on more activation of the amygdala to provide sufficient motivation.

4.3. Girls with ADHD. TD girls demonstrated widespread cerebral activation and there were no differences found for the ADHD girls > TD girls contrast. TD girls activated large portions of the cerebellum (culmen), a region activated in response to temporally unexpected stimuli [18]. There is mounting evidence that the basal ganglia and the cerebellum might project directly to one another [40, 41]. Interestingly, both regions were activated in TD girls, but not in ADHD girls. Moreover, hypoactivation of the frontocerebellar network in girls with ADHD might have negatively impacted their ability to predict "when" events are going to occur and affect detection of violations of these predictions as suggested by previous studies [42, 43]. Because of its outputs to both the PFC and the basal ganglia, the cerebellum is in position to influence activity in circuits implicated in ADHD [42]. Moreover, because of its protracted development and sexual dimorphism, the cerebellum could play a crucial role in the neuropathology of girls with ADHD [44]. TD girls also activated the middle temporal gyrus (BA 21), a region activated in controls in the Durston et al. (2007) study [18], which investigated expectancy violation in ADHD, a condition similar to the incongruent situation of forethought.

TD girls also activated the claustrum, a region highlighted by Dickstein et al. (2006) [11] as being more activated in controls compared to participants with ADHD during EF performance. According to Crick and Koch (2005) [45], this part of basal ganglia plays a regulatory role in consciousness and cognition. Implication of the basal ganglia in conjunction with other regions might have helped TD girls in selecting the appropriate action and reject an incongruent action. Indeed the basal ganglia is believed to help in deciding among several possible behaviors at any given time [46, 47].

However, to fully establish the primacy of cerebral dysfunction in ADHD, future studies will need to employ a more comprehensive examination of executive function, using tasks known to produce consistent patterns of activity in other regions considered putative sources of dysfunction. Because the forethought task produced specific patterns of activity in boys and girls, our paradigm seems promising in further exploration of sex differences in the neural correlates of ADHD. Recent advances in brain imaging technology (e.g., diffusion tensor imaging and magnetoencephalography) allow us to examine more precisely and directly the relationships between brain regions during a cognitive task. A closer examination of the brain functional and anatomical connectivity would help in identifying entire neural networks underlying cognitive deficits in ADHD. Future research, including girls in the field of ADHD, promises exciting results linking the genomic, structural, and functional changes in the brain of individuals with ADHD. Advances in understanding of the ADHD neurobiology will hopefully help in developing new psychotherapeutic interventions and in identifying more targeted pharmacotherapies so that child psychiatrists can better manage their patients.

In conclusion, the present findings point to greater EF deficits in boys compared to girls with ADHD. Moreover, boys with ADHD exhibited cerebral hypoactivation in the frontoparietal network. On the other hand, they hyperactivated cerebral regions linked to motivation. Taken together, these findings indicate that boys with ADHD show decreased attention processing that seems compensated by the use of supplemental motivation to perform as accurately as their TD counterparts. However, this compensation comes with a time cost. Girls with ADHD displayed more dispersed decreased neural activation in the frontocerebellar and frontoparietal systems compared to the TD girls. This suggests that they rely on different circuits to make decisions about incongruent situations with a related time cost. Overall, the present study supports the hypothesis of different neuropsychological and neurofunctional profiles in boys and girls with ADHD. This brings to light the importance of considering both genders while investigating ADHD in order to better understand the disorder and propose clinical intervention more specific to the gender.

Competing Interests

The authors declare that they have no competing interests.

References

[1] American Psychiatric Association, *Diagnostic and Statistical Manual of Mental Disorders*, American Psychiatric, Arlington, Va, USA, 2013.

[2] E. M. Valera, S. V. Faraone, K. E. Murray, and L. J. Seidman, "Meta-analysis of structural imaging findings in attention-deficit/hyperactivity disorder," *Biological Psychiatry*, vol. 61, no. 12, pp. 1361–1369, 2007.

[3] R. A. Barkley, *Attention-Deficit Hyperactivity Disorder: A Handbook for Diagnosis and Treatment*, Guilford, New York, NY, USA, 3rd edition, 2005.

[4] J. Gershon, "A meta-analytic review of gender differences in ADHD," *Journal of Attention Disorders*, vol. 5, no. 3, pp. 143–154, 2002.

[5] E. W. Skogli, M. H. Teicher, P. N. Andersen, K. T. Hovik, and M. Øie, "ADHD in girls and boys—gender differences in co-existing symptoms and executive function measures," *BMC Psychiatry*, vol. 13, no. 1, article 298, 2013.

[6] J. J. Rucklidge, "Gender differences in attention-deficit/hyperactivity disorder," *Psychiatric Clinics of North America*, vol. 33, no. 2, pp. 357–373, 2010.

[7] S. L. Andersen and M. H. Teicher, "Sex differences in dopamine receptors and their relevance to ADHD," *Neuroscience & Biobehavioral Reviews*, vol. 24, no. 1, pp. 137–141, 2000.

[8] S. Hosenbocus and R. Chahal, "A review of executive function deficits and pharmacological management in children and adolescents," *Journal of the Canadian Academy of Child and Adolescent Psychiatry*, vol. 21, no. 3, pp. 223–229, 2012.

[9] J. E. Schreiber, K. L. Possin, J. M. Girard, and C. Rey-Casserly, "Executive function in children with attention deficit/hyperactivity disorder: the NIH EXAMINER battery," *Journal of the International Neuropsychological Society*, vol. 20, no. 1, pp. 41–51, 2014.

[10] R. Martinussen, J. Hayden, S. Hogg-Johnson, and R. Tannock, "A meta-analysis of working memory impairments in children with attention-deficit/hyperactivity disorder," *Journal of the American Academy of Child & Adolescent Psychiatry*, vol. 44, no. 4, pp. 377–384, 2005.

[11] S. G. Dickstein, K. Bannon, F. Xavier Castellanos, and M. P. Milham, "The neural correlates of attention deficit hyperactivity disorder: an ALE meta-analysis," *Journal of Child Psychology and Psychiatry and Allied Disciplines*, vol. 47, no. 10, pp. 1051–1062, 2006.

[12] K. Rubia, A. B. Smith, R. Halari et al., "Disorder-specific dissociation of orbitofrontal dysfunction in boys with pure conduct disorder during reward and ventrolateral prefrontal dysfunction in boys with pure ADHD during sustained attention," *The American Journal of Psychiatry*, vol. 166, no. 1, pp. 83–94, 2009.

[13] U. P. Ramtekkar, A. M. Reiersen, A. A. Todorov, and R. D. Todd, "Sex and age differences in attention-deficit/hyperactivity disorder symptoms and diagnoses: implications for DSM-V and ICD-11," *Journal of the American Academy of Child and Adolescent Psychiatry*, vol. 49, no. 3, pp. 217.e3–228.e3, 2010.

[14] E. M. Valera, A. Brown, J. Biederman et al., "Sex differences in the functional neuroanatomy of working memory in adults with ADHD," *The American Journal of Psychiatry*, vol. 167, no. 1, pp. 86–94, 2010.

[15] M. A. Sheridan, S. Hinshaw, and M. D'Esposito, "Efficiency of the prefrontal cortex during working memory in attention-deficit/hyperactivity disorder," *Journal of the American Academy of Child & Adolescent Psychiatry*, vol. 46, no. 10, pp. 1357–1366, 2007.

[16] F. E. Dupuy, R. J. Barry, A. R. Clarke, R. McCarthy, and M. Selikowitz, "Sex differences between the combined and inattentive types of attention-deficit/hyperactivity disorder: an EEG perspective," *International Journal of Psychophysiology*, vol. 89, no. 3, pp. 320–327, 2013.

[17] R. A. Barkley, "Attention-deficit/hyperactivity disorder, self-regulation, and executive functioning," in *Handbook of Self-Regulation: Research, Theory, and Applications*, K. D. Vohs and F. B. Roy, Eds., pp. 551–564, Guilford, New York, NY, USA, 2011.

[18] S. Durston, M. C. Davidson, M. J. Mulder et al., "Neural and behavioral correlates of expectancy violations in attention-deficit hyperactivity disorder," *Journal of Child Psychology and Psychiatry and Allied Disciplines*, vol. 48, no. 9, pp. 881–889, 2007.

[19] H. Poissant, A. Mendrek, and N. Senhadji, "Neural correlates of forethought in ADHD," *Journal of Attention Disorders*, vol. 18, no. 3, pp. 258–267, 2014.

[20] H. Poissant and S. Lecomte, "Risk factors in families of children with attention deficit/hyperactivity disorders: Quebec data," *Journal of the Canadian Academy of Child and Adolescent Psychiatry*, vol. 16, no. 1, pp. 9–17, 2007.

[21] C. K. Conners, J. N. Epstein, A. Angold, and J. Klaric, "Continuous performance test performance in a normative epidemiological sample," *Journal of Abnormal Child Psychology*, vol. 31, no. 5, pp. 555–562, 2003.

[22] R. K. Heaton, W. Miller, M. J. Taylor, and I. Grant, *Wisconsin Card Sorting Test*, PAR Staff, 2004.

[23] C. Paniak, H. B. Miller, D. Murphy, A. Andrews, and J. Flynn, "Consonant trigrams test for children: development and norms," *Clinical Neuropsychologist*, vol. 11, no. 2, pp. 198–200, 1997.

[24] A. S. Kaufman and N. L. Kaufman, *Kaufman Brief Intelligence Test*, John Wiley & Sons, New York, NY, USA, 2004.

[25] R. C. Wolf, M. M. Plichta, F. Sambataro et al., "Regional brain activation changes and abnormal functional connectivity of the ventrolateral prefrontal cortex during working memory processing in adults with attention-deficit/hyperactivity disorder," *Human Brain Mapping*, vol. 30, no. 7, pp. 2252–2266, 2009.

[26] K. P. Schulz, J. Fan, C. Y. Tang et al., "Response inhibition in adolescents diagnosed with attention deficit hyperactivity disorder during childhood: an event-related fMRI study," *The American Journal of Psychiatry*, vol. 161, no. 9, pp. 1650–1657, 2004.

[27] S. J. Suskauer, D. J. Simmonds, S. Fotedar et al., "Functional magnetic resonance imaging evidence for abnormalities in response selection in attention deficit hyperactivity disorder: differences in activation associated with response inhibition but not habitual motor response," *Journal of Cognitive Neuroscience*, vol. 20, no. 3, pp. 478–493, 2008.

[28] S. Cortese, C. Kelly, C. Chabernaud et al., "Toward systems neuroscience of ADHD: a meta-analysis of 55 fMRI studies," *The American Journal of Psychiatry*, vol. 169, no. 10, pp. 1038–1055, 2012.

[29] J. M. Shine, G. M. Halliday, S. L. Naismith, and S. J. G. Lewis, "Visual misperceptions and hallucinations in Parkinson's disease: dysfunction of attentional control networks?" *Movement Disorders*, vol. 26, no. 12, pp. 2154–2159, 2011.

[30] A. Bischoff-Grethe, K. M. Goedert, D. T. Willingham, and S. T. Grafton, "Neural substrates of response-based sequence learning using fMRI," *Journal of Cognitive Neuroscience*, vol. 16, no. 1, pp. 127–138, 2004.

[31] C. Ranganath, M. K. Johnson, and M. D'Esposito, "Prefrontal activity associated with working memory and episodic long-term memory," *Neuropsychologia*, vol. 41, no. 3, pp. 378–389, 2003.

[32] A. C. Nobre, G. N. Sebestyen, D. R. Gitelman, M. M. Mesulam, R. S. J. Frackowiak, and C. D. Frith, "Functional localization of

the system for visuospatial attention using positron emission tomography," *Brain*, vol. 120, no. 3, pp. 515–533, 1997.

[33] A. Solodkin, P. Hlustik, E. E. Chen, and S. L. Small, "Fine modulation in network activation during motor execution and motor imagery," *Cerebral Cortex*, vol. 14, no. 11, pp. 1246–1255, 2004.

[34] M. J. Catalan, M. Honda, R. A. Weeks, L. G. Cohen, and M. Hallett, "The functional neuroanatomy of simple and complex sequential finger movements: a PET study," *Brain*, vol. 121, no. 2, pp. 253–264, 1998.

[35] M. Corbetta, G. Patel, and G. L. Shulman, "The reorienting system of the human brain: from environment to theory of mind," *Neuron*, vol. 58, no. 3, pp. 306–324, 2008.

[36] P. Helenius, M. Laasonen, L. Hokkanen, R. Paetau, and M. Niemivirta, "Neural correlates of late positivities associated with infrequent visual events and response errors," *NeuroImage*, vol. 53, no. 2, pp. 619–628, 2010.

[37] E. J. S. Sonuga-Barke, "Editorial: ADHD as a reinforcement disorder—moving from general effects to identifying (six) specific models to test," *Journal of Child Psychology and Psychiatry*, vol. 52, no. 9, pp. 917–918, 2011.

[38] L. Tamm, M. E. Narad, T. N. Antonini, K. M. O'Brien, L. W. Hawk Jr., and J. N. Epstein, "Reaction time variability in ADHD: a review," *Neurotherapeutics*, vol. 9, no. 3, pp. 500–508, 2012.

[39] E. J. S. Sonuga-Barke and F. X. Castellanos, "Spontaneous attentional fluctuations in impaired states and pathological conditions: a neurobiological hypothesis," *Neuroscience & Biobehavioral Reviews*, vol. 31, no. 7, pp. 977–986, 2007.

[40] A. C. Bostan, R. P. Dum, and P. L. Strick, "The basal ganglia communicate with the cerebellum," *Proceedings of the National Academy of Sciences of the United States of America*, vol. 107, no. 18, pp. 8452–8456, 2010.

[41] E. Hoshi, L. Tremblay, J. Féger, P. L. Carras, and P. L. Strick, "The cerebellum communicates with the basal ganglia," *Nature Neuroscience*, vol. 8, no. 11, pp. 1491–1493, 2005.

[42] S. Durston, J. van Belle, and P. de Zeeuw, "Differentiating frontostriatal and fronto-cerebellar circuits in attention-deficit/hyperactivity disorder," *Biological Psychiatry*, vol. 69, no. 12, pp. 1178–1184, 2011.

[43] R. B. Ivry and R. M. C. Spencer, "The neural representation of time," *Current Opinion in Neurobiology*, vol. 14, no. 2, pp. 225–232, 2004.

[44] H. Tiemeier, R. K. Lenroot, D. K. Greenstein, L. Tran, R. Pierson, and J. N. Giedd, "Cerebellum development during childhood and adolescence: a longitudinal morphometric MRI study," *NeuroImage*, vol. 49, no. 1, pp. 63–70, 2010.

[45] F. C. Crick and C. Koch, "What is the function of the claustrum?" *Philosophical Transactions of the Royal Society B: Biological Sciences*, vol. 360, no. 1458, pp. 1271–1279, 2005.

[46] A. Stocco, C. Lebiere, and J. R. Anderson, "Conditional routing of information to the cortex: a model of the basal Ganglia's role in cognitive coordination," *Psychological Review*, vol. 117, no. 2, pp. 541–574, 2010.

[47] V. S. Chakravarthy, D. Joseph, and R. S. Bapi, "What do the basal ganglia do? A modeling perspective," *Biological Cybernetics*, vol. 103, no. 3, pp. 237–253, 2010.

21

Patients' Experience of Winter Depression and Light Room Treatment

Cecilia Rastad,[1,2] Lennart Wetterberg,[3] and Cathrin Martin[1]

[1]*Department of Neuroscience, Uppsala University, Uppsala, Sweden*
[2]*Center for Clinical Research Dalarna (CKF), Falun, Sweden*
[3]*Department of Clinical Neuroscience, Karolinska Institute, St. Göran, Stockholm, Sweden*

Correspondence should be addressed to Cecilia Rastad; cecilia.rastad@ltdalarna.se

Academic Editor: Ulrich Schweiger

Background. There is a need for more knowledge on the effects of light room treatment in patients with seasonal affective disorder and to explore patients' subjective experience of the disease and the treatment. *Methods.* This was a descriptive and explorative study applying qualitative content analysis. A purposeful sample of 18 psychiatric outpatients with a major depressive disorder with a seasonal pattern and a pretreatment score ≥12 on the 9-item Montgomery-Åsberg Depression self-rating scale was included (10 women and 8 men, aged 24–65 years). All patients had completed light room treatment (≥7/10 consecutive weekdays). Data was collected two weeks after treatment using a semistructured interview guide. *Results.* Patients described a clear seasonal pattern and a profound struggle to adapt to seasonal changes during the winter, including deterioration in sleep, daily rhythms, energy level, mood, activity, and cognitive functioning. Everyday life was affected with reduced work capacity, social withdrawal, and disturbed relations with family and friends. The light room treatment resulted in a radical and rapid improvement in all the major symptoms with only mild and transient side effects. *Discussion.* The results indicate that light room treatment is essential for some patients' ability to cope with seasonal affective disorder.

1. Introduction

The clinical features of seasonal affective disorder (SAD) were first described in 1984 in the classic study by Rosenthal et al. [1]. In the Diagnostic and Statistical Manual of Mental Disorders (DSM-5) [2], depression with a seasonal pattern is classified as a subtype of major depressive disorder or bipolar disorder. A diagnosis requires having these experiences for at least two years, a depression that regularly begins and ends during a specific season, no episodes of depression during the season in which the patient experiences normal mood (past two years), and more seasons with than seasons without depression over the lifetime of the illness. In this study, the concept winter depression is used interchangeably with SAD-winter type.

The prevalence of SAD varies between 1% and 2.4% in general population samples [3, 4]. A number of studies have shown that approximately 10–20% of the general population in northern countries report similar but less impairing symptoms [5, 6]. These persons suffer from subsyndromal SAD (winter fatigue) and not major depression [7]. Winter fatigue is associated with lower ratings of health-related quality of life [8, 9]. Reviews on the neurobiology of SAD are published elsewhere [10–13].

A nonpharmacological treatment for SAD is light therapy (LT) [1, 14]. Despite a number of studies over the years, the evidence for LT remains an unresolved issue. Some maintain that it is the first-line therapy for SAD [15, 16], but in Sweden it is not approved as an evidence-based treatment [17]. In a review of randomized placebo-controlled trials, eight studies of LT in SAD and two studies of LT in nonseasonal depression were included [18]. In all these studies, only light boxes were used and the treatment effects were restricted to short-term effects. In conclusion, the authors considered the evidence "not unequivocal" [18]. A recent randomized, double-blind, placebo- and sham-controlled trial of patients with nonseasonal depression (n = 122) reported that LT was an effective treatment both as a monotherapy and in combination with

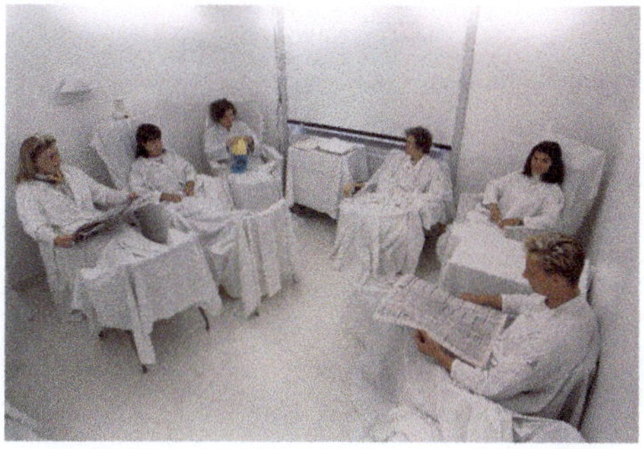

FIGURE 1: Illustration of light treatment in a room comparable to those used in the present study. Volunteers from the medical staff have in the photograph replaced the patients to keep the participants' privacy (by consent of the photographer Stig-Göran Nilsson).

antidepressant medication [19]. In one study by Lam et al., LT and antidepressant medication in patients with SAD were equally effective in reducing depressed mood [20].

Most clinical studies evaluating the effects of LT have used light boxes and portable devices used for treatment in patients' home [14]. In Swedish public health care, light therapy is also provided in light rooms (Figure 1). The light room was designed by professor Wetterberg and colleagues at the Karolinska Institute in Stockholm during the 1970s primarily for research of endocrine responses to light in humans [21]. This setting was further developed into light rooms for treatment studies in the 1980s and 1990s. The advantages of light rooms were improved control of treatment compliance and the ability to treat several patients at the same time and under similar light conditions [7, 22, 23]. Light rooms for research purposes of SAD were also introduced in Finland during the same time period [24].

There are some differences in the setting between treatment at home using a light box and treatment in a light room that is situated in a health care environment [7], which is why the results of clinical trials with light boxes cannot automatically be transferred to the light room settings [8, 22, 25, 26]. In a study with a factorial experimental design by Thalén and coworkers, the effects of light room treatment were compared in two diagnostic subgroups under the same light conditions [26]. The treatment effect in patients with SAD was larger compared to those with non-SAD, suggesting a more explicit effect of light room treatment in patients with SAD [26]. In a controlled clinical study by Rastad and coauthors, patients with SAD were randomized to light room treatment or a three-week waiting list followed by light room treatment [25]. A total of 54% in the experimental condition improved ≥50%, while no such improvement was seen in the control condition. After merging the two groups at the one-month follow-up, 83% had improved ≥50% and 64% were within the normal range in depression scores [25].

In a Cochrane review 2015, it was concluded that comparative evidence regarding LT versus other treatment options for preventing winter depression is limited [27]. The authors therefore recommend that the selection of treatment should be strongly based on patient preferences. What do we know about the patients' perspective on light treatment? One way to explore the subject of patient preferences is to use qualitative research designs. When this study was planned, there were no previous publications exploring the patients' subjective experience of light room treatment.

A starting point for the study was the biopsychosocial model [28]. This model, in addition to a biomedical model, includes a combination of biological, psychological, and social factors in order to obtain a broader description and understanding of the patients' perspective.

The aim of this study was to explore and to describe the patients' subjective experience of the disease seasonal affective disorder and the treatment in a light room.

2. Method

2.1. Design. This was a descriptive and explorative study applying qualitative content analysis in accordance with the procedures described by Graneheim and Lundman [29].

2.2. Participants and Procedure. A purposeful sample of 19 patients with seasonal affective disorder (SAD) referred to a psychiatric outpatient clinic in Stockholm was included. The clinic is situated at latitude 60°N. One patient left the study for personal reasons. Thus, the final sample consisted of 18 patients: 10 women and 8 men, aged 24–65 years (Md = 41 years) (Table 1).

Inclusion criteria were a history of major depressive disorder with a winter seasonal pattern (subtype) according to the diagnostic manual DSM-IV [30], ≥18 years of age, being able to participate in an interview conducted in Swedish, a pretreatment scoring ≥12 on the Montgomery-Åsberg Depression Rating Scale self-rating version (MADRS-S), and having completed treatment in the light room (≥7–10 consecutive weekdays). Four patients scheduled for preventative treatment were included (N = 4/18) and, for these patients, the inclusion criteria regarding depressed mood (MADRS-S) were not applied. Patients with a bipolar disorder, delusional disorder, severe personality, or eating disorder or with current abuse were excluded.

A registered nurse (RN) at the psychiatric outpatient clinic gave oral and written information about the project and asked possible informants about participation in the study. An experienced psychiatrist (LW) made the final inclusion of informants based on information from the referral, the patient record, and the total score on the pretreatment MADRS-S. The RN was responsible for the treatment in the light rooms and the registration of attendance at each session. The interviews (conducted by CR) were carried out during the two winter seasons (Oct–Feb) 2012-2013 and (Nov–March) 2013-2014. The self-report questionnaires were filled out during the first day and the last day of the treatment at the psychiatric outpatient clinic. The demographic background data were collected at the first day of the treatment. The two-week posttreatment questionnaires and a prepaid return envelope were sent by mail to the informant's home address at the time of the interview with a letter requesting the informants to fill out the form and return it by mail within a week.

Table 1: Overview of the informants' background characteristics: sex, civil status, employment, sick leave, medication, previous number of years with winter depression, previous light therapy, preventative treatment or not, and scores on the Montgomery-Åsberg Depression Rating Scale, self-rating version (MADRS-S) before treatment, at posttreatment, and at two weeks after treatment ($N = 18$).

Age (y)	Sex	Civil status[1]	Employment[2] (%)	Sick leave[3] (%)	Antidepressants[4] (Yes/No)	Other current medications[5] (Nb)	Previous winter depression[6] (y)	Previous light therapy[7] (y)	Preventative treatment[8] (Yes/No)	Pretreatment MADRS-S[8] (total)	Posttreatment MADRS-S[8] (total)	2 weeks after treatment MADRS-S[8] (total)
62	Male	Live apart	100	0	No	0	5-6	2	Yes	0	0	3
64	Female	Live apart	Retired	0	Yes	9	20–30	0	No	24	23	3
24	Male	Married	100	0	No	0	6	0	Yes	10	9	x[9]
60	Female	Married	No	75	Yes	2	8–10	0	No	25	18	3
48	Male	Married	Student	0	Yes	3	29	4	No	15	3	1
28	Female	Married	100	0	No	0	14	0	No	12	4	9
65	Female	Single	Retired	0	No	2	26	0	No	30	0	10
58	Male	Single	Retired	0	Yes	2	24	0	No	30	10	8
41	Female	Married	100	0	No	0	20	5	No	22	7	1
41	Male	Married	100	0	Yes	1	2	0	No	23	8	1
47	Male	Single	Job-seeker	0	Yes	0	10–12	6–8	Yes	0	1	0
37	Female	Married	50	0	Yes	1	20	0	Yes	1	2	x[9]
30	Female	Live apart	100	0	No	0	15	0	No	13	10	4
29	Male	Single	Student	0	Yes	1	13	0	No	16	3	0
44	Male	Married	25	75	Yes	4	15	0	No	20	25	x[9]
41	Female	Single	No	100	Yes	4	24	5-6	No	21	20	7
38	Female	Single	No	75	Yes	3	24	0	No	17	17	x[9]
33	Female	Single	50	0	No	0	4	0	No	14	9	9

[1]Married/cohabitant, single/divorced, or living apart.
[2]Employment full-time 75–100%, part-time ≤50%, job-seeker, retired, or student.
[3]On sick leave full-time 75–100%, part-time <50%, or no sick leave.
[4]Current antidepressive medication.
[5]Other current psychiatric and/or somatic medications.
[6]Informants' retrospective estimate of number of years with winter depression.
[7]Previous experience of bright light treatment (number of years).
[8]The Montgomery-Åsberg Depression Rating Scale, self-rating version (MADRS-S), Svanborg and Åsberg (2001).
[9]Data missing.

Sampling was stopped when a preliminary evaluation suggested that adding more informants would not elicit any fundamentally new information not already provided by previous informants [31]. The Regional Ethical Review Board in Stockholm, Sweden, approved this study (Dnr 2012/1-31/3) before its start. The study was conducted in accordance with the Declaration of Helsinki (1964).

2.3. Measures. In this study, the 9-item patient-administered self-rating version of the MADRS (MADR-S) [32–34] was used. The items concern sadness, inner tension, reduced sleep and appetite, concentration difficulties, lassitude, inability to feel, pessimistic thought, and suicidal thought. Each item is scored between 0 (no symptoms) and 6 (severe symptoms). The total score ranges between 0 and 54. *Attrition.* The few single missing values ($N = 2$) on the pretreatment MADRS-S were imputed using the median value. There were no missing values on the posttreatment MADRS-S. The few single missing values ($N = 3$) in the two weeks after treatment MADRS-S were imputed with the value from the previous measurement (the posttreatment MADRS-S). There was a total of 4/18 missing MADRS-S at two weeks after treatment.

2.4. The Light Room Treatment. The light room treatment was provided at a psychiatric outpatient clinic in the western part of Stockholm. The walls in the light rooms were painted in white/light colors and the furniture was covered with white sheets. Patients rested comfortably in armchairs in small groups reading, talking, or just relaxing (Figure 1). Treatment was given daily for 2 h on weekdays (between 8 and 12 am) during the period from October to March. A minority of informants preferred shorter treatments between 1 and 2 h. Shaded fluorescent tubes with 6500 Kelvin, $R_0$94 rendering average, reflecting the light on the ceiling and on the walls provided the configuration of the light source. Light intensity was 350 candela/m^2 (1500 lux at eye level, measured 0.8 meters above the floor).

2.5. The Interview. A semistructured interview guide (The Interview Guide) was used during the telephone interviews (CR) covering the two areas of interest. Follow-up questions (e.g., "can you tell more" and "can you give an example") were used to clarify or to go in more depth on the experiences related to the research objectives. A pilot interview was included in the analysis with only minor changes in the interview guide. The interviews lasted between 20 and 60 min (Md 33 min).

The Interview Guide

Light room treatment:

(1) Is this the first time you have had light therapy or have you tried it before?

(2) Can you explain in as much detail as possible how you experienced the treatment?

(3) What is the best thing and worst thing about light therapy in your experience?

(4) Do you remember any time in the past when you felt that you really benefited from light therapy?

(5) Describe an occasion when you had a negative experience of the treatment.

(6) Do you think your life and everyday activities are affected by the treatment?

Seasonal affective disorder:

(7) Can you describe how you feel affected by the different seasons of the year?

(8) Can you describe an occasion when you found winter depression was especially hard?

(9) Can you do anything yourself to affect how you feel and cope during the winter months?

(10) Do you have winter depression in your own opinion?

2.6. Data Analysis. The interviews were transcribed verbatim [35] and analyzed with qualitative content analysis [29]. First, all interviews were read repeatedly to obtain a general impression of the content. Second, the parts of the interviews related to the research objectives were marked, extracted, and labeled with a condensed description of the meaning (meaning unit). Third, the meaning units were divided into subcategories and categories. The division into subcategories and categories was repeated and rearranged several times by the first author in collaboration with the coauthors until agreement was obtained [29]. Through this process of reflection and discussion, the final themes, categories, and subcategories were agreed upon (Tables 2 and 3). For the purpose of illustration, citations in the form of condensed meaning units, that is, excluding repeats, were used in Results [29]. Interviews and content analysis were performed in Swedish. An experienced, bilingual translator translated the citations into English.

2.7. Trustworthiness. In order to increase credibility and transferability, we strived to capture a variety of experiences by heterogeneity among participants regarding sex, severity of depression, and previous experience of light room treatment. The rich variation in the data suggests that the sampling procedure was relevant. The presentation of the informants' background characteristics (Table 1) makes it possible for the reader to evaluate the extent to which the findings can be transferable to another sample. Trustworthiness was increased through dialogue with subsequent agreement between coresearchers (researcher triangulation) [29]. The clinical and research experience among the authors was considered of importance for the planning of the study and the analysis. The first author (CR) has more than 20 years of experience from clinical work as a registered physiotherapist in psychiatric outpatient health care and 9 years of clinical experience with light room treatment. The second author (LW) is a psychiatrist with extensive research experience and is the founder of the light room treatment. The third author's (CM) research area has been primarily in social sciences and qualitative method.

TABLE 2: Overview of the results regarding patients' experience of seasonal affective disorder: one main theme, three categories, and 19 subcategories ($N = 18$).

Theme	Categories	Subcategories
Struggling to adapt to the inevitable	A clear seasonal pattern	The shift, early signals Discover the pattern Fall into the black hole and be trapped in the darkness Problems with sleep and daily rhythms Lack of energy, overwhelming tiredness, and inactivity Depressed mood Changes in food habits and weight To feel "alive" only half of the year
Struggling to adapt to the inevitable	Consequences for everyday life	Difficulties to meet the expectations of everyday life Disturbed relationships with family and friends Reduced work capacity The dilemma, lack of a legitimate diagnosis and treatment
Struggling to adapt to the inevitable	Coping strategies	Wait and see and hope for the best Maintain physical and outdoor activities, helpful but difficult Give priority to work and reduce social contacts and recreational activities Travel abroad Consider the pros and cons of antidepressants Psychotherapy Light room treatment

TABLE 3: Overview of the results regarding the patients' experience of the light room treatment: three categories and 11 subcategories ($N = 18$).

Categories	Subcategories
Positive treatment effects	A radical and sudden transformation Increased energy and activity Improvement in mood and thinking Improvement in sleep and daily rhythms Positive changes in food habits
The importance of a good environment	A calming and relaxing experience The need for mutual respect and silence The physical environment
Negative experiences	Initial side effects Insufficient treatment effects Treatment is time-consuming

3. Results

3.1. Patients' Experience of Winter Depression. The analysis of patients' experience of seasonal affective disorder resulted in one main theme, *"struggling to adapt to the inevitable,"* three categories, and 19 subcategories (Table 2). Categories and subcategories are described below and illustrated with quotations. The numeral following each quotation refers to the informants. An overview of the informants is presented in Table 1.

3.1.1. A Clear Seasonal Pattern. In the late summer or beginning of the fall, informants described that they *became aware of the seasonal shift in the form of a signal, a personal symptom that functioned as a marker* for worse times soon to come. It was described as a sudden recognition of a thought, a feeling, or a change in behavior. "It creeps up on you when it starts getting cold outside or when the nights start drawing in. Sometimes it just takes someone to say, 'Oh, how lovely now that autumn is on the way' to make me think, 'ugh, it's soon autumn.' I'm engulfed in a feeling of unease for a few moments, a feeling which then creeps up on me more and more." (3)

It is the experience of a clear difference in feelings, thoughts, and behavior between the summer season and the winter season over longer periods that constitute the pattern. To *discover the pattern* therefore takes several years. "I manage to do much more in the summer, especially after work. I have more energy. That is the most obvious difference. Things like meeting friends, taking exercise or just being outdoors and going for a walk and enjoying the light of an evening. Those are things I don't do in the winter." (13) The depressions vary over the years. "I've felt the change of season for some thirty years. But I've not been depressed for thirty years; rather, it's been the last eight to ten years that I've found every autumn really difficult." (2) Some of the informants experienced seasonal depressions that continued for 1 or 2 months, while other informants were depressed for 6 or 7 months each year. "It starts September, October time. But January, February... February is my absolute worst month. It's like I have no go in me, there's no ray of hope anywhere." (6)

During the summer when feeling well, the informants "forgot" about the winter depression. When it came back, it was described as hitting a wall or *falling into a black hole and being trapped in the darkness*. "This winter was like hitting a damn wall when the darkness set in. It's pitch black when you wake up, pitch black when you go to work, pitch black when you come home. I get panicky. It feels like someone's pulled a bag down over my head and I can't breathe. I feel completely enclosed in darkness." (18)

Some of the informants described severe *sleep problems and disturbance of daily rhythms* during the winter period. The problems with sleep often preceded the depressive symptoms. Sleep problems included difficulties going to sleep, maintaining sleep, frequent arousals, and having major difficulties getting up in the morning. Others suffered mainly from hypersomnia; however, sleeping for 10–12 h did not relieve daytime fatigue. "Worst of all is the extreme tiredness, and the feeling that more than anything I want to sleep like a bear until I come out of hibernation in April." (16) The informants described a feeling that internal and external time was poorly synchronized during the winter period, being more alert in the late evening and extremely tired in the afternoon. "My rhythm is completely at odds with the actual time." (13)

A pronounced lack of energy, an overwhelming feeling of tiredness, and inactivity were major problems for the informants during the winter. The feelings of energy, vitality, and joie de vivre experienced during the summer season flowed away and were lost. This pronounced lack of energy resulted in difficulties initiating and completing ordinary, daily activities. "It's much harder to deal with things and get them done. Everything is a huge effort. I really have to force myself to do things that need doing." (2)

Depressed Mood. Lowered mood and anxiety increased during the winter. There were severe depressions. "I just cried. It was the only thing I did in principle for a period of two months, every day. Complete hopelessness." (18) Thoughts came that life was not worth living this way. "I don't want to live, but I don't want to die either. Or I don't have the energy to live, but nor do I want to die. I don't want to live through this winter." (4) Participants with a milder depression described low energy and increased irritability and sensitivity to stress rather than depressed mood. "I have a stress threshold that is so low, so low. I react really badly to all kinds of stress. And when I react badly to stress I get mad and angry." (9) These informants were able to continue their work but described a low quality of life during the winter season.

Some participants described clear *seasonal changes in food habits and weight*. During the winter period, informants preferred eating warm, more robust, and "heavy" food (e.g., pasta). In the summertime, the preference was for cold and "lighter" food (e.g., salads). Some experienced craving sweets. Sweets were used as an attempt to increase a low energy level. One informant described a significant seasonal weight gain. "I notice that with my dog. She goes up in weight during the winter. And that's because I don't take her out for exercise. It's a bit awkward because people can see she's become fat. Yes, it's the same for me, although people don't mention it." (5)

Informants described *a feeling of being "alive" only half of the year*. During the winter, there was a feeling of not being able to participate in life: a feeling of mental hibernation. In the summer, on the other hand, the participants felt they were coming back to normal and coming back to "oneself." (6) "With the arrival of spring and lighter days, that's when I feel alert, I've got energy, I really enjoy living." (1)

3.1.2. Consequences for Everyday Life. The informants experienced *difficulties to meet the expectations of everyday life* during the winter season. "It's a source of stress during that entire part of the year, having to perform while not actually having the energy." (16) There were descriptions of *disturbed relationship with family and friends* during the winter season. It was the inactivity, irritability, and depressed mood that made it difficult for other members of the family. "What happens is that I sleep and don't do anything of my own volition. I have no contact with my friends during those periods. I lie on the sofa and watch TV and don't take the initiative to do the housework. So naturally that affects the entire family." (5) "What was so difficult was that my depression affected my daughter so much. Finally we ended up at the Child and Adolescent Psychiatry Clinic because her day care center rang the alarm. She was being unruly and playing up." (18) Informants experienced a *reduced capacity for work*. The lack of initiative was especially difficult for students who missed classes and for entrepreneurs because they were at risk of losing their income. "It was difficult because I didn't have a boss who said that I had to work." (5)

Some informants experienced *a dilemma because they knew the diagnosis and the treatment were not considered legitimate in the Swedish health care*. "It may be a placebo. Quite honestly, it doesn't matter. If anything has this effect on me which means I don't need pills, then I will happily continue with it." (6) There was a fear of not being able to receive the treatment in the future because they knew that light rooms had been closed down during recent years and only few were still in use.

3.1.3. Coping Strategies. Some informants used *passive coping strategies like "wait and see" or "hope for the best next year".* "It's got worse over the years, but I don't want to talk about it very much because I wish it weren't so. Next year it won't happen, that's what one always believes, thinks and wants." (5) Other informants used more *active coping strategies and tried to maintain physical and outdoor activities, which was considered helpful but difficult.* "I should force myself to go to some sort of keep fit during the winter. But it doesn't happen because I don't have the energy." (17) Informants with jobs *prioritize work in front of all other activities.* "I cried a huge amount from exhaustion, but I still went to work. Because I was used to going to work even if I didn't feel well." (7) As the depression got worse during the winter season, the informants refrained from social contacts and recreational activities. "This last winter, I couldn't face meeting up with anyone and had no energy to call anyone. I have quite a large network of friends, but it's like I just hide away, I don't have the energy." (18) Those informants who could afford it used *travelling abroad* during the late autumn as a way of coping with the winter depression. "A trip around October-November time is almost like going for light treatment." (9)

For informants with severe depressions, taking *antidepressants* was considered necessary. Some were taking antidepressants semiannually or changed the dose depending on the season. For informants with milder depression, antidepressants were not considered an option. Some had tried medication but stopped because it did not help them or they experienced side effects. "I have tried a lot of things, above all antidepressants and sleeping pills, but I haven't experienced any great improvement as a result. I've had a lot of side-effects which were so worrying that I finally decided that it wasn't worth it." (13) One informant had tried *psychotherapy* but with no major effect on the seasonal symptoms. "I've had psychodynamic therapy and also CBT. But despite trying hard in therapy, this feeling still came over me. It's like I've understood that it's a matter of something else, something biological." (12) In addition to travelling south to sunny latitudes and taking antidepressants, only *light room treatment* was considered helpful. "There's not much I can do, there's very little that makes a difference. I haven't found anything. What I think has been most noticeable is the light treatment." (13)

3.2. Patients' Experience of the Light Room Treatment. The analysis of the patients' experience of the light room treatment resulted in three categories and 11 subcategories (Table 3).

3.2.1. Positive Treatment Effects. The informants described the overall treatment effect as *a radical, sudden, and profound transformation.* Metaphors as "awakening," "illumination," "coming back to normal and to oneself," "to climb from the basement up to the roof," "like a conversion," or "like becoming a new person" were used. "I felt really good straight after the first ten sessions. I still remember the almost physical relief I felt throughout my body. I was speechless and totally amazed at what had happened. It was as though a yoke had been lifted from my shoulders, a purely physical feeling that I was now free of something." (9)

The change was described in "energy" terms: a physical sensation of something happening in the brain and with the body and mind feeling electrified and more energetic. "During the first days in the light room I don't notice that much difference. But during the second week, when I sit there for the final half hour, that's when this feeling comes over me. And then when I go out on to the street and it's grey weather, I still feel a sort of charge of energy in my being, or whatever you can call it. I feel it in my legs and body and arms like an electric charge." (5) "I felt straight away that some sort of change had taken place. I felt something happen inside me... a very distinct change... it feels like a little "ping" in my brain. Something is brought to life, and it happens after the second session of treatment. What I notice is that I'm given energy." (1) The informants reported *increased feelings of energy and activity*, being able to achieve more during the day. "I came home and set about making dinner and baking bread in the evenings, as opposed to just lying down and crashing out." (6)

Mood and thinking improved following treatment. Anxiety, irritability, and rumination were reduced and feelings of joy increased: "... and it's not as difficult thinking and keeping a lot of thoughts in my head when I'm at work. I feel in a lighter mood, I don't brood quite as much. It feels as though I don't have this cap fixed on to my head the way I do when I get depressed, which prevents me from trying to do things or trying to think differently. I felt as though I became lighter both physically and mentally." (13) "It's like a weight on my shoulders. Like a bloody millstone round my neck. It was so strange, having had that millstone round my neck and then suddenly having it lifted from me. Despite it being just as dark and miserable outside, it was somehow not as dark and miserable any more. It wasn't as oppressive." (9)

Informants described that *problems with sleep and daily rhythms improved* following treatment. "Before that I'd had trouble sleeping, I slept an hour or two. But now it's completely different. Now I don't wake up, I sleep all night, and around seven o'clock I wake up of my own accord." (8) "At this time of year my daily rhythm goes totally haywire, my body doesn't really know when it's time to be awake and when it's time to sleep. I have quite a lot of trouble sleeping; I can lie awake for a long time before getting to sleep at night. And things got better as a result of the light treatment. I then became more awake while I was sitting there. And felt more tired and found it easier to wind down in the evening." (13) The informants reported that improvement in their sleep and daily rhythm often preceded improvement in other symptoms. Informants reported *positive changes in food habits*, a normalization of eating habits following treatment. "As soon as I have had my light therapy I notice that I have far more energy, and my appetite is restored." (16)

3.2.2. The Importance of a Good Environment in the Light Room. The treatment was a *calming and relaxing experience* for the informants, albeit some initial feelings of stress or boredom. "The first day I found utterly boring. When I took a book with me to read, and then began to feel it was enjoyable."

(4) Informants stressed *the importance of mutual respect and silence* in the light room. This was especially important at the beginning of the treatment when feeling depressed. Mobile phones were accepted if all sounds were turned off and when not used for talking during the treatment. Other patients talking too much were considered disturbing. There were some problems in relation to *the physical environment* in the light room, for example, bad air quality and the temperature being too high or too low.

3.2.3. Negative Experiences Related to the Light Room Treatment. Some informants experienced *side effects during the first (but not the second) week* of the treatment, for example, mild headaches, increased tiredness, or difficulties going to sleep in the evening. "I got really tired during the first week especially. The second week wasn't quite as bad. But the first week I was completely washed out." (18) Some informants were disappointed because of *insufficient treatment effects* or because the treatment effect was not the same each year. Some described that the effect lasted only a few days or weeks, which made it necessary to continue the light treatment during the winter. "I think I felt the effect quite quickly and then I had to sustain it to ensure it took hold properly. And my idea is to continue going twice a week." (13) The *treatment was considered time-consuming* because of travelling time to and from the psychiatric outpatient clinic and for some stressful because of having to get up earlier than usual to participate in the treatment.

4. Discussion

This is the first study with a qualitative method investigating patients' experiences of seasonal affective disorder (SAD) and of light room treatment. The overall finding was a description of a profound struggle by the patients to adapt to a recurring situation experienced as inevitable and apparently difficult to escape. The winter depression affected not only the patients' subjective well-being but all important aspects of everyday life, that is, work capacity, recreational activities, and relations with family and friends. There were feelings of being "alive" only half of the year (summer) and feeling like a robot the other half (winter).

In a phenomenological study of the differences between nonseasonal depression and grief, depression was described as a place of darkness, beyond the person's control, and leading to secondary losses [36]. This is similar to the results in the present study. The descriptions of the symptoms are congruent to previous descriptions of symptoms in SAD [2, 37, 38]. Our results are also congruent with studies showing that patients with SAD experience low quality of life during the winter season which changes for the better in the summer [9], after light box treatment [39], and following light room treatment [8].

The effects of the light room treatment were described as a radical and sudden change for the better, usually within the first week. Improvement occurred in all the major symptoms, mood, sleep, daily rhythms, and thinking, energy, activity, and food habits. The light room treatment was described as one of the most important available coping strategies for the patients to improve the situation and regain a sense of control and hope.

The physical and psychological environment was of importance for the experience of the light room treatment. The treatment was described as a calming, positive, and relaxing experience. There were some descriptions of negative experiences; the treatment was considered time-consuming; the treatment effect was sometimes described as insufficient and, at times, other patients in the light room were described as slightly disturbing. There were some initial side effects, but these were experienced as mild and transient. Most patients tolerated the treatment in the light room well, which is similar to findings from treatment studies with light boxes [12, 20, 40, 41].

One finding of special interest is the description of *a "sign,"* a signal that functioned as a personal marker for the beginning of the seasonal depression. It was described as a sudden recognition of a thought, a feeling, or a change in behavior and was accompanied by an almost instantaneous reaction of uneasiness or aversion.

Another new finding in this study was the description of *a dilemma* between the personal experience of an effective treatment and the awareness that this treatment is not endorsed (evidence-based) in the Swedish health care system [17]. The patients worried about not being able to receive the treatment in future depressive relapses. Whether the positive treatment was due to a placebo effect or not did not matter much to the patients. The "proof" the patients needed was that of their own experience of renewed energy, better mood, and increased activity.

Another finding was that the deterioration of *sleep and daily rhythms* in the autumn preceded the experience of depressed mood and inactivity. The sleep problems (insomnia and hypersomnia) and delayed circadian rhythms described by the patients in this study are well known in SAD [10]. In a study using 24 h actigraph recordings of patients with SAD, total daytime activity was reduced by almost 1/3 in SAD patients compared with healthy controls. After 4 weeks of LT in that study, there were no differences between groups [42]. The authors concluded that the findings suggested that LT increased blunted activity levels, restored circadian rhythms, and improved sleep in SAD patients. These findings are congruent with how the patients in the present study described how activity, sleep, and daily rhythms improved following light room treatment. There is strong evidence that the human circadian system is entrained by exposure to light and darkness [43]. There is some evidence that patients with SAD become depressed in the winter because of internal circadian misalignment [44, 45]. Researchers try to find a firm association of genetic markers for gene based analysis of circadian genes and seasonal pattern in bipolar disorders as recently reported by Geoffroy et al. [46].

Light and the seasons obviously have strong effects on our biology. But are there also psychological factors associated with seasonal affective disorder? The concept *illness cognitions* is defined as patient's own beliefs about their illness [47]. These cognitions constitute a personal framework for understanding and dealing with illness. There are five dimensions related to illness cognitions: identity (symptoms and diagnosis), perceived cause (biological, psychosocial, or stress), the time line ("how long will it last?"), consequences (physical, emotional, and social) and curability/controllability ("can it be cured?") [47]. The first part of the results from the present study is a description of illness cognitions in patients with SAD: the perception of symptoms, perceived cause, consequences for everyday life, and coping strategies used. The impact of the different aspects of illness cognitions is only partially known in SAD. In cognitive-behavioral therapy (CBT), dysfunctional cognitions are a focus of the treatment and there is some evidence that CBT is effective for patients with SAD [48–50]. In the present study, however, psychotherapy was not described by the patients as effective for alleviating the seasonal symptoms. This may be an effect of "sample bias," since only patients who completed light room treatment were included. It is reasonable to assume that some patients with SAD benefit more from CBT, while others benefit more from LT or a combination. Who benefits from the light room treatment (moderators) and what parts of the treatment is effective (mediators) require further investigation.

Is the dark season a stressor for vulnerable individuals? Psychological factors are central to the stress response and coexist with the physiological changes. The *transactional model of stress and coping* describes how individuals deal with stressful experiences [51]. When facing a stressor, the individual evaluates the situation through primary ("is it stressful, harmful?") and secondary appraisal ("can I cope?"). The primary appraisal includes the perception of personal susceptibility and severity of the stressor. In this study, the informants described a clear perception of personal susceptibility and a strong negative reaction to the early signals of the winter depression (that is, a strong negative primary appraisal). The "secondary appraisal" is the individual's perceived ability to manage the situation, to alter the situation, and/or to handle negative emotions (coping strategies). The patients were very clear in their descriptions of effective means to handle the seasons. For some, antidepressants were necessary; for others they were not considered an option. Physical activity was considered helpful but difficult to achieve during depression. All patients described social withdrawal and reduction of activity as necessary. Travelling abroad to sunny countries was an important coping strategy in addition to light treatment, but not all could afford to travel. Active, approach, and acceptance coping strategies result in better health outcomes for the individual, compared to avoidant or passive strategies [52]. Patients with depression use more avoidant coping strategies compared to the healthy controls [53]. The patients in this study used avoidant strategies during the summer ("wait and see," "hope for the best") and active, approach strategies during the winter (travel abroad, take antidepressants, or light room treatment). The results from this study indicate that patients with SAD considered light room treatment one of their most important, active coping strategies. This may be of importance, since a positive association between perception of control and improved well-being and adjustment has been observed across a variety of disorders [52].

4.1. Methodological Considerations. The informants provided rich, colorful, and elaborate descriptions of their subjective reality and lived experience, that is, using metaphors and figurative descriptions of symptoms and treatment effects. The sample is well described and presented with extensive background data (Table 1). This, together with the large variation in experiences obtained, facilitates the readers' evaluation of transferability of the results to other contexts [29]. In qualitative analysis, there is no single interpretation of the meaning of a text. Therefore, methods to increase trustworthiness are necessary. Triangulation is a common method to achieve this and was used in the present study; the authors discussed all steps in the analysis until agreement was obtained. Furthermore, four patients who received preventative treatment were included in the study, which contributed to more variation in experiences.

4.2. Limitations. A limitation of this study is the inclusion process, which for practical reasons was not based on complete clinical information but on a judgment of the referral in combination with self-report measures of depression. Another limitation is related to side effects. Only patients who completed ≥7 treatments in the light room were included, which is why there may be side effects experienced by patients who discontinued treatment at an early state and were not included in this study.

5. Conclusions

The results from this study show that patients with winter depression experience a clear seasonal pattern including deterioration in sleep, daily rhythms, energy level, mood, activity, and cognitive functioning. The disorder affected major aspects of everyday life, with reduced work capacity, social withdrawal, and disturbed relations with family and friends. Light room treatment was described as one of the most effective and personally important coping strategies, with improvement in all the major symptoms and with mild and transient side effects. Considering the 2015 recommendations from the Cochrane Collaboration that the selection of treatment for preventing winter depression should be strongly based on patient preferences, the results of the present study may be used in the clinical evaluation and discussion with the patient and considering possible treatment options. Further studies about the specific individual signs and symptoms profile which mark the beginning of repeated seasonal depressive episodes are called for [54].

Competing Interests

The authors declare that there are no competing interests regarding the publication of this manuscript.

Acknowledgments

Special thanks are due to participating patients and personnel at the psychiatric outpatient clinic West in Stockholm and to RN Eva-Maria Fast who assisted in recruiting informants and collecting the data. The research was financially supported by a research grant at the Karolinska Institute, Stockholm, Sweden.

References

[1] N. E. Rosenthal, D. A. Sack, J. C. Gillin et al., "Seasonal affective disorder: a description of the syndrome and preliminary findings with light therapy," *Archives of General Psychiatry*, vol. 41, no. 1, pp. 72–80, 1984.

[2] APA, *Diagnostic and Statistical Manual of Mental Disorders (DSM-V)*, American Psychiatric Association, Arlington, Va, USA, 5th edition, 2013.

[3] D. G. Blazer, R. C. Kessler, and M. S. Swartz, "Epidemiology of recurrent major and minor depression with a seasonal pattern. The national comorbidity survey," *British Journal of Psychiatry*, vol. 172, pp. 164–167, 1998.

[4] E. E. Michalak, C. Wilkinson, C. Dowrick, and G. Wilkinson, "Seasonal affective disorder: prevalence, detection and current, treatment in North Wales," *British Journal of Psychiatry*, vol. 179, pp. 31–34, 2001.

[5] S. Kasper, T. A. Wehr, J. J. Bartko, P. A. Gaist, and N. E. Rosenthal, "Epidemiological findings of seasonal changes in mood and behavior: a telephone survey of Montgomery county, Maryland," *Archives of General Psychiatry*, vol. 46, no. 9, pp. 823–833, 1989.

[6] C. Rastad, P.-O. Sjöden, and J. Ulfberg, "High prevalence of self-reported winter depression in a Swedish county," *Psychiatry and Clinical Neurosciences*, vol. 59, no. 6, pp. 666–675, 2005.

[7] C. Rastad, *Winter fatigue and winter depression. Prevalence and treatment with bright light [thesis]*, Uppsala University, Uppsala, Sweden, 2009.

[8] C. Rastad, J. Ulfberg, and P. Lindberg, "Improvement in fatigue, sleepiness, and health-related quality of life with bright light treatment in persons with seasonal affective disorder and subsyndromal SAD," *Depression Research and Treatment*, vol. 2011, Article ID 543906, 10 pages, 2011.

[9] E. E. Michalak, E. M. Tam, C. V. Manjunath, A. J. Levitt, R. D. Levitan, and R. W. Lam, "Quality of life in patients with seasonal affective disorder: summer vs winter scores," *Canadian Journal of Psychiatry*, vol. 50, no. 5, pp. 292–295, 2005.

[10] C.-H. Sohn and R. W. Lam, "Update on the biology of seasonal affective disorder," *CNS Spectrums*, vol. 10, no. 8, pp. 635–646, 2005.

[11] R. D. Levitan, "The chronobiology and neurobiology of winter seasonal affective disorder," *Dialogues in Clinical Neuroscience*, vol. 9, no. 3, pp. 315–324, 2007.

[12] G. Pail, W. Huf, E. Pjrek et al., "Bright-light therapy in the treatment of mood disorders," *Neuropsychobiology*, vol. 64, no. 3, pp. 152–162, 2011.

[13] D. A. Oren, M. Koziorowski, and P. H. Desan, "SAD and the not-so-single photoreceptors," *American Journal of Psychiatry*, vol. 170, no. 12, pp. 1403–1412, 2013.

[14] R. W. Lam and E. M. Tam, *A Clinician's Guide to Using Light Therapy*, Cambridge University Press, New York, NY, USA, 2009.

[15] R. N. Golden, B. N. Gaynes, R. D. Ekstrom et al., "The efficacy of light therapy in the treatment of mood disorders: a review and meta-analysis of the evidence," *American Journal of Psychiatry*, vol. 162, no. 4, pp. 656–662, 2005.

[16] A. V. Ravindran, R. W. Lam, M. J. Filteau et al., "Canadian Network for Mood and Anxiety Treatments (CANMAT) Clinical guidelines for the management of major depressive disorder in adults. V. Complementary and alternative medicine treatments," *Journal of Affective Disorders*, vol. 117, supplement 1, pp. S54–S64, 2009.

[17] SBU, Light therapy in depression and other treatments of seasonal affective disorder, A systematic literature review, The Swedish County on Health Technology and Assessment (In Swedish: Ljusterapi vid depression samt övrig behandling av årstidsbunden depression, En systematisk litteraturöversikt, SBU. Statens beredning för medicinsk utvärdering), Stockholm, Sweden, vol. 186, 2007.

[18] B. Mårtensson, A. Pettersson, L. Berglund, and L. Ekselius, "Bright white light therapy in depression: a critical review of the evidence," *Journal of Affective Disorders*, vol. 182, pp. 1–7, 2015.

[19] R. W. Lam, A. J. Levitt, R. D. Levitan et al., "Efficacy of bright light treatment, fluoxetine, and the combination in patients with nonseasonal major depressive disorder: a randomized clinical trial," *JAMA Psychiatry*, vol. 73, no. 1, pp. 56–63, 2016.

[20] R. W. Lam, A. J. Levitt, R. D. Levitan et al., "The can-SAD study: a randomized controlled trial of the effectiveness of light therapy and fluoxetine in patients with winter seasonal affective disorder," *American Journal of Psychiatry*, vol. 163, no. 5, pp. 805–812, 2006.

[21] L. Wetterberg, "Melatonin in humans physiological and clinical studies," *Journal of Neural Transmission, Supplement*, no. 13, pp. 289–310, 1978.

[22] L. Wetterberg, B. Kjellman, B. E. Thalén et al., "Ljusbehandling vid depression," *Läkartidningen*, vol. 88, no. 5, pp. 310–312, 1991 (Swedish).

[23] L. Wetterberg, "Light therapy of depression; basal and clinical aspects," *Pharmacology & Toxicology*, vol. 71, supplement 1, pp. 96–106, 1992.

[24] T. Partonen, B. Appelberg, and M. Partinen, "Effects of light treatment on sleep structure in seasonal affective disorder," *European Archives of Psychiatry and Clinical Neuroscience*, vol. 242, no. 5, pp. 310–313, 1993.

[25] C. Rastad, J. Ulfberg, and P. Lindberg, "Light room therapy effective in mild forms of seasonal affective disorder—a randomised controlled study," *Journal of Affective Disorders*, vol. 108, no. 3, pp. 291–296, 2008.

[26] B.-E. Thalén, B. F. Kjellman, L. Mørkrid, R. Wibom, and L. Wetterberg, "Light treatment in seasonal and nonseasonal depression," *Acta Psychiatrica Scandinavica*, vol. 91, no. 5, pp. 352–360, 1995.

[27] B. Nussbaumer, A. Kaminski-Hartenthaler, C. A. Forneris et al., "Light therapy for preventing seasonal affective disorder," *The Cochrane Database of Systematic Reviews*, no. 11, Article ID CD011269, 2015.

[28] G. L. Engel, "The need for a new medical model: a challenge for biomedicine," *Science*, vol. 196, no. 4286, pp. 129–136, 1977.

[29] U. H. Graneheim and B. Lundman, "Qualitative content analysis in nursing research: concepts, procedures and measures to achieve trustworthiness," *Nurse Education Today*, vol. 24, no. 2, pp. 105–112, 2004.

[30] APA, *Diagnostic and Statistical Manual of Mental Disorders (DSM-IV)*, American Psychiatric Association, Washington, DC, USA, 4th edition, 1994.

[31] G. Guest, A. Bunce, and L. Johnson, "How many interviews are enough? An experiment with data saturation and variability," *Field Methods*, vol. 18, no. 1, pp. 59–82, 2006.

[32] J. B. W. Williams and K. A. Kobak, "Development and reliability of a structured interview guide for the Montgomery-Åsberg Depression Rating Scale (SIGMA)," *British Journal of Psychiatry*, vol. 192, no. 1, pp. 52–58, 2008.

[33] P. Svanborg and M. Åsberg, "A comparison between the Beck Depression Inventory (BDI) and the self-rating version of the Montgomery Åsberg Depression Rating Scale (MADRS)," *Journal of Affective Disorders*, vol. 64, no. 2-3, pp. 203–216, 2001.

[34] J. L. Cunningham, L. Wernroth, L. Von Knorring, L. Berglund, and L. Ekselius, "Agreement between physicians' and patients' ratings on the Montgomery-Åsberg Depression Rating Scale," *Journal of Affective Disorders*, vol. 135, no. 1–3, pp. 148–153, 2011.

[35] P. Nikander, "Working with transcripts and translated data," *Qualitative Research in Psychology*, vol. 5, no. 3, pp. 225–231, 2008.

[36] G. Parker, S. McCraw, and A. Paterson, "Clinical features distinguishing grief from depressive episodes: a qualitative analysis," *Journal of Affective Disorders*, vol. 176, pp. 43–47, 2015.

[37] T. Partonen and N. Rosenthal, "Symptoms and course of illness," in *Seasonal Affective Disorder, Practice and Research*, T. Partonen and A. Magnusson, Eds., pp. 19–30, Oxford University Press, New York, NY, USA, 2001.

[38] A. J. Lewy, J. S. Emens, J. B. Songer et al., "Winter depression: integrating mood, circadian rhythms, and the sleep/wake and light/dark cycles into a bio-psycho-social-environmental model," *Sleep Medicine Clinics*, vol. 4, no. 2, pp. 285–299, 2009.

[39] E. E. Michalak, G. Murray, A. J. Levitt et al., "Quality of life as an outcome indicator in patients with seasonal affective disorder: results from the Can-SAD study," *Psychological Medicine*, vol. 37, no. 5, pp. 727–736, 2007.

[40] Y. Botanov and S. S. Ilardi, "The acute side effects of bright light therapy: a placebo-controlled investigation," *PLoS ONE*, vol. 8, no. 9, Article ID e75893, 2013.

[41] M. Terman and J. S. Terman, "Bright light therapy: side effects and benefits across the symptom spectrum," *Journal of Clinical Psychiatry*, vol. 60, no. 11, pp. 799–808, 1999.

[42] D. Winkler, E. Pjrek, N. Praschak-Rieder et al., "Actigraphy in patients with seasonal affective disorder and healthy control subjects treated with light therapy," *Biological Psychiatry*, vol. 58, no. 4, pp. 331–336, 2005.

[43] J. F. Duffy and K. P. Wright Jr., "Entrainment of the human circadian system by light," *Journal of Biological Rhythms*, vol. 20, no. 4, pp. 326–338, 2005.

[44] K. A. Roecklein, P. M. Wong, P. L. Franzen et al., "Melanopsin gene variations interact with season to predict sleep onset and chronotype," *Chronobiology International*, vol. 29, no. 8, pp. 1036–1047, 2012.

[45] A. J. Lewy, "Circadian misalignment in mood disturbances," *Current Psychiatry Reports*, vol. 11, no. 6, pp. 459–465, 2009.

[46] P. A. Geoffroy, M. Lajnef, F. Bellivier et al., "Genetic association study of circadian genes with seasonal pattern in bipolar disorders," *Scientific Reports*, vol. 5, article 10232, 2015.

[47] J. Ogden, "Illness cognitions," in *Health Psychology: A Textbook*, pp. 47–72, Open University Press, Berkshire, UK, 2007.

[48] K. J. Rohan, K. A. Roecklein, K. T. Lindsey et al., "A randomized controlled trial of cognitive-behavioral therapy, light therapy, and their combination for seasonal affective disorder," *Journal of Consulting and Clinical Psychology*, vol. 75, no. 3, pp. 489–500, 2007.

[49] L. Sitnikov, K. J. Rohan, M. Evans, J. N. Mahon, and Y. I. Nillni, "Cognitive predictors and moderators of winter depression treatment outcomes in cognitive-behavioral therapy vs. light therapy," *Behaviour Research and Therapy*, vol. 51, no. 12, pp. 872–881, 2013.

[50] K. J. Rohan, J. N. Mahon, M. Evans et al., "Randomized trial of cognitive-behavioral therapy versus light therapy for seasonal affective disorder: acute outcomes," *American Journal of Psychiatry*, vol. 172, no. 9, pp. 862–869, 2015.

[51] R. Lazarus and S. Folkman, *Stress, Appraisal and Coping*, Springer, New York, NY, USA, 1984.

[52] K. Glanz, B. K. Rimer, and K. Viswanath, "Stress, coping, and health behavior," in *Health Behavior and Health Education. Theory, Research, and Practice*, K. Glanz, B. K. Rimer, and K. Viswanath, Eds., pp. 211–236, Jossey-Bass, San Francisco, Calif, USA, 2008.

[53] S. T. Sigmon, J. J. Pells, J. G. Schartel et al., "Stress reactivity and coping in seasonal and nonseasonal depression," *Behaviour Research and Therapy*, vol. 45, no. 5, pp. 965–975, 2007.

[54] A. E. Tyrer, R. D. Levitan, S. Houle et al., "Serotonin transporter binding is reduced in seasonal affective disorder following light therapy," *Acta Psychiatrica Scandinavica*, vol. 134, no. 5, pp. 410–419, 2016.

22

Prevalence and Factors Associated with Undernutrition among Adults with Major Depressive Disorder in Northwest Ethiopia

Edmialem Gezahegn,[1] Melkie Edris,[2] and Berihun Assefa Dachew[3]

[1]*Psychiatric Clinic, University of Gondar Hospital, Gondar, Ethiopia*
[2]*Departmpent of Human Nutrition, Institute of Public Health, University of Gondar, Gondar, Ethiopia*
[3]*Department of Epidemiology and Biostatistics, Institute of Public Health, University of Gondar, Gondar, Ethiopia*

Correspondence should be addressed to Berihun Assefa Dachew; berihunassefa21@gmail.com

Academic Editor: Ulrich Schweiger

Background. Undernutrition and major depressive disorder are frequently co-occurring. Patients with impaired mental health are strongly vulnerable to the risks of having involuntary weight loss or deficiency of essential nutrients. However, there is no study which assesses undernutrition among major depressive patients in Ethiopia. *Method.* A total of 422 clients were included in the study. Structured questionnaires and anthropometric measurements were used for collecting the data. Bivariate and multivariate logistic regression model was fitted to identify factors associated with undernutrition. Odds ratio with 95% confidence interval was computed to determine the level of significance. *Results.* The prevalence of undernutrition was 31.4% [95% CI: 27.2–36.0]. Being in a rural residence [AOR = 1.84, 95% CI (1.18–2.85)], taking multiple medication [AOR = 1.77, 95% CI (1.03–3.05)], taking prescribed diet [AOR = 1.90, 95% CI (1.06–3.41)], and current use of alcohol [AOR = 2.96, 95% CI (1.34–6.55)] were factors significantly associated with undernutrition among depressive patients. *Conclusion.* The prevalence of undernutrition among adults with major depressive disorder was found to be higher than the general population. Appropriate nutritional education and nutritional assessment are recommended during the course of major depressive disorder.

1. Background

Mental health problems account for 13% of the total burden of disease [1, 2]. Malnutrition and major depressive disorder are common health problems [3, 4]. According to World Health Organization (WHO) estimate, major depressive disorder is projected to become the leading cause of disability and the second leading contributor to the global burden of disease by the year 2020 and the impact of this burden of disease is thought to be worse in developing countries [5].

Malnutrition is a major public health problem in developing countries including Ethiopia. According to the 2011 Ethiopian Demographic and Health Survey, the prevalence of moderately/severely malnutrition among Ethiopian men aged 15–59 years was 13.4% and the prevalence is 11.8% (women) and 17% (men) in Amhara region where the study is conducted [6]. It is also the most important risk factor for the burden of many diseases like TB [7], pneumonia [8], visceral leishmaniasis [9], and mental disorders [10].

Malnutrition and major depressive disorder are frequently cooccurring among adults with their interrelated effects and exacerbate one another in a vicious cycle. In developed countries malnourished persons have a 55% increased risk of major depression over time and depressed persons have a 58% increased risk of becoming malnutrition but far less known in developing country [11]. Moreover, impaired mental health is strongly vulnerable to the risks of being involuntary weight gain, weight loss, or deficiency of essential nutrients [12–14]. This is because of poor self-care, being unable to shop or prepare foods, poor balanced diet, and unhealthy lifestyle. In addition, loss of appetite, being unable to eat regularly, and energy expenditure contribute for this association [4, 13].

The sociodemographic characteristics of the respondents (such as sex, age, race/ethnicity, education status, and area of residence), dieting for medical reasons, use of psychiatric medicines, use of alcohol, and use of substances were factors associated with nutritional status of adults with major depressive disorder [12, 15, 16].

Although there are an abundance of research about the underlying conditions that ultimately lead to undernutrition and major depressive disorder individually, little is known about the burden of undernutrition among depressive patients in developing countries [17]. In Ethiopia, many studies have been conducted to identify the magnitude and consequence of undernutrition in different population groups. However, the issue of undernutrition was not well addressed among adults with major depressive disorder. Therefore, assessing the nutritional status of major depressive patients is crucial for identifying the multidimensional conditions where management requires a holistic approach by several methods of assessment and intervention, including nutrition-related health indicators, dietary intake, and energy expenditure [15].

Thus, this study was able to disclose the prevalence and associated factors of undernutrition among adults with major depressive disorder at the University of Gondar Teaching Hospital and Bahir Dar Felege Hiwot Referral Hospital. The findings of this study will be useful for policy makers, program managers, and other concerned bodies to design appropriate strategies.

2. Methods and Materials

2.1. Study Design and Setting. Institutional based cross-sectional study design was conducted to determine prevalence of undernutrition and associated factors among adults with major depressive disorder. The study was conducted in psychiatry outpatient clinic at University of Gondar (UOG) Teaching Hospital and Bahir Dar Felege Hiwot Referral Hospital. University of Gondar teaching Hospital is located in Gondar town, 738 km way form Addis Ababa, capital city of Ethiopia, to Northwest direction and Felege Hiwot Referral Hospital is found in Bahir Dar town Ethiopia, the capital city of Amhara Regional State, and situated 565 Km away from Addis Ababa to Northwest direction. Approximately, 8,000 adult patients per year have enrolled in chronic care from psychiatry outpatient clinics in both hospitals, of which, a total of 4500 patients per year with major depressive disorder (MDD) have been attending in both outpatient clinics (2,500 from UOG teaching hospital and 2,000 from Felege Hiwot Referral Hospital).

2.1.1. Source and Population. All psychiatry clinic outpatient adults with MDD who attend in the University of Gondar Teaching Hospital and Felege Hiwot Referral Hospital Bahir Dar were the source population for this study.

2.1.2. Inclusion and Exclusion Criteria. All adults with major depressive disorder were included, whereas pregnant and lactating women (<6 months) were excluded from the study.

2.1.3. Sample Size, Sampling Technique, and Sampling Procedures. The sample size of the study was calculated using the formula for the estimation of single proportion with the assumptions of 95% confidence interval (z), 5% marginal error (d), and taking proportion undernutrition among depressive patients as 50%.

$$n = \frac{z^2 (p(1-P))}{d^2}, \quad n = \frac{1.96^2 (0.5(1-0.5))}{0.05^2} = 384. \tag{1}$$

With this assumption, the sample size becomes 384. Considering 10% nonresponse rate the final sample size becomes 422. Proportional allocation is used to maintain proportionality among the two hospitals and then study participants from each hospital were selected by using systematic random sampling methods. Thus, 235 were from UOG Hospital and the rest 188 were from Bahir Dar Felege Hiwot Hospital.

2.2. Data Collection Instrument. Data were collected by using interviewer administered structured questionnaire and anthropometric measurements. The questionnaire contains sociodemographic characteristics, clinical factors, dietary-related factors, behavioral factors, and psychosocial factors. The questionnaires were prepared in English and then translated to Amharic (local language) and again back translated to English to check its consistency. Major depressive disorder and sleep disorder were diagnosed based on DSM-IV criteria [18]. Study subjects are considered as current use of alcohol or cigarette smoker, when they use specified substance at least once in the last three months and respondents who were taking ≥4 types of medication per day were considered as taking multiple medications.

2.3. Anthropometric Measurements. A studio meter was used to measure the height of the study subjects. Each study subject was asked to stand on the surface, with weight distributed evenly on both feet, heels together against the studio meter, and the head positioned so that the line of vision was perpendicular to the body. The movable headboard was brought to the topmost point on the head with sufficient pressure to compress the hairs. The well-calibrated scale was used to weigh the study participants. To avoid the variability among the data collectors, the same measurement was employed for a given anthropometric measurement more than one time. Finally, BMI was calculated as kg/m^2 to determine the nutritional status of the respondents. A score less than 18.5 is considered as having undernutrition. It can be further classified as mild (17–18.4), moderate (16–16.9), and severe undernutrition (<16).

2.4. Data Processing and Analysis. The data were coded and entered into Epi-Info version 7 and exported to SPSS version 20.0 software packages for analysis. Both descriptive and analytical statistical procedures were utilized. Binary logistic regression was used to identify factors associated with undernutrition among the depressive patients. Variables with a bivariate P value < 0.20 were further fitted into multivariate models for controlling the possible effect of confounders, and finally the variables that had significant association with depression were identified on the basis of odds ratio (OR), with 95% confidence interval (CI) and P value ($P < 0.05$). The variables were entered to the multivariate model using the Backward Stepwise (Likelihood Ratio) regression method. Model fitness was checked using Hosmer and Lemeshow goodness-of-fit test ($P = 0.6$). Multicollinearity was checked using variance inflation factor (VIF = 1.5–2.5).

2.5. Ethical Considerations. Ethical clearance was obtained from Institutional Review Board (IRB) of the University of Gondar. Written informed consent was obtained from respondents who were selected to participate in the study.

3. Results

3.1. Sociodemographic Characteristics. A total of 405 respondents were included in the study with a response rate of 95.5%. Among those 228 (56.3%) were females. About 40% of the respondents were married and 63% of the respondents were rural dwellers (Table 1).

3.2. Clinical Characteristics of Respondents. Nearly half 206 (50.9%) of the respondents were under Amitriptyline medication. About 24% of the respondents were taking multiple (4 or more) medication per day.

From a total of 405 respondents only 98 (24.2%) had known previous psychiatric disorder and 37 (9.1%) of them had known previous medical disorders like TB, pneumonia, malaria, and acute gastritis. Two hundred and twelve (52.3%) of the respondents had no sleep problem (Table 2).

3.3. Dietary and Behavioral Characteristics of Respondents. Among respondents 56 (13.8%) of the participants were taking prescribed diet due to different medical reason in their dietary habit. The commonest food eaten by the majority (76.6%) of the respondents was injera (Ethiopian traditional food).

Regarding to their behavioral characteristics 55 (13.6%) participants used alcoholic beverages in the past three months and about 47% of them used greater than once per day (Table 3).

3.4. Prevalence of Undernutrition. The overall prevalence of undernutrition among adults with major depression disorder was 31.4% [95% CI: 27.2–36.0] and 23.7% [95% CI: 18.4–28.6] were mild, 4.7% [95% CI: 1.6–7.8] were moderate, and 3.0% [95% CI: 1.2–4.3] were severe undernutrition cases.

Table 1: Sociodemographic characteristics of adults with major depressive disorder (MDD) in University of Gondar and Felege Hiwot Referral Hospital ($n = 405$).

Variables	Frequency	Percent
Sex		
Male	177	43.7
Female	228	56.3
Age in years		
18–26	105	25.9
27–35	112	27.7
36–45	98	24.2
>45	90	22.2
Marital status		
Married	161	39.8
Single	157	38.8
Separate/divorced	60	14.8
Widowed	27	6.7
Living condition		
With family	342	84.4
Alone	63	15.4
Educational status		
Cannot read and write	107	26.4
Primary school	129	31.9
Secondary school	106	26.2
Higher education	63	15.6
Occupation		
No job	126	31.1
Private employee	93	23.0
Governmental employee	56	13.8
Farmer	52	12.8
Merchant	51	12.6
Daily laborers	27	6.7
Monthly income (USD)		
<50	146	36.0
50–100	139	34.3
>100	120	29.6
Residence		
Rural	254	62.7
Urban	151	37.3

3.5. Factors Associated with Undernutrition. In multivariate analysis, residence, multiple medication intake, taking prescribed diet, and current use of alcohol were significantly associated with undernutrition among patients with major depressive disorder.

Participants who live in rural areas were nearly two times more likely [AOR = 1.84, 95% CI (1.18–2.85)] to have undernutrition as compared to participants who live in urban areas. On the other hand, participants who have used multiple medications per day were 1.70 times more likely [AOR = 1.70, 95% CI (1.01–2.87)] to have undernutrition as compared to nonusers.

Participants who were not taking the prescribed diet due to medical reasons were nearly two times more likely to have undernutrition than those who had taken prescribed diet [AOR = 1.90, 95% CI (1.06–3.41)]. Moreover, participants who were using alcoholic beverages in the past three months were three times more likely to have undernutrition as compared to participants who had not used [AOR = 2.96, 95% CI (1.34–6.55)] (Table 4).

TABLE 2: Clinical characteristics of respondents with major depressive disorder in University of Gondar Referral Teaching Hospital and Felege Hiwot Referral Hospital, Northwest Ethiopia, 2015 (n = 405).

Variable	Frequency	Percent
Length of treatment for MDD in month		
<3	114	28.1
3–8	101	24.9
9–27	89	22.0
>27	101	24.9
Type of medication for MDD		
Only amitriptyline	206	50.9
Only fluoxetine	146	36.0
Amitriptyline & Chlorpromazine	25	6.2
Fluoxetine & Chlorpromazine	14	3.5
Imipramine or others	14	3.5
Food intake declined		
Yes	170	42
No	230	58
Past psychiatric disorders		
Yes	98	24.2
No	307	75.8
Known past medical disorders		
Yes	37	9.1
No	368	90.9
Known current comorbidity		
Yes	30	7.2
No	375	89.5
Under multiple medication		
Yes	99	24.4
No	306	75.6
Sleep problem		
Yes	122	47.6
No	212	52.3

TABLE 3: Individual characteristics related to dietary and behavioral characteristics of respondents with major depressive disorder in University of Gondar Referral Teaching Hospital and Felege Hiwot Referral Hospital, Northwest Ethiopia, 2015 (n = 405).

Variable	Number	Percent
Taking prescribed diet		
Yes	56	13.8
No	349	86.2
Food commonly eaten		
Injera	311	76.6
Bread/Kita	69	17
Qolo (cereals)	25	6.2
Frequency of meal per day		
Two times	135	33.3
Three times	241	59.5
Four times	29	7.2
Taking breakfast		
Yes	253	62.5
No	152	37.5
Fruit & vegetable per day		
Yes	132	32.6
No	273	67.4
Water or fluid intake/day		
<3 litters	282	69.9
3–5 litters	95	23.5
>5 litters	28	6.9
Current smoker		
Yes	33	14.6
No	372	85.4
Current use of alcohol		
Yes	55	13.6
No	350	86.4
Frequency alcohol use		
Once per day	21	38.2
>1 per day	26	47.3
Once per week	8	12.7

4. Discussion

The prevalence of undernutrition in this study was found to be 31.4% (95% CI: 27.2–36.0). This finding is relatively high as compared to similar cross-sectional studies conducted in Taiwan [13], Portugal [19], and Bangladesh [20], in which 11%, 12%, and 26% of patients with major depressive disorder had undernutrition, respectively.

Moreover, this prevalence was also much higher than the previous study done in Iran (1.43%) [21] and Boston (1.6%) [22]. The difference might be due to socioeconomic difference, difference in dietary habits, and type of medication intake.

The findings of multivariate analysis revealed that the likelihood of being undernutrition was found to be higher among patients who come from rural area as compared to urban [AOR = 1.84, 95% CI (1.18–2.85)]. This finding was in line with the finding reported from Nepal [16]. This could be due to the fact that patients coming from rural area were engaged in high energy expending activities as compared to urban dwellers. Moreover, those study subjects from rural area might not be aware of healthy eating due to poor educational status or might not get the required amount of diet due to low income [21].

The current study, respondents who took multiple medications (≥4 medications per day) were 1.70 times more likely to have undernutrition as compared to those who had not. This finding is supported by the previous studies done in Portugal [19], Boston [22], and Taiwan [13]. This could be due to the fact that medical comorbid illnesses could be associated with increased side effects and treatment resistance related to metabolic dysfunction which in turn leads to undernutrition [19, 22].

Moreover, a depressive patient who was not taking prescribed diet was two times more likely to have undernutrition as compared to those who had taken prescribed diet. This could be due to the fact that patients who had not take prescribed diet might be prone to different diseases and highly

TABLE 4: Bivariate and multivariate analysis of factors associated with undernutrition among adults with major depressive disorder at University of Gondar Referral Teaching Hospital & Felege Hiwot Referral Hospital.

Characteristics	Undernutrition		COR (95% CI)	AOR (95%)
	Yes	No		
Sex				
Male	62	115	1	1
Female	65	163	1.35 (0.89–2.06)	1.42 (0.92–2.21)
Living condition				
Alone	25	38	0.65 (0.37–1.13)	0.76 (0.40–1.44)
With family	102	240	1	1
Residence				
Rural	66	188	1.93 (1.26–2.97)*	1.84 (1.18–2.85)*
Urban	61	90	1	1
Medication for MDD				
Only amitriptyline	63	143	0.66 (0.33–1.32)	0.87 (0.41–1.88)
Only fluoxetine	52	94	0.53 (0.26–1.10)	0.60 (0.28–1.31)
Other	12	41	1	1
Known comorbid disease				
Yes	6	24	1.91 (0.76–4.76)	1.51 (0.50–4.57)
No	121	254	1	1
Taking multiple medication				
Yes	51	119	1.77 (1.03–3.05)*	1.70 (1.01–2.87)*
No	76	159	1	1
Sleep problem				
Yes	53	140	1.19 (0.96–2.59)	1.5 (0.78–2.50)
No problem	22	49	1	1
Taking prescribed diet				
Yes	25	31	1	1
No	102	247	1.95 (1.09–3.47)*	1.09 (1.06–3.41)*
Alcohol use				
Yes	8	47	3.03 (1.39–6.61)*	2,96 (1.34–6.55)*
No	119	231	1	1

*Statistically significant at $P < 0.05$.

predisposed to different comorbidities, which in turn leads to undernutrition [16].

In addition, current use of alcohol was significantly associated with undernutrition among depressive patients. Those participants who used alcoholic beverages were nearly 3 times more likely to have undernutrition as compared to participants who had not drunk in the past three months. This is due to the fact that alcohol use interferes with the absorption and storage micronutrients. In addition, alcohol irritates the gastrointestinal system; it increases acid secretion by the stomach which can injure the lining of the small intestine and interferes with the ability to absorb vital nutrients. Furthermore, alcohol is a toxin that has to be deactivated by the liver, during the detoxification process the body uses thiamin, zinc, and other important nutrients and this can deplete the investments of healthy metabolism and also cause low mood, irritability, and/or aggressive behavior as well as more serious and long-term mental health problems which further predispose to undernutrition [4, 23].

The cross-sectional nature of the study design does not show the temporal relationship. Moreover, recall bias and reporting bias are the potential limitations of this study. However, interviewers allowed sufficient time for adequate recall of long-term memory.

5. Conclusion

The prevalence of undernutrition was found to be high in this study. Residences, multiple medications, taking prescribed diet, and current use of alcohol were factors associated with undernutrition among depressive patients. Therefore, prevention as well as early detection and treatment of undernutrition is mandatory for patients with major depressive disorders with special emphasis among patients who come from a rural area and patient taking multiple medications. Furthermore, awareness creation on the prevention of alcohol use among depressive patient is also recommended.

Abbreviations

AOR: Adjusted odds ratio
BMI: Body mass index
COR: Crude odds ratio
DSM-IV: Diagnostic and Statistical Manual of Mental Disorders 4th edition
Kg/m^2: Kilogram per meter square
MDD: Major depressive disorder
OR: Odds ratio
SPSS: Statistical package for the social sciences
WHO: World Health Organization.

Competing Interests

The authors declare that they have no competing interests.

Authors' Contributions

Edmialem Gezahegn originated the idea and wrote the proposal, participated in data collection, analyzed the data, and drafted the paper. Edmialem Gezahegn, Melkie Edris, and Berihun Assefa Dachew approved the proposal and participated in data analysis. Berihun Assefa Dachew wrote the manuscript. All authors read and approved the final version of the manuscript.

Acknowledgments

The authors would like to acknowledge the University of Gondar for ethical clearance and providing financial support. The authors would also like to thank study participants, data collectors, and all staffs working at the University of Gondar and Bahir Dar Felege Hiwot Referral Hospital Psychiatric Clinic for their dedicated cooperation.

References

[1] B. Gelaye, S. Lemma, N. Deyassa et al., "Prevalence and correlates of mental distress among working adults in Ethiopia," *Clinical Practice and Epidemiology in Mental Health*, vol. 8, pp. 126–133, 2012.

[2] B. Gelaye, M. A. Williams, S. Lemma et al., "Validity of the patient health questionnaire-9 for depression screening and diagnosis in East Africa," *Psychiatry Research*, vol. 210, no. 2, pp. 653–661, 2013.

[3] L. Payahoo, Y. Khaje-Bishak, B. Pourghassem Gargari, M. B. Kabir-Alavi, and M. AsghariJafarabadi, "Assessment of nutritional and depression status in free-living elderly in Tabriz, Northwest Iran," *Health Promotion Perspectives*, vol. 3, no. 2, pp. 288–293, 2013.

[4] L. Harbottle, *Healthy Eating and Depression. How Diet May Help Protect Your Mental Health*, Mental Health Group of the British Dietetic Association, 2007.

[5] World Health Organization, *Mental Health: New Understanding, New Hope*, World Health Organization, Geneva, Switzerland, 2001.

[6] Central Statistical Agency, *Ethiopia Demographic and Health Survey 2011*, pp. 182–183, 2012.

[7] L. J. Podewils, T. Holtz, V. Riekstina et al., "Impact of malnutrition on clinical presentation, clinical course, and mortality in MDR-TB patients," *Epidemiology and Infection*, vol. 139, no. 1, pp. 113–120, 2011.

[8] A. S. Ginsburg, R. Izadnegahdar, J. A. Berkley, J. L. Walson, N. Rollins, and K. P. Klugman, "Undernutrition and pneumonia mortality," *The Lancet Global Health*, vol. 3, no. 12, pp. e735–e736, 2015.

[9] G. Malafaia, "Protein-energy malnutrition as a risk factor for visceral leishmaniasis: a review," *Parasite Immunology*, vol. 31, no. 10, pp. 587–596, 2009.

[10] I. Naidoo, K. E. Charlton, T. M. Esterhuizen, and B. Cassim, "High risk of malnutrition associated with depressive symptoms in older South Africans living in KwaZulu-Natal, South Africa: a cross-sectional survey," *Journal of Health, Population and Nutrition*, vol. 33, article 19, 2015.

[11] F. S. Luppino, L. M. de Wit, P. F. Bouvy et al., "Overweight, obesity, and depression: a systematic review and meta-analysis of longitudinal studies," *Archives of General Psychiatry*, vol. 67, no. 3, pp. 220–229, 2010.

[12] A. Bilgiç, A. İbis, E. Tutal, S. Koç, S. Sezer, and N. Özdemir, "Association of nutritional status with depression and sleep disorders in elderly end stage renal disease patients—does chronic inflammation cause it all?" *Turkish Nephrology, Dialysis and Transplantation Journal*, vol. 21, no. 2, pp. 148–155, 2012.

[13] A. C. Tsai, Y.-T. Chou, and T.-L. Chang, "Usefulness of the Mini Nutritional Assessment (MNA) in predicting the nutritional status of people with mental disorders in Taiwan," *Journal of Clinical Nursing*, vol. 20, no. 3-4, pp. 341–350, 2011.

[14] J. A. Solomon, Z. Zukier, and M. J. Hamadeh, *The Role of Nutrition in Mental Health: Depression*, Nutrition and Depression, 2010.

[15] C. U. Onyike, R. M. Crum, H. B. Lee, C. G. Lyketsos, and W. W. Eaton, "Is obesity associated with major depression? Results from the third national health and nutrition examination survey," *American Journal of Epidemiology*, vol. 158, no. 12, pp. 1139–1147, 2003.

[16] Z. Vafaei, H. Mokhtari, Z. Sadooghi, R. Meamar, A. Chitsaz, and M. Moeini, "Malnutrition is associated with depression in rural elderly population," *Journal of Research in Medical Sciences*, vol. 18, supplement 1, pp. S15–S19, 2013.

[17] C. Hadley, A. Tegegn, F. Tessema, J. A. Cowan, M. Asefa, and S. Galea, "Food insecurity, stressful life events and symptoms of anxiety and depression in east Africa: evidence from the Gilgel Gibe growth and development study," *Journal of Epidemiology and Community Health*, vol. 62, no. 11, pp. 980–986, 2008.

[18] American Psychiatric Association, *Diagnostic and Statistical Manual of Mental Disorders*, DSM-IV, 4th edition, 2000.

[19] J. Correia and P. Ravasco, "Weight changes in Portuguese patients with depression: which factors are involved?" *Nutrition Journal*, vol. 13, article 117, 2014.

[20] T. Ferdous, Z. N. Kabir, Å. Wahlin, K. Streatfield, and T. Cederholm, "The multidimensional background of malnutrition

among rural older individuals in Bangladesh—a challenge for the Millennium Development Goal," *Public Health Nutrition*, vol. 12, no. 12, pp. 2270–2278, 2009.

[21] B. Pourghassem Gargari, M. Saboktakin, S. Mahboob, and N. Pourafkari, "Nutritional status in patients with major depressive disorders: a pilot study in Tabriz, Iran," *Health Promotion Perspectives*, vol. 2, no. 2, pp. 145–152, 2012.

[22] M. S. P. Toups, A. K. Myers, S. R. Wisniewski et al., "Relationship between obesity and depression: characteristics and treatment outcomes with antidepressant medication," *Psychosomatic Medicine*, vol. 75, no. 9, pp. 863–872, 2013.

[23] C. S. Lieber and N. Spritz, "Effects of prolonged ethanol intake in man: role of dietary adipose, and endogenously synthesized fatty acids in the pathogenesis of the alcoholic fatty liver," *Journal of Clinical Investigation*, vol. 45, no. 9, pp. 1400–1411, 1966.

23

Towards a Standard Psychometric Diagnostic Interview for Subjects at Ultra High Risk of Psychosis: CAARMS versus SIPS

P. Fusar-Poli,[1,2] M. Cappucciati,[1] G. Rutigliano,[1] T. Y. Lee,[3] Q. Beverly,[4] I. Bonoldi,[1,2] J. Lelli,[5] S. J. Kaar,[2] E. Gago,[2] M. Rocchetti,[1] R. Patel,[1,2] V. Bhavsar,[1,2] S. Tognin,[1,2] S. Badger,[1,2] M. Calem,[1,2] K. Lim,[3] J. S. Kwon,[3] J. Perez,[4,6] and P. McGuire[1,2]

[1] *Institute of Psychiatry Psychology and Neuroscience (IoPPN), King's College London, London SE5 8AF, UK*
[2] *OASIS Service, South London and Maudsley NHS Foundation Trust, London SE11, UK*
[3] *Department of Psychiatry, Seoul National University College of Medicine, Seoul 08826, Republic of Korea*
[4] *Cambridgeshire and Peterborough NHS Foundation Trust, Cambridge CB21 5HH, UK*
[5] *Real-Time Systems Laboratory, Scuola Superiore Sant'Anna, 56124 Pisa, Italy*
[6] *Department of Psychiatry, University of Cambridge, Cambridge CB2 0SZ, UK*

Correspondence should be addressed to P. Fusar-Poli; p.fusar@libero.it

Academic Editor: Lenin Pavon

Background. Several psychometric instruments are available for the diagnostic interview of subjects at ultra high risk (UHR) of psychosis. Their diagnostic comparability is unknown. *Methods.* All referrals to the OASIS (London) or CAMEO (Cambridgeshire) UHR services from May 13 to Dec 14 were interviewed for a UHR state using both the CAARMS 12/2006 and the SIPS 5.0. Percent overall agreement, kappa, the McNemar-Bowker χ^2 test, equipercentile methods, and residual analyses were used to investigate diagnostic outcomes and symptoms severity or frequency. A conversion algorithm (CONVERT) was validated in an independent UHR sample from the Seoul Youth Clinic (Seoul). *Results.* There was overall substantial CAARMS-versus-SIPS agreement in the identification of UHR subjects ($n = 212$, percent overall agreement = 86%; kappa = 0.781, 95% CI from 0.684 to 0.878; McNemar-Bowker test = 0.069), with the exception of the brief limited intermittent psychotic symptoms (BLIPS) subgroup. Equipercentile-linking table linked symptoms severity and frequency across the CAARMS and SIPS. The conversion algorithm was validated in 93 UHR subjects, showing excellent diagnostic accuracy (CAARMS to SIPS: ROC area 0.929; SIPS to CAARMS: ROC area 0.903). *Conclusions.* This study provides initial comparability data between CAARMS and SIPS and will inform ongoing multicentre studies and clinical guidelines for the UHR psychometric diagnostic interview.

"The comparability of measurements made in differing circumstances by different methods and investigators is a fundamental precondition for all of science"
Dorans and Holland (2000)

1. Introduction

The development of psychometric tools to prospectively identify subjects at ultra high clinical risk (UHR hereafter) of psychosis has allowed preventative screening [1], diagnosis [2], and interventions [3] to be feasible in psychiatry. In 1991, Jackson and McGorry were the first to initiate reliability studies to psychometrically assess first-episode subjects via a semistructured interview in order to ascertain the presence of prodromal symptoms [4]. On the basis of their results, in 1995 Yung and colleagues set up the first clinical service for UHR individuals and conceived the first comprehensive UHR psychometric instrument [5]. The Comprehensive Assessment of At-Risk Mental States (CAARMS hereafter) was developed at the Personal Assessment and Crisis Evaluation (PACE) Clinic in Melbourne [6] and has been widely used in Australia, Asia, and Europe to interview for "At-Risk Mental State, ARMS," criteria. Their pivotal work resulted in the formulation of three UHR criteria: attenuated psychotic symptoms (APS hereafter), brief limited intermittent psychotic symptoms (BLIPS hereafter), and trait vulnerability plus a marked decline in psychosocial functioning (Genetic Risk and Deterioration syndrome: GRD hereafter). A few years later, in 1999, based on these criteria, Miller et al. (1999) [7] developed a similar psychometric instrument for quantitatively rating symptoms in patients at UHR of psychosis [8], in the Prevention through Risk Identification, Management and Education (PRIME) Clinic in New Haven (USA): the Structured Interview for Psychosis-Risk Syndrome (SIPS hereafter) [8] (for a detailed genealogy of the CAARMS and SIPS see [9, 10]).

The CAARMS and the SIPS address the same construct and use similar criteria, and they can deliver comparable positive predictive values over follow-up time [11, 12]. However, their operationalization differs [10], with substantial changes over different versions of the instruments [10]. Operationalization differences include disparity in psychopathological definitions of the APS, time and frequency criteria, functional decline criterion, BLIPS criteria, assessment of comorbidities, and substance misuse (see Tables 1 and 2 and eTable 1 (in Supplementary Material available online at http://dx.doi.org/10.1155/2016/7146341) for a detailed comparison of CAARMS 12/2006 and SIPS 5.0).

The resulting overall weight of similarities and differences between the two instruments on UHR identification is unknown. Psychometric diagnostic uncertainty questions validity of the UHR diagnostic interview, creating inconsistencies between clinicians or researchers and misunderstandings in patients [13]. Comparability of current clinical, neurobiological, cognitive, and therapeutic UHR research findings may be also questionable and compromised, with the risk of "a profusion of statistically significant, but minimally differentiating" [14] results of limited clinical utility. Psychometric uncertainty may significantly impact the development of future large-scale UHR multicentre studies, by amplifying heterogeneity across individual sites. These concerns and speculations have never been tested empirically. To resolve the "current confusion" [13], research studies allowing "a thorough evaluation of the comparability of samples" [13] have been urgently advocated [10, 15].

We present here the first study addressing the psychometric comparability of the CAARMS 12/2006 [16] versus SIPS 5.0 [8]. Our principal aim was to test if the CAARMS 12/2006 and the SIPS 5.0 can equally identify UHR subjects in a large pool of individuals referred to high-risk services for potential UHR symptoms. Our second aim was to qualitatively investigate potential discrepancies and to link the severity and frequency of symptoms with equipercentile-linking tables. Our third aim was to develop a pragmatic algorithm to convert individual cases across the two instruments, to implement it in an automated conversion package (CONVERT), and to validate it in an independent UHR sample.

2. Methods

2.1. Samples. We included all referrals to the OASIS (Outreach And Support In South London; http://www.slam.nhs.uk/oasis) and CAMEO (Cambridgeshire and Peterborough Assessing Managing and Enhancing Outcomes, http://www.cameo.nhs.uk/) clinics assessed for a UHR state in the period May 2013–December 2014. The OASIS team was started in 2001 [17] and it is specialized in detecting and treating subjects at UHR of psychosis aged 16–35 [17]. CAMEO was started in 2007 and it is an early intervention in psychosis service which offers management for UHR people aged 17–35 in Cambridgeshire, UK, and provides initial assessments to those under 17. Referrals for both services are accepted from multiple sources including general practitioners, other mental health services, school and college counselors, relatives, and self-referrals [18]. The validation sample for CONVERT included all referrals to the Seoul Youth Clinic assessed for a UHR state with the CAARMS 12/2006 and the SIPS 5.0 as part of the standard clinical practice. The Seoul Youth Clinic was started in 2004 and offers assessment and treatment for UHR people aged 15–35 in Seoul, South Korea [19]. Subjects are recruited from Seoul National University Hospital and other psychiatric clinics and public mental health centers or they can contact the clinic by telephone or an Internet homepage.

2.2. Procedure. The study samples were designed to reflect at-risk populations as they are encountered in day-to-day practice: all subjects were drawn from the same pool of people referred to high-risk services because of suspect prodromal signs and symptoms of psychosis. Avoiding the use of external and non-help-seeking control groups who do not reflect the clinical composition of people actually assessed in high risk is essential to properly compare the diagnostic abilities of the two instruments. Furthermore, we only included subjects who were directly assessed with both psychometric instruments during face-to-face interviews, excluding those who declined the full assessment or who were unable to complete it. Responsible clinicians interviewed the participants with the CAARMS 12/2006 [16] and with the SIPS 5.0 [8]. The training procedure and the interrater reliability of the OASIS and CAMEO clinicians have been fully detailed in Supplementary eMethod 1. Subjects accessing the Seoul Youth Clinic are usually assessed with both CAARMS 12/2006 and SIPS 5.0 instruments as part of standard clinical practice, and further details are provided in an independent publication [19].

2.3. Clinical Measures. The primary outcome measure was the psychometric diagnosis under the CAARMS 12/2006 [16] versus SIPS 5.0 [8] at the end of the diagnostic interview assessment: at risk of psychosis (UHR+ hereafter), not at risk of psychosis (UHR− hereafter), and Psychosis. Secondary outcome measures included the severity and frequency of UHR as measured on the diagnostic subscales: P1–P4 on the CAARMS 12/2006 and P1–P5 on the SIPS 5.0 (eTable 1). Additional variables recorded were subgroup of UHR+ (APS, BLIPS, and GRD), age, gender, ethnicity, baseline comorbid diagnosis, duration of follow-up, and functional status (GAF in the SIPS 5.0 and SOFAS in the CAARMS 12/2006).

2.4. Statistical Analysis. The primary aim of the study was investigated by comparing the diagnostic outcomes

Table 1: UHR criteria: similarities and differences between the SIPS 5.0 and the CAARMS 12/2006 (see also eTable 1 for details on the psychopathological dimensions investigated by P1–P5 and P1–P4).

(a) Rating system

	SIPS *version 5.0* [8]	CAARMS *version 12/2006* [16]
Subscales	P1: Unusual Thought Content/Delusional Ideas P2: Suspiciousness/Persecutory Ideas P3: Grandiose Ideas P4: Perceptual Abnormalities/Hallucinations P5: Disorganized Communication	P1: Unusual Thought Content P2: Non-Bizarre Ideas P3: Perceptual Abnormalities P4: Disorganized Speech
Frequency	1: at least several min per d at least 1/mo 2: several min/d at least once/wk in the past mo 3: at least 1 h/d for at least 4 d/wk over 1 mo	0: absent 1: less than 1/mo 2: 1/mo to 2/wk, <1 h per occasion 3: 1/mo to 2/wk, >1 h per occasion, OR 3 to 6/wk, <1 h per occasion 4: 3 to 6/wk, > 1 h per occasion, OR daily, <1 h per occasion 5: daily, >1 h per occasion, OR several times/d 6: continuous
Substance use	Exclusion criterion if strongly intertwined with symptoms	0: no relation to substance use noted 1: occurs in relation to substance use and at other times as well 2: noted only in relation to substance use
Distress	Subjective qualifier Not used to determine an individual's UHR status	Rated on scale 0–100 Not used to determine an individual's UHR status

(b) Attenuated psychotic symptoms

	Attenuated positive symptom psychosis-risk syndrome SIPS *version 5.0* [8]	Attenuated psychosis group CAARMS *version 12/2006* [16]
Inclusion criteria	Severity score of 3–5 on at least one of P1–P5 *PLUS* Frequency score of 2 on P1, P2, P3, P4, and/or P5	*Subthreshold intensity* Severity score of 3–5 on P1, 3–5 on P2, 3-4 on P3, and/or 4-5 on P4 *PLUS* Frequency score of 3–6 on P1, P2, P3, and/or P4 *Subthreshold frequency* Severity score of 6 on at least one of P1, P2, and P4 and/or 5-6 on P3 *PLUS* Frequency score of 3 on P1, P2, P3, and/or P4
Onset	Symptoms should have begun within the past year *OR* currently rate one or more scale points higher compared to 12 months before Symptoms that occurred over the past month only are rated	Symptoms should have been present in the previous 12 mo *AND* for not longer than 5 y
Level of functioning	No social/occupational dysfunction requirement	30% drop in SOFAS score from premorbid level, sustained for a mo, within the past 12 mo *OR* SOFAS score <50 for the past 12 mo or more
Exclusion criteria	Symptoms are strongly intertwined temporally with substance use episodes (substance-induced psychosis may be considered)	Symptoms occur only during peak intoxication from a substance known to be associated with psychotic experiences (e.g., hallucinogens, amphetamines, and cocaine)
	Symptoms are better accounted for by another DSM diagnosis	—
	Past psychosis ruled in according to information obtained through the initial screen and evaluated using the POPS	The person has had a previous psychotic episode (treated or untreated)

(c) Brief limited intermittent psychotic symptoms

	Brief intermittent psychotic symptom psychosis-risk syndrome SIPS *version 5.0* [8]	Brief limited intermittent psychotic symptoms group CAARMS *version 12/2006* [16]
Inclusion criteria	Severity score of 6 on at least one of P1–P5 *PLUS* Frequency score of 1 on P1, P2, P3, P4, and/or P5	Severity score of 6 on at least one of P1, P2, and P4 and/or 5-6 on P3 *PLUS* Frequency score of 4–6 on P1, P2, P3, and/or P4
Onset	Symptoms should have reached a psychotic level of intensity in the previous 3 mo	Symptoms should have been present in the previous 12 mo and for not longer than 5 y
Duration	Up to 3 mo	Up to 7 d
Level of functioning	No social/occupational dysfunction requirement	30% drop in SOFAS score from premorbid level, sustained for a mo, within the past 12 mo *OR* SOFAS score <50 for the past 12 mo or more
Exclusion criteria	Symptoms are strongly intertwined temporally with substance use episodes (substance-induced psychosis may be considered)	Symptoms occur only during peak intoxication from a substance known to be associated with psychotic experiences (e.g., hallucinogens, amphetamines, and cocaine)
	Symptoms are better accounted for by another DSM diagnosis	—
	Past psychosis ruled in according to information obtained through the initial screen and evaluated using the POPS	The person has had a previous psychotic episode (treated or untreated)
	Symptoms are seriously disorganizing and dangerous	—
	—	Symptoms do not resolve spontaneously (without antipsychotic medication)

(d) Genetic risk and deterioration syndrome

	Genetic risk and deterioration psychosis-risk syndrome SIPS *version 5.0* [8]	Vulnerability group CAARMS *version 12/2006* [16]
Inclusion criteria	The patient meets criteria for Schizotypal Personality Disorder *OR* The patient has a first-degree relative with a psychotic disorder	Schizotypal Personality Disorder in identified patient *OR* Family history of psychosis in a first-degree relative
Level of functioning	30% drop in GAF score over the last mo as compared to 12 mo before	30% drop in SOFAS score from premorbid level, sustained for a mo, within the past 12 mo *OR* SOFAS score <50 for the past 12 mo or more

CAARMS, Comprehensive Assessment of At-Risk Mental States; d, day; GAF, Global Assessment of Functioning; h, hour; min, minute; mo, month; SIPS, Structured Interview for Psychosis-Risk Syndrome; SOFAS, Social and Occupational Functioning Assessment Scale; UHR, ultra high risk; wk, week.

TABLE 2: Psychosis threshold: similarities and differences between the SIPS 5.0 and the CAARMS 12/2006.

	Presence of psychotic syndrome SIPS *version 5.0*	Psychosis threshold CAARMS *version 12/2006*
Inclusion criteria	Severity score of 6 on at least one of P1–P5 *PLUS* Frequency score of 3 on P1, P2, P3, P4, and/or P5	Severity score of 6 on at least one of P1, P2, and P4 and/or 5-6 on P3 *PLUS* Frequency score of 4–6 on P1, P2, P3, and/or P4
Urgency	Symptoms are seriously disorganizing and dangerous (a)	—

CAARMS, Comprehensive Assessment of At-Risk Mental States; SIPS, Structured Interview for Psychosis-Risk Syndrome.
(a) "'Dangerous' is taken to mean physically dangerous, for example, risk of death or serious physical injury, and 'disorganizing' means potentially psychosocially dangerous, for example, risk of seriously damaging work relations, social relations, family relations, or personal dignity." Personal communication from the authors of the SIPS, published with permission (see Acknowledgments).

(i.e., UHR+, UHR−, and Psychosis) under CAARMS 12/2006 versus SIPS 5.0 in OASIS and CAMEO samples, using IBM SPSS Statistics 22 and STATA 13 software. Specifically, we calculated percent overall agreement, kappa (with its 95% CI), and the exact McNemar-Bowker χ^2 test to assess marginal errors. Given evidence that baseline functional status is a strong predictor of longitudinal outcome [20], we further performed a weighted kappa analysis, weighting the three groups according to their relative baseline functional level, as established in our previous meta-analysis (i.e., UHR− = 1, UHR+ = 0.84, and Psychosis = 0, eFigure 1, adapted from [20]). We additionally estimated the prevalence and bias adjusted kappa (PABAK) [21] which adjusts the kappa for imbalances caused by differences in prevalence and bias [22]. Interpretation of the kappa values varies, but some guidelines were provided by Landis and Koch (1977) for kappa coefficients suggesting that kappa of 0.01 indicates "poor" agreement; kappa values from 0.01 to 0.20 indicate "slight" agreement; kappa values from 0.21 to 0.40 indicate "fair" agreement; kappa values from 0.41 to 0.60 indicate "moderate" agreement; kappa values from 0.61 to 0.80 indicate "substantial" agreement; kappa values from 0.81 to 1.00 indicate "almost prefect" agreement [23].

The secondary aim of the study was investigated using post hoc explorative residual analyses comparing different subgroups (i.e., UHR−, GRD, APS, BLIPS, and Psychosis), Bonferroni-corrected for multiple comparisons. Qualitative analyses of discrepancies across the two instruments were also conducted, to better elucidate the impact of each specific cell on the overall results. We further converted the severity and frequency of symptoms by employing a linking method, using equate 2.0-3 [24] under R 3.1.2 software. This method is detailed in eMethod 2.

The third aim of the study was investigated with qualitative a priori comparisons of a priori operationalization differences between the CAARMS 12/2006 and SIPS 5.0, as detailed in Tables 1 and 2. Equipercentile linking, percent overall agreement, and kappa estimated above here in the OASIS and CAMEO services were not used for the development of this pragmatic algorithm. A software engineer (JL) then implemented the conversion algorithm in an automated package. CONVERT is a Python application which implements the conversions of individual outcomes (UHR−, UHR+ [GRD, APS, and BLIPS], and Psychosis) between the CAARMS 12/2006 and SIPS 5.0 as proposed by the conversion algorithm. CONVERT takes as input a ∗.xls file and produces as output a ∗.xls file. To freely download the tool and the template ∗.xls input file and get further details please visit https://bitbucket.org/ioppn/convert. We first piloted CONVERT in the OASIS and CAMEO dataset and then validated it in an independent UHR sample recruited at the Seoul Youth Clinic. Diagnostic accuracy measures of CONVERT were analysed with respect to both CAARMS 12/2006-to-SIPS 5.0 and SIPS 5.0-to-CAARMS 12/2006 conversions and included percent overall agreement, kappa (with its 95% CI), PABAK, sensitivity, specificity, and nonparametric Receiver Operating Characteristic (ROC) analyses.

3. Results

3.1. Samples and Raters Characteristics. The OASIS and CAMEO sample consisted of 212 consecutive help-seeking subjects recruited between May 2013 and December 2014 (OASIS = 128, CAMEO = 84). Of the 212 subjects, 82 were females (38.7%). The mean age was of 24.13 years (SD = 4.98, range = 16–35 years). The majority of subjects were white British (50%), followed by black British (26.1%) and subjects from Asia (4.1%), Africa (4.3%), and South America (1.1%) and from other European countries (11.4%). The mean SOFAS score was of 51.51 (SD = 17.26, median = 48, and range = 18–95). Sociodemographic characteristics of referrals across OASIS and CAMEO are detailed in the Supplementary Material (eTable 2). Each rater interviewed on average 35.33 (SD 31.1) subjects. The IRR for the principal diagnostic outcome (n = 21) was of kappa = 0.902 for the CAARMS 12/2006 and kappa = 0.854 for the SIPS 5.0. The IRRs for each subscale were in the excellent range: CAARMS 12/2006 kappa from 0.863 to 0.915 and SIPS 5.0 kappa from 0.815 to 0.923 (eMethod 1).

The validation sample from the Seoul Youth Clinic included 93 UHR subjects, with a mean age of 20.24 years (SD = 4.00, range = 15–33), mostly males (29% females), of Asian ethnicity [19].

3.2. Diagnostic Comparison of CAARMS 12/2006 and SIPS 5.0 in OASIS and CAMEO. The percent overall agreement was 86.32% (expected agreement by chance 37.42%) and the kappa was substantial 0.781 (Z = 15.83, $p < 0.001$, and 95% CI from 0.684 to 0.878) with the McNemar-Bowker χ^2 (7.087) resulting in p = 0.069. The prevalence and bias adjusted kappa was 0.795 (95% CI from 0.731 to 0.856). The kappa remained substantial when it was estimated in the subset of subjects rated by independent raters (overall agreement 92.86%, expected agreement by chance 76.08%, kappa = 0.701, Z = 3.87, and p = 0.001). Full details of the main diagnostic comparison are appended in Table 3. When the analysis was weighted for the relative functional impairment of the three groups the results were very similar: the percent overall agreement was 88.43% (expected agreement 45.44%) and the kappa was 0.788 (Z = 16.22, $p < 0.001$, and 95% CI from 0.693 to 0.883).

3.3. Qualitative Analysis and Equipercentile Linking of CAARMS 12/2006 and SIPS 5.0. Post hoc analyses (see eTable 3) confirmed an overall substantial agreement across the two instruments with the exception of the cell [2,5: CAARMS 12/2006-BLIPS versus SIPS 5.0-Psychosis, adjusted residual = 3.7]. This indicates that, out of the 25 subjects diagnosed with BLIPS by the CAARMS 12/2006, 14 were diagnosed as psychotic by the SIPS 5.0 (eTable 3). The count in this cell was statistically higher than the count expected by chance. To better elucidate these differences we have conducted a qualitative analysis of psychopathological characteristics of these 14 patients, which is appended in eTable 4. The equipercentile linking between severity and frequency scores of the two instruments is detailed in Table 4.

3.4. Development and Validation of an Automatized Conversion Algorithm (CONVERT). The pragmatic algorithm to convert individual cases across the SIPS 5.0 and the CAARMS 12/2006 is depicted in Figure 1.

The steps illustrated in Figure 1 have been fully automatized in the CONVERT tool, which is appended online (https://bitbucket.org/ioppn/convert) with further information for users. The tool was first piloted on the OASIS and CAMEO sample and it was able to correctly convert all cases between the two instruments. External validation was performed in an independent sample assessed for suspicion of UHR symptoms at the Seoul Youth Clinic (see eTable 5). For the SIPS 5.0-to-CAARMS 12/2006 CONVERT

TABLE 3: Diagnostic comparison between CAARMS 12/2006 and SIPS 0.5 outcomes in subjects seeking help from high-risk services ($p < 0.001$).

			SIPS outcome			
			UHR−	UHR+	Psychotic	Total
CAARMS outcome	UHR−	Count	51	0	0	51
		%	24.1%	0.0%	0.0%	24.1%
		Adj Res	13.5	−7.8	−4.8	
	UHR+	Count	5	92	14	111
		%	2.4%	91.1%	6.6%	52.4%
		Adj Res	−7.7	10.8	−4.5	
	Psychotic	Count	1	9	40	50
		%	0.5%	4.2%	18.9%	23.6%
		Adj Res	−4.5	−4.8	10.1	
	Total	Count	57	101	54	212
		%	29.6%	47.6%	25.5%	100.0%

CAARMS, Comprehensive Assessment of At-Risk Mental States; SIPS, Structured Interview for Psychosis-Risk Syndrome; UHR, ultra high risk; Adj Res, adjusted residuals; adjusted residuals lower than −3.29 or greater than 3.29 indicate that the number of cases in that cell is significantly larger or small than expected under the null hypothesis at $p < 0.001$ corrected for multiple comparisons. No cells have expected count less than 5. The minimum expected count is 12.74.

conversion, the percent overall agreement was of 92.47% (expected agreement 56.63%), kappa = 0.826 (95% CI from 0.623 to 1), PABAK = 0.85, sensitivity = 83.87%, specificity = 96.77%, and ROC area = 0.903 (95% CI from 0.833 to 0.972). For the CAARMS 12/2006-to-SIPS 5.0 CONVERT conversion, the percent overall agreement was of 98.92% (expected agreement 86.99%), kappa = 0.917 (95% CI from 0.714 to 1), PABAK = 0.98, sensitivity = 100%, specificity = 85.7%, and ROC area = 0.929 (95% CI from 0.789 to 1).

4. Discussion

This is the first pilot study addressing comparability of the two psychometric instruments most frequently used to interview subjects seeking help from high-risk services for psychosis. Strengths of this study include enrolment of a relatively large sample size inclusive of UHR+, UHR−, and psychotic patients, the use of kappa analyses and equipercentile-linking methods, the development of automatized algorithms, and the use of external validation samples of different ethnic background. We found an overall substantial agreement between CAARMS 12/2006 and SIPS 5.0 in the identification of UHR subjects, with the exception of BLIPS. These findings however may be influenced by the type of recruitment strategies adopted by the high-risk services. Residual and qualitative analyses and equipercentile-linking tables provided additional comparability data. The automated conversion algorithm (CONVERT) to convert individual cases was validated in an independent sample and showed an excellent accuracy.

Our first aim was to test the diagnostic comparability of CAARMS 12/2006 versus SIPS 5.0 in a large sample of more than 200 subjects referred for psychometric diagnostic interview to high-risk services. We found an overall substantial agreement (kappa) between the CAARMS 12/2006 and SIPS 5.0. Such a substantial agreement is not completely surprising. First, the two instruments show similar psychometric parameters, such as excellent reliability properties (overall IRR agreement for the SIPS 0.95 [25], for the CAARMS 0.85 [6]). Second, independent authors not involved with the development of the two instruments argue that the development of the SIPS was influenced by the CAARMS. Specifically, they claimed that the SIPS was developed at the PRIME Clinic "to evaluate the severity of ARMS, as defined by [9]." Third, in our previous meta-analysis we found that the CAARMS and the SIPS can identify a similar proportion of true positives over time (transition risk by 31 months with the CAARMS = 27.4%, 95% CI from 24.6% to 30.4%; transition risk by 31 months with the SIPS = 28.1%, 95% CI from 25.1% to 31.3%; $p = 0.73$) [12]. Finally, in a recent meta-analysis we specifically confirmed that, in help-seeking samples, the two instruments share similar excellent prognostic accuracy in ruling out psychosis risk, with no significant differences [26]. On the basis of the above substantial agreement, our findings are the first to address the "Babylonian confusion" of UHR diagnostic interview, making it easier to overall compare the results of UHR research, which had formerly been difficult and risky [9]. Indeed, the definition of case (i.e., whether or not a subject has the condition of interest) is highly problematic across the entirety of clinical psychiatry, where no objectively assessable measures/markers/tests/exams other than clinical impression usually exist to establish the presence or absence of a given condition. Our results are thus highly relevant to permit overall meaningful comparisons of clinical, neurobiological, neurocognitive, and cost-effectiveness UHR studies worldwide, with potential beneficial impact for ongoing large-scale multicentre UHR projects such as the PRONIA (http://www.pronia.eu/), NAPLS (http://napls.commons.yale.edu/), and PSYSCAN (http://www.psyscan.eu/).

Our secondary aim was to qualitatively investigate potential discrepancies across the two instruments and to provide equipercentile-linking comparisons. The

Table 4: Equipercentile-linking table comparing symptoms severity and frequency across CAARMS 12/2006 and SIPS 5.0 in the OASIS and CAMEO sample.

Domain	Severity scores				Frequency scores			
	CAARMS to	SIPS	SIPS to	CAARMS	CAARMS to	SIPS	SIPS to	CAARMS
P1 CAARMS to P1 SIPS & P1 SIPS to P1 CAARMS	0	0.012	0	0.011	0	0.019	0	0.017
	1	1.092	1	0.916	1	0.718	1	1.690
	2	2.212	2	1.816	2	1.163	2	3.321
	3	3.258	3	2.759	3	1.781	3	5.282
	4	4.180	4	3.799	4	2.481		
	5	5.019	5	4.976	5	2.899		
	6	5.965	6	6.033	6	3.289		
P2 CAARMS to P2 SIPS	0	0.026			0	0.028		
	1	1.059			1	0.602		
	2	2.234			2	1.001		
	3	3.216			3	1.669		
	4	4.105			4	2.406		
	5	5.956			5	2.861		
	6	5.961			6	3.271		
P2 CAARMS to P3 SIPS	0	0.041			0	0.004		
	1	0.124			1	0.027		
	2	0.178			2	0.071		
	3	0.112			3	0.106		
	4	0.297			4	0.237		
	5	0.464			5	0.469		
	6	2.692			6	2.462		
P2/P3 SIPS* to P2 CAARMS			0	0.007			0	0.062
			1	0.919			1	1.779
			2	1.778			2	3.541
			3	2.735			3	5.478
			4	3.806				
			5	4.991				
			6	6.025				
P3 CAARMS to P4 SIPS & P4 SIPS to P3 CAARMS	0	0.012	0	0.013	0	0.007	0	0.007
	1	0.893	1	1.112	1	0.625	1	1.984
	2	1.891	2	2.106	2	1.001	2	3.347
	3	2.953	3	3.045	3	1.701	3	4.899
	4	3.944	4	4.059	4	2.537		
	5	4.861	5	5.153	5	3.034		
	6	5.876	6	6.099	6	3.530		
P4 CAARMS to P5 SIPS & P5 SIPS to P4 CAARMS	0	0.067	0	0.079	0	0.080	0	0.095
	1	0.855	1	1.126	1	0.594	1	1.743
	2	1.981	2	2.017	2	1.133	2	3.612
	3	3.032	3	2.968	3	1.666	3	5.234
	4	4.064	4	3.936	4	2.193		
	5	5.158	5	4.844	5	2.798		
	6	6.090	6	5.889	6	3.472		

P1–P4 on the CAARMS and P1–P5 on SIPS are defined in Table 1; *using the highest score across P2 and P3 SIPS. For analytical purposes in this table the SIPS frequency was coded as follows: 1: ≥1 h/d, ≥4 d/wk; 2: ≥several minutes/d, ≥1x/mo; 3: ≥1x/wk; 0: none of the above.

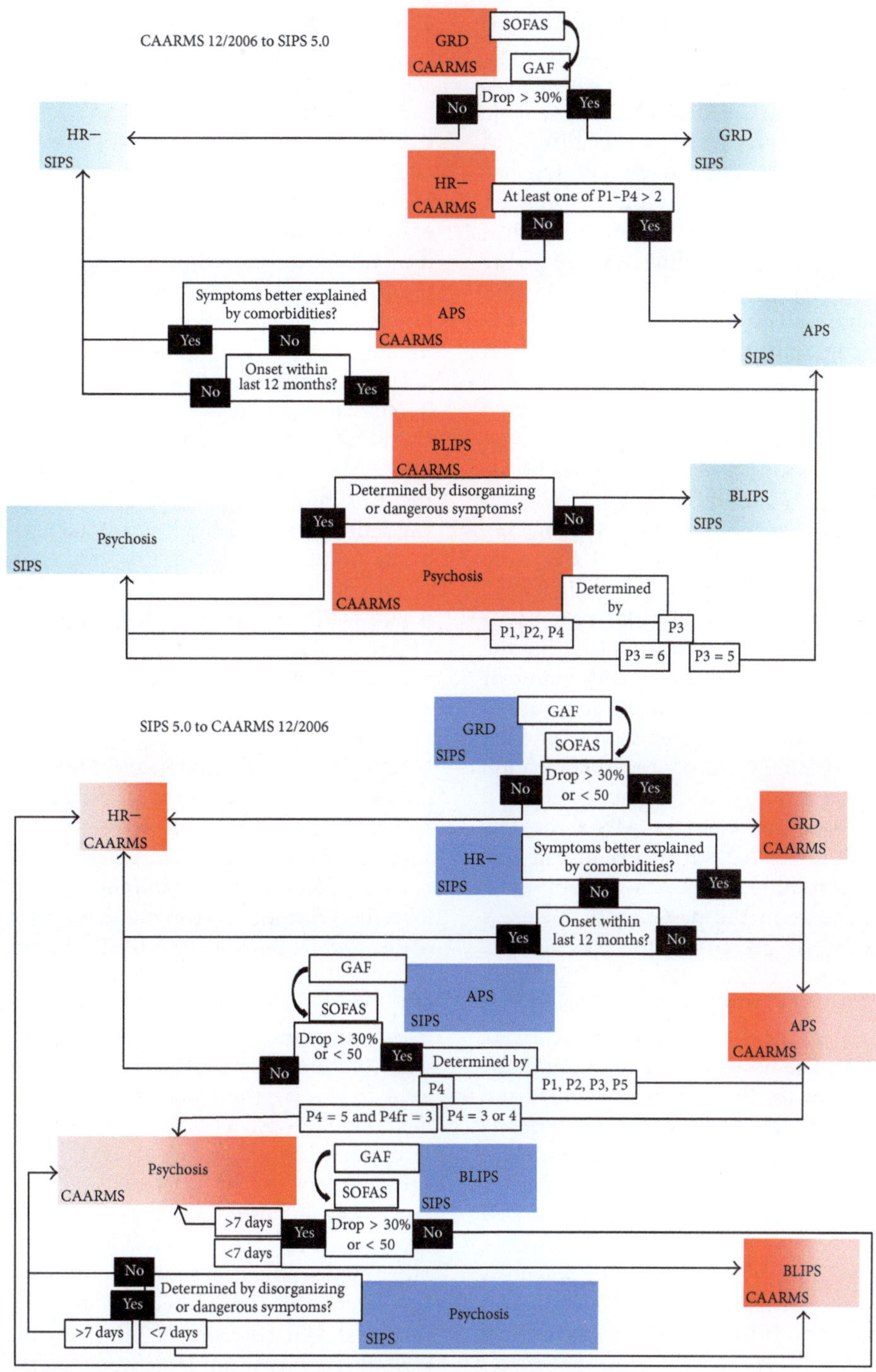

FIGURE 1: Pragmatic algorithms to convert CAARMS 12/2006-versus-SIPS 5.0 individual cases, automatized in the package CONVERT, which is appended online at https://bitbucket.org/ioppn/convert.

equipercentile-linking table (Table 4) suggests a close relationship between the symptoms severity and frequency scores of the CAARMS 12/2006 and SIPS 5.0, as also confirmed by equipercentile-linking analyses of SOFAS and GAF measures [27]. However, we also found some sources of disagreement, in particular, with respect to the diagnosis of BLIPS subjects. Indeed 14 out of the 25 BLIPS subjects diagnosed by the CAARMS 12/2006 were diagnosed as already psychotic by the SIPS 5.0 (eTable 4). There are significant differential operationalizations of the BLIPS across the two instruments. On one side the psychosis threshold is higher in the SIPS 5.0 than in the CAARMS 12/2006 (psychotic symptoms may last more than 7 days); on the other it is lower since the symptoms should not have urgency features [28] ("*urgency is any positive psychotic symptom that is seriously disorganizing or dangerous no matter what the duration*" (*SIPS 5.0 manual page 15* [8])). To elucidate this difference we conducted a qualitative analysis of the medical records of these 14 subjects. We confirmed that all of them were presenting with disorganized or dangerous symptoms (see definition in Table 2), which were meeting BLIPS criteria under the CAARMS 12/2006 (eTable 3) while at the same time being regarded as over threshold for psychosis with the SIPS 5.0. Since South London has one of the highest rates of psychosis in the world [17], BLIPS subjects alone represent about 9% of OASIS patients, with an additional 9% meeting conjointly APS or GRD criteria (Figure 6 from [17]). Conversely, operationalization differences in BLIPS duration (i.e., less than 7 days on the CAARMS 12/2006) affected only 4 subjects in our database (eTable 3). This may be partially due to the fact that our referrers are trained to refer only BLIPS subjects defined by the CAARMS 12/2006 criteria. Similarly, differences on psychosis threshold in the Perceptual Abnormalities subscale (i.e., severity of 6 on the SIPS 5.0 and 5 on the CAARMS 12/2006) affected only 6 subjects in our database (eTable 3).

Conversely, operationalization differences of the APS, which includes four domains (P1–P4) in the CAARMS 12/2006 and five in the SIPS 5.0 (P1–P5), did not play a significant role (eTable 3). It is possible to speculate that the additional SIPS 5.0 domain, Grandiose Ideas, with manic or hypomanic features is not particularly frequent or severe in UHR subjects (4 subjects only had higher scores on SIPS 5.0 P3 as compared to SIPS 5.0 P2). Also, operationalization differences in APS onset criteria did not impact the overall consistency of the diagnostic interview for APS across the two instruments. This is somewhat surprising giving that CAARMS 12/2006 permits positive symptoms to qualify even if they are no longer present in the past month, whereas SIPS 5.0 requires them to be present in the past month. Also, the functional decline criterion (i.e., SOFAS drop), which is explicitly used in the CAARMS 12/2006 but not in the SIPS 5.0, did not impact the diagnostic agreement (see limitations below). This finding however is also supported by our recent meta-analysis showing that both SIPS-defined and CAARMS-defined UHR samples display consistent baseline functional impairments as compared to matched controls [20]. Similarly, there was no effect for the assessment of differential diagnoses associated with comorbidities [29] between the CAARMS 12/2006 (which does not consider comorbidities) and SIPS 5.0 (in which the UHR+ diagnosis should not be made if the symptoms are better explained by other comorbid disorders; this affected only 5 subjects in our database; see eTable 3). However, the notion "better explained" is poorly coded and may therefore be subject to arbitrary clinical judgment: no studies have ever addressed the impact of this criterion on subjects identified by the SIPS. Because of this, comorbid disorders may be highly prevalent in both the CAARMS 12/2006 and the SIPS 5.0. Indeed in our meta-analysis specifically investigating comorbid affective disorders in UHR subjects, we found a similar prevalence of anxiety or depressive disorders in SIPS [30, 31] and CAARMS [32] studies.

Our third aim was to develop an automated algorithm to convert individual cases and to validate it in an external sample. Therefore, on the basis of the CAARMS 12/2006 and SIPS 5.0 differences in operationalizations detailed in Tables 1 and 2, we were finally able to develop and propose a pragmatic algorithm to convert the main clinical outcomes across the two instruments (see Figure 1). This algorithm has been implemented in the CONVERT tool, which has been made freely available for the use of future researchers and clinicians and externally validated in an independent sample. We found that CONVERT performed in the excellent range of accuracy in both directions: the ROC area was 0.903 for the SIPS 5.0-to-CAARMS 12/2006 conversion and 0.929 for the CAARMS 12/2006-to-SIPS 5.0 conversion. The ROC area serves as a global measure of test performance and values in the range of 0.9–1 are considered excellent, between 0.8 and 0.9 very good, between 0.7 and 0.8 good, between 0.6 and 0.7 sufficient, and between 0.5 and 0.6 bad [33]. Of relevance, CONVERT was developed on a priori differences between CAARMS 12/2006 and SIPS 5.0 operationalizations (Tables 1 and 2), and its performance was tested against an external validation sample that was characterized by a different ethnic background. Because of this, we expect that CONVERT could perform well in other UHR samples and we hope that it will facilitate data merging across UHR sites employing different diagnostic instruments. This may support large-scale multicentre UHR analyses across PRONIA, PSYSCAN, or NAPLS or replication studies to consolidate the current UHR findings.

This study had limitations. First, we did not perform a follow-up. Second, the type of recruitment adopted in OASIS and CAMEO services may have impacted the observed substantial agreement between CAARMS 12/2006 and SIPS 5.0. For example, the close link of the OASIS or CAMEO with the local first-episode services may have increased the proportion of disorganizing/dangerous BLIPS or the clinical composition of subjects referred for UHR assessment to our services [34]. Also, our referrers underwent a long-standing training to identify and signpost subjects meeting the functional deterioration criterion according to the CAARMS 12/2006 intake criteria. Therefore, it is possible that UHR patients meeting SIPS 5.0 criteria (e.g., with attenuated psychotic symptoms but without functional deterioration) may have been undetected by referrers and not assessed at all by our teams, inflating the observed agreement. Indeed, when the CAARMS 12/2006 was compared with the SIPS 5.0 in other epidemiological samples of non-help-seeking subjects, significant differences between the two instruments were observed [35] (the use of UHR instruments in non-help-seeking samples is not recommended however [11]). There is also recent meta-analytical evidence indicating that samples referred to high-risk services are highly heterogeneous and that their actual composition may reflect the type of outreach campaigns adopted [36, 37]. Future studies should investigate the likely possibility of a lower agreement between CAARMS 12/2006 and SIPS 5.0 in high-risk services employing SIPS-based outreach campaigns. Third, our procedure involving a unique rater scoring both instruments in an uncontrolled order may have significantly inflated agreement across instruments. However, assessing subjects referred for suspicion of UHR symptoms at the time of the first contacts with high-risk services (who may be already psychotic or eventually deemed not at risk of psychosis) with independent raters poses severe logistic difficulties for the patients. It may also paradoxically create additional biases because the most severe patients may be more likely to decline lengthy assessments. To control for this we performed an independent analysis in a subset of patients ($n = 21$) assessed with independent raters and we confirmed that magnitude of agreement remained substantial (see results in eMethod 1). Interrater reliability of the original instruments has been investigated in even smaller samples ($n = 14$) [25]. Fourth, given the differences in the two instruments' development itself [10], our findings and the CONVERT tool may not be applied to older versions of the instruments. Fifth, psychometric reconciliation of the CAARMS versus SIPS is not sufficient to mitigate the differences between the various UHR research teams. Differences remain between the characteristics of the basic population, the recruitment of patients, the follow-up, and the specific treatments provided [9].

5. Conclusions

There is overall substantial diagnostic agreement between the CAARMS 12/2006 and SIPS 5.0 towards identification of UHR subjects. Disagreement was mostly due to differential operationalization of BLIPS. However, type of recruitment strategies may have inflated the observed agreement and future studies should repeat these analyses in high-risk services adopting different outreach campaigns. The conversion algorithm, CONVERT, had excellent performance characteristics even in samples of different ethnic background. The results of the current investigation may be highly relevant to the field, as they may inform future multicentre studies as well as international consensus conferences aiming at standardizing the UHR diagnostic interview.

Acronyms and Abbreviations

UHR+:	At ultra high risk of psychosis
UHR–:	Not at ultra high risk of psychosis
CAARMS:	Comprehensive Assessment of At-Risk Mental States
SIPS:	Structured Interview for Psychosis-Risk Syndrome
APS:	Attenuated psychotic symptoms
BLIPS:	Brief limited intermittent psychotic symptoms
GRD:	Genetic Risk and Deterioration syndrome
ROC:	Receiver Operating Characteristic
fr:	Frequency
d:	Day
GAF:	Global Assessment of Functioning
h:	Hour
min:	Minute
mo:	Month
SOFAS:	Social and Occupational Functioning Assessment Scale
wk:	Week.

Competing Interests

The authors declare that they have no competing interests.

Acknowledgments

The authors thank Professor Scott Woods for his external advice on the use of the SIPS and on his personal comments on the disorganized and dangerous symptoms. The research leading to these results has received funding from the European Community's Seventh Framework Programme under Grant Agreement HEALTH-F2-2013-603196 (project PSYSCAN [translating neuroimaging findings from research into clinical practice]). This study was supported in part by a 2014 NARSAD Young Investigator Award to P. Fusar-Poli.

References

[1] J. Addington, J. Stowkowy, and M. Weiser, "Screening tools for clinical high risk for psychosis," *Early Intervention in Psychiatry*, vol. 9, no. 5, pp. 345–356, 2015.

[2] P. Fusar-Poli, W. T. Carpenter, S. W. Woods, and T. H. McGlashan, "Attenuated psychosis syndrome: ready for DSM-5.1?" *Annual Review of Clinical Psychology*, vol. 10, pp. 155–192, 2014.

[3] M. R. Stafford, H. Jackson, E. Mayo-Wilson, A. P. Morrison, and T. Kendall, "Early interventions to prevent psychosis: systematic review and meta-analysis," *BMJ*, vol. 346, no. 7892, article f185, 2013.

[4] H. J. Jackson, P. D. McGorry, and D. McKenzie, "The reliability of DSM-III prodromal symptoms in first-episode psychotic patients," *Acta Psychiatrica Scandinavica*, vol. 90, no. 5, pp. 375–378, 1994.

[5] A. R. Yung, P. D. McGorry, C. A. McFarlane, H. J. Jackson, G. C. Patton, and A. Rakkar, "Monitoring and care of young people at incipient risk of psychosis," *Schizophrenia Bulletin*, vol. 22, no. 2, pp. 283–303, 1996.

[6] A. R. Yung, H. P. Yuen, P. D. McGorry et al., "Mapping the onset of psychosis: the comprehensive assessment of At-Risk Mental States," *Australian and New Zealand Journal of Psychiatry*, vol. 39, no. 11-12, pp. 964–971, 2005.

[7] T. J. Miller, T. H. McGlashan, S. W. Woods et al., "Symptom assessment in schizophrenic prodromal states," *Psychiatric Quarterly*, vol. 70, no. 4, pp. 273–287, 1999.

[8] T. McGlashan, B. Walsh, and S. Woods, *The Psychosis-Risk Syndrome: Handbook for Diagnosis and Follow-Up*, Oxford University Press, Oxford, UK, 2010.

[9] J.-G. Daneault, E. Stip, M. Villeneuve et al., "Genealogy of instruments for prodrome evaluation of psychosis," *Frontiers in Psychiatry*, vol. 4, article 25, 2013.

[10] F. Schultze-Lutter, B. G. Schimmelmann, S. Ruhrmann, and C. Michel, "'A rose is a rose is a rose', but at-risk criteria differ," *Psychopathology*, vol. 46, no. 2, pp. 75–87, 2013.

[11] F. Schultze-Lutter, C. Michel, S. J. Schmidt et al., "EPA guidance on the early detection of clinical high risk states of psychoses," *European Psychiatry*, vol. 30, no. 3, pp. 405–416, 2015.

[12] P. Fusar-Poli, I. Bonoldi, A. R. Yung et al., "Predicting psychosis: meta-analysis of transition outcomes in individuals at high clinical risk," *Archives of General Psychiatry*, vol. 69, no. 3, pp. 220–229, 2012.

[13] F. Schultze-Lutter, B. G. Schimmelmann, and S. Ruhrmann, "The near babylonian speech confusion in early detection of psychosis," *Schizophrenia Bulletin*, vol. 37, no. 4, pp. 653–655, 2011.

[14] S. Kapur, A. G. Phillips, and T. R. Insel, "Why has it taken so long for biological psychiatry to develop clinical tests and what to do about it?" *Molecular Psychiatry*, vol. 17, no. 12, pp. 1174–1179, 2012.

[15] N. J. Dorans and P. W. Holland, "Population invariance and the equatability of tests: basic theory and the linear case," *Journal of Educational Measurement*, vol. 37, no. 4, pp. 281–306, 2000.

[16] A. R. Yung, L. J. Phillips, H. P. Yuen, and P. D. McGorry, *Comprehensive Assessment of at Risk Mental State*, The PACE Clinic, ORYGEN Research Centre, University of Melbourne, Department of Psychiatry, Parkville, Australia, 2006.

[17] P. Fusar-Poli, M. Byrne, S. Badger, L. R. Valmaggia, and P. K. McGuire, "Outreach and support in South London (OASIS), 2001–2011: ten years of early diagnosis and treatment for young individuals at high clinical risk for psychosis," *European Psychiatry*, vol. 28, no. 5, pp. 315–326, 2013.

[18] J. Zimbrón, S. Ruiz de Azúa, G. M. Khandaker et al., "Clinical and sociodemographic comparison of people at high-risk for psychosis and with first-episode psychosis," *Acta Psychiatrica Scandinavica*, vol. 127, no. 3, pp. 210–216, 2013.

[19] J. S. Kwon, M. S. Byun, T. Y. Lee, and S. K. An, "Early intervention in psychosis: insights from Korea," *Asian Journal of Psychiatry*, vol. 5, no. 1, pp. 98–105, 2012.

[20] P. Fusar-Poli, M. Rocchetti, A. Sardella et al., "Disorder, not just state of risk: meta-analysis of functioning and quality of life in people at high risk of psychosis," *British Journal of Psychiatry*, vol. 207, no. 3, pp. 198–206, 2015.

[21] K. J. Vannest, R. I. Parker, and O. Gonen, *Single Case Research: Web Based Calculators for SCR Analysis*, (Version 1.0) WordPress, 2011, http://www.singlecaseresearch.org.

[22] T. Byrt, J. Bishop, and J. B. Carlin, "Bias, prevalence and kappa," *Journal of Clinical Epidemiology*, vol. 46, no. 5, pp. 423–429, 1993.

[23] J. R. Landis and G. G. Koch, "The measurement of observer agreement for categorical data," *Biometrics*, vol. 33, no. 1, pp. 159–174, 1977.

[24] A. Albano, *Equate: Observed-Score Linking and Equating*, R Package Version 2.0-3, 2014, http://cran.r-project.org/web/packages/equate/index.html.

[25] T. J. Miller, T. H. McGlashan, J. L. Rosen et al., "Prodromal assessment with the structured interview for prodromal syndromes and the scale of prodromal symptoms: predictive validity, interrater reliability, and training to reliability," *Schizophrenia Bulletin*, vol. 29, no. 4, pp. 703–715, 2003.

[26] P. Fusar-Poli, M. Cappucciati, G. Rutigliano et al., "At risk or not at risk? A meta-analysis of the prognostic accuracy of psychometric interviews for psychosis prediction," *World Psychiatry*, vol. 14, no. 3, pp. 322–332, 2015.

[27] M. T. Samara, R. R. Engel, A. Millier, J. Kandenwein, M. Toumi, and S. Leucht, "Equipercentile linking of scales measuring functioning and symptoms: examining the GAF, SOFAS, CGI-S, and PANSS," *European Neuropsychopharmacology*, vol. 24, no. 11, pp. 1767–1772, 2014.

[28] P. Fusar-Poli and J. Van Os, "Lost in transition: setting the psychosis threshold in prodromal research," *Acta Psychiatrica Scandinavica*, vol. 127, no. 3, pp. 248–252, 2013.

[29] G. Modinos, P. Allen, M. Frascarelli et al., "Are we really mapping psychosis risk? Neuroanatomical signature of affective disorders in subjects at ultra high risk," *Psychological Medicine*, vol. 44, no. 16, pp. 3491–3501, 2014.

[30] S. Ruhrmann, F. Schultze-Lutter, R. K. R. Salokangas et al., "Prediction of psychosis in adolescents and young adults at high risk: results from the prospective European prediction of psychosis study," *Archives of General Psychiatry*, vol. 67, no. 3, pp. 241–251, 2010.

[31] S. W. Woods, J. Addington, K. S. Cadenhead et al., "Validity of the prodromal risk syndrome for first psychosis: findings from the North American Prodrome Longitudinal Study," *Schizophrenia Bulletin*, vol. 35, no. 5, pp. 894–908, 2009.

[32] P. Fusar-Poli, B. Nelson, L. Valmaggia, A. R. Yung, and P. K. McGuire, "Comorbid depressive and anxiety disorders in 509 individuals with an at-risk mental state: impact on psychopathology and transition to psychosis," *Schizophrenia Bulletin*, vol. 40, no. 1, pp. 120–131, 2014.

[33] N. A. Obuchowski, M. L. Lieber, and F. H. Wians Jr., "ROC curves in clinical chemistry: uses, misuses, and possible solutions," *Clinical Chemistry*, vol. 50, no. 7, pp. 1118–1125, 2004.

[34] J. Rietdijk, R. Klaassen, H. Ising et al., "Detection of people at risk of developing a first psychosis: comparison of two recruitment strategies," *Acta Psychiatrica Scandinavica*, vol. 126, no. 1, pp. 21–30, 2012.

[35] I. Kelleher, A. Murtagh, C. Molloy et al., "Identification and characterization of prodromal risk syndromes in young adolescents in the community: a population-based clinical interview study," *Schizophrenia Bulletin*, vol. 38, no. 2, pp. 239–246, 2012.

[36] P. Fusar-Poli, F. Schultze-Lutter, M. Cappucciati et al., "The dark side of the moon: meta-analytical impact of recruitment strategies on risk enrichment in the clinical high risk state for psychosis," *Schizophrenia Bulletin*, vol. 42, no. 3, pp. 732–743, 2016.

[37] P. Fusar-Poli, F. Schultze-Lutter, and J. Addington, "Intensive community outreach for those at ultra high risk of psychosis: dilution, not solution," *The Lancet Psychiatry*, vol. 3, no. 1, article 18, 2016.

24

The Brief Symptom Inventory and the Outcome Questionnaire-45 in the Assessment of the Outcome Quality of Mental Health Interventions

Aureliano Crameri,[1] Christopher Schuetz,[2] Andreas Andreae,[2] Margit Koemeda,[3] Peter Schulthess,[3] Volker Tschuschke,[4,5] and Agnes von Wyl[1]

[1] *Zurich University of Applied Sciences, Zurich, Switzerland*
[2] *Integrated Psychiatric Services Winterthur and Zurich Unterland (ipw), Winterthur, Switzerland*
[3] *Swiss Charter of Psychotherapy, Stäfa, Switzerland*
[4] *University Hospital of Cologne, Cologne, Germany*
[5] *Sigmund Freud University, Berlin, Germany*

Correspondence should be addressed to Aureliano Crameri; aureliano.crameri@zhaw.ch

Academic Editor: Yvonne Forsell

Self-report questionnaires are economical instruments for routine outcome assessment. In this study, the performance of the German version of the Outcome Questionnaire-45 (OQ-45) and the Brief Symptom Inventory (BSI) was evaluated when applied in analysis of the outcome quality of psychiatric and psychotherapeutic interventions. Pre-post data from two inpatient samples ($N = 5711$) and one outpatient sample ($N = 239$) were analyzed. Critical differences (reliable change index) and cut-off points between functional and dysfunctional populations were calculated using the Jacobson and Truax method of calculating clinical significance. Overall, the results indicated that the BSI was more accurate than the OQ-45 in correctly classifying patients as clinical subjects. Nonetheless, even with the BSI, about 25% of inpatients with schizophrenia attained a score at admission below the clinical cut-off. Both questionnaires exhibited the highest sensitivity to psychopathology with patients with personality disorders. When considering the differences in the prescores, both questionnaires showed the same sensitivity to change. The advantage of using these self-report measures is observed primarily in assessing outpatient psychotherapy outcome. In an inpatient setting two main problems—namely, the low response rate and the scarce sensitivity to psychopathology with severely ill patients—limit the usability of self-report questionnaires.

1. Introduction

Along with accessibility to services, appropriateness of treatment, and perception of care, outcome is an important quality indicator in mental health care [1]. A widely used approach to assess outcome quality is measuring symptom reduction through rating scales, either clinician-administered or self-reported. Self-report scales are widely used in outcome evaluation of psychotherapies [2]. Their standardized form allows easy administration by clinicians without additional training and also guarantees a high level of reliability. On the other hand, for patients with a high degree of psychopathology, clinician-administered scales are preferred [3], for with these scales, the psychological status of each patient can be assessed independently of the person's capability or willingness to accurately describe their relevant symptoms and behaviors. However, achieving good rating quality requires clinician training in the application of these instruments plus subsequent assessment of interexaminer reliability. Given that in general psychiatric hospitals it has been proven to be quite difficult to routinely involve clinicians in training courses, the question arises as to whether clinician-rated assessments can be substituted by similar scales filled out by psychotherapy patients themselves (self-report) [4].

For general assessment of mental health symptoms, one of the frequently suggested multidimensional self-report instruments is the Symptom Checklist (SCL-90R) or its short form, the Brief Symptom Inventory (BSI) [5–7]. However, based on the number of published studies implementing these questionnaires, it can be asserted that in the field of mental health they have been used predominantly with outpatients and far less frequently with inpatients or, more generally, with patients with severe mental illness [8–10]. Nevertheless, these instruments seem promising in assessing the mental health status of the latter patient group, because they also contain specific scales for measuring psychotic and schizotypal symptoms, such as the Psychoticism or the Paranoid Ideation scale. However, the validity of these scales has not as yet been unequivocally confirmed. Wood [11] found no evidence that patients with schizophrenia score higher on the Psychoticism scale than patients without schizophrenia. Johnson et al. [12] found no differences on the Paranoid Ideation and Psychoticism scales between patients diagnosed with or without schizophrenia. In contrast, Preston and Harrison [13] demonstrated in a sample of 69 patients presenting their first psychotic episode that responses on the BSI items could discriminate between patients with weak and with marked positive symptoms.

Another instrument recommended for assessment of individuals seeking mental health treatment is the Outcome Questionnaire-45 (OQ-45) [14–16]. It is a newer, self-report outcome measure created primarily for psychotherapy patients, which has already been used in psychiatric inpatient care [17, 18].

In the context of quality assurance programs, quantitative data collected via mental health questionnaires find their application in the analysis of pre-post differences, which reflect the intraindividual changes attained during the treatment. One widely used analysis method is the calculation of clinical significance proposed by Jacobson and Truax [19]. The aim of the method is to identify which patients move outside the range of the dysfunctional population and consequently attain "normal" functioning. Patients who improve significantly and cross a well-defined cut-off score between dysfunctional and functional distributions are classified as "remitted." However, patients can only be consistently classified in this way if the self-report measurement at the beginning of the treatment correctly identifies them as dysfunctional.

The objective of this study was to evaluate *the German versions of the OQ-45 and the BSI when applied in the analysis of outcome quality of inpatient and outpatient treatments*. The analyses focused on three aspects of usability:

(1) *Response Rate*. How many patients fill out the questionnaires? To produce a representative outcome estimation, the majority of the patients should be able to fill out the self-report forms. A high rate of nonresponse increases the risk of bias in the results.

(2) *Sensitivity to Psychopathology*. Applying the cut-off scores calculated with the Jacobson and Truax method, what percentages of patients are correctly classified by the self-report measures at admission as belonging to the dysfunctional population?

(3) *Sensitivity to Change*. Do the two questionnaires have the same sensitivity to change? The equivalence of the two measures is not obvious, since compared to the BSI, the OQ-45 contains fewer symptom-specific items and focuses partially on social functioning (e.g., work), which requires more time for change to occur than the time required to see change in acute symptoms.

2. Methods

2.1. Samples. Three different samples, two inpatient samples and one outpatient sample, were used for this study. Both inpatient samples were treated at an inpatient clinic in Switzerland, the Integrated Psychiatric Services of Winterthur, and Zurich Unterland (ipw).

At the ipw, the OQ-45 was implemented as a self-report measure of outcome quality from 2008 to 2010; it was replaced by the BSI starting in 2012. For samples 1 and 2, inpatient treatments from 2008 to 2009 (OQ-45) and from 2012 and 2013 (BSI) were selected from the database using the following inclusion criteria:

(i) A principal diagnosis belonging to one of these major groups: F1 (substance abuse), F2 (schizophrenia or other psychotic disorders), F3 (mood disorders), F4 (anxiety or stress related disorders), and F6 (personality disorders).

(ii) Age of at least 18 years.

(iii) Hospitalization of at least 7 days.

Sample 3 was recruited in a project on outpatients promoted by the Swiss Charta for Psychotherapy. The aim of this nonrandomized field study is to investigate various process-outcome aspects of outpatient treatments carried out with different experiential or psychodynamic therapy methods [26–28]. Cases from this sample were selected using the following criteria:

(i) At least one Axis I disorder according to the criteria of DSM-IV.

(ii) Age of at least 18 years.

(iii) Minimum of 10 treatment sessions.

Both studies above were carried out in accordance with the ethical principles of the Declaration of Helsinki. For the Swiss Charta project, a research application was submitted to the ethics committee of each of the Swiss cantons in which the projects were carried out; all of the applications were approved. All patients gave informed written consent for their participation in the study. Data from the ipw were collected within an internal quality measurement system for which, according to Swiss federal and cantonal law, no ethical approval was required. For this reason, the present study was granted an exemption from the requirement for ethics approval by the Cantonal Ethics Committee of Zurich

TABLE 1: Descriptive statistics of the analyzed samples.

	Sample 1 (N_1 = 2894)	Sample 2 (N_2 = 2877)	Sample 3 (N_3 = 239)
Sex			
Female	1424 (49.2%)	1532 (53.2%)	162 (67.8%)
Male	1470 (50.8%)	1345 (46.8%)	77 (32.2%)
Education			
Low	1005 (34.7%)	895 (31.1%)	24 (10.0%)
Middle	1461 (50.5%)	1488 (51.7%)	86 (36.0%)
High	428 (14.8%)	494 (17.2%)	129 (54.0%)
Income			
Salary	729 (25.2%)	687 (23.9%)	185 (77.4%)
Sickness/disability benefit	1060 (36.6%)	1147 (39.9%)	23 (9.6%)
Social welfare payments	425 (14.7%)	373 (13.0%)	3 (1.3%)
Old age insurance	232 (8.0%)	292 (10.1%)	7 (2.9%)
Other	448 (15.5%)	378 (13.1%)	21 (8.8%)
GAF	47.0 (17.2)	38.5 (14.3)	60.5 (13.1)
Principal diagnosis (ICD-10/DSM-IV)	F1: 884 (30.6%) F2: 681 (23.5%) F3: 706 (24.4%) F4: 386 (13.3%) F6: 237 (8.2%)	F1: 594 (20.6%) F2: 649 (22.6%) F3: 927 (32.2%) F4: 461 (16.0%) F6: 246 (8.6%)	Mood: 107 (44.8%) Anxiety: 65 (27.2%) Adjustment: 45 (18.8%) Other: 22 (9.2%)
Duration of treatment	36.7 days (38.1)	36.0 days (31.7)	41.3 sessions (34.2)
Type of discharge			
Mutual consent	2327 (80.4%)	2489 (86.5%)	180 (75.3%)
Decided by the patient	221 (7.6%)	117 (4.1%)	46 (19.2%)
Decided by the treating person	215 (7.4%)	181 (6.3%)	11 (4.6%)
Other	131 (4.6%)	90 (3.1%)	2 (0.1%)

(Waiver number 09-2016). Participating patients at the ipw gave informed verbal consent for the use of the data.

Table 1 presents the characteristics of the three samples. In the inpatient samples 1 and 2 the most frequent substance-related disorder (F1) was associated with alcohol consumption (71.5% of the patients with an F1 diagnosis in sample 1 and 56.2% in sample 2, resp.). In the F2 group paranoid schizophrenia was prominent (61.8% and 59.3%, resp., of the F2 group). Most of the patients with a mood disorder had either a depressive episode (53.2% and 51.0% within the F3 group) or a recurrent depressive disorder (40.3% and 45.4% within the F3 group). The most frequently diagnosed personality disorder was of the Borderline type (64.6% and 53.6% within the F6 group). In the outpatient setting, 69.2% of diagnosed mood disorders were major depressions. The most frequent anxiety disorders in this setting were social phobia, panic disorder/agoraphobia, and generalized anxiety disorder.

2.2. Measures. The following self-report and clinician-administered instruments were used for this analysis:

(i) *Basic Documentation.* Important clinical information and sociodemographic characteristics were recorded on a form. These data were collected by the treating psychiatrists (for inpatients) and the treating psychotherapists (for outpatients).

(ii) *ICD-10.* Diagnoses based on this system were available for the inpatient samples and had been assigned by the treating psychiatrists.

(iii) *Structured Clinical Interviews for DSM-IV (SCID-I/-II) [29].* These interviews, which were available only for sample 3, served in assessing Axis I and II disorders (clinical syndromes and personality disorders) according to the DSM-IV criteria. Trained psychologists (not involved in treatment of the patients) were engaged to carry out the two clinical interviews.

(iv) *Clinical Global Impressions (CGI) [30].* This instrument gathers the clinician's view of the severity of psychopathology (CGI-S) and of the improvements from the initiation point of the treatment (CGI-I). The two aspects are each rated on a 7-point scale. Ratings with this instrument were available only for the inpatient samples and were provided by the treating psychiatrists.

(v) *Global Assessment of Functioning (GAF) [31].* On this scale psychological, social, and occupational functioning are rated on a hypothetical continuum from severe mental illness (0) to mental health (100).

(vi) *OQ-45.* The questionnaire consists of 45 items grouped in the three scales Symptom Distress (SD), Interpersonal Relations (IR), and Social Role (SR), which add up to a total score (OQ Total Score). The scale structure of the original version is supported by confirmatory factor analysis [14]. The single scales in the German version exhibit good internal consistency [20].

(vii) *BSI.* This questionnaire is the short version of the SCL-90R [6]. The 53 items assess nine primary symptom dimensions: Somatization (SOM), Obsessive-Compulsiveness (OBS), Interpersonal Sensitivity (INS), Depression (DEP), Anxiety (ANX), Hostility (HOS), Phobic Anxiety (PHOB), Paranoid Ideation (PAR), and Psychoticism (PSY). Additional global indices of distress can be obtained, for example, the General Symptom Index (GSI), which is the mean score of all items. In the analysis carried out by Derogatis and Melisaratos [5] seven of the primary scales showed a clear convergence with their counterparts among the MMPI scales. All scales in the German version exhibit satisfactory test-retest reliability [22].

2.3. Statistical Analysis

2.3.1. Missing Data. Nonresponse is a common problem in surveys and can occur for single items or for the entire examination. Analyzing only data of patients that responded to every item on the self-report measures at admission as well as at discharge would lead to a substantial loss of information, especially for the analyses for the inpatient setting. To include as many cases as possible, we defined different inclusion criteria for each analysis (Figure 1). First, we defined the minimal number of answered items to calculate scale scores. In a previous unpublished study we tested (through simulations) the impact of incomplete item values in the calculation of scores for the OQ-45 scales. Our results showed that if, for the three scales, namely, SD, IR, and SR, at least 8, 6, and 6 items, respectively, had a valid value, then the generated scale scores preserved a correlation of $r > 0.90$ with the corresponding scores based on completely observed values. In this study, we considered as evaluable only data records that fulfilled the rule mentioned above. Concerning the BSI, we analyzed only returned questionnaires with at least 40 valid item values [32].

We calculated the response rate on the basis of the number of returned questionnaires that fulfilled the above-mentioned criteria of completeness. Patients who completed a sufficient number of items at admission were included in the analysis of sensitivity to psychopathology. Patients who additionally did the same at discharge were included in the analysis of sensitivity to change.

2.3.2. Parameters of Clinical Significance. For the analysis of intraindividual changes we applied Jacobson and Truax's method of calculating clinical significance [19], with which the proportions of improved and recovered cases can be calculated [2]. To determine these proportions, two parameters are needed: (1) a critical difference D, which allows identification of individual pre-post differences that are sufficiently large to be considered statistically significant (reliable change) and (2) a cut-off C, which distinguishes scores that are a variation of normal functioning from scores indicating a psychopathological state. Therefore, patients exhibiting a reduction of at least D points from their initial impairment score are considered "improved." If their score additionally falls below the cut-off C, then they are considered "remitted."

The critical difference, for example, at a confidence level of 95%, is obtained by using the standard deviation and the reliability coefficients of the measure:

$$D_{95\%} = 1.96 \cdot \mathrm{SD}_{\text{patient}} \cdot \sqrt{2(1-r)}, \tag{1}$$

whereas the cut-off is calculated as a weighted midpoint between the means of a patient and a nonpatient population as follows:

$$C = \frac{\mathrm{SD}_{\text{patient}} \cdot M_{\text{nonpatient}} + \mathrm{SD}_{\text{nonpatient}} \cdot M_{\text{patient}}}{\mathrm{SD}_{\text{patient}} + \mathrm{SD}_{\text{nonpatient}}}. \tag{2}$$

We additionally compared our parameter values with those published in other studies on the basis of samples from Germany.

2.3.3. Outcome Comparisons. To compare sensitivity to change, measured with two different questionnaires within three different samples, the following analysis techniques were used: propensity score matching and linear mixed modeling. Given that within the inpatient setting OQ-45 and BSI data were collected in two different samples, we matched sample 1 and sample 2 using the propensity score technique proposed by Rosenbaum and Rubin [33]. It is primarily used in nonrandomized studies in order to build equivalent samples for causal inference, but it can also be applied to compare different survey samples [34]. In our analysis treatment modalities were defined as the two different questionnaires presented to the patient (BSI versus OQ-45), and outcome was defined as the scale scores measured at intake and at discharge and then converted either in categories of clinical significance or in z values. As a matching algorithm we applied the nearest neighbor matching with a logistic regression-based propensity score [35]. The following covariates were used in the regression equation: sex, age, marital status, educational level, GAF and CGI, respectively, at intake and at discharge, principal diagnosis, compulsory treatment order, duration of treatment, and type of discharge. Matches were formed on a 1 : 1 ratio within a caliper size of 0.1 standard deviations of the propensity score. The adequacy of the matching procedure was checked using graphical visualizations of the propensity score distribution; the quality of the balance in the matched groups was examined through the standardized difference of means of each covariate [36, 37].

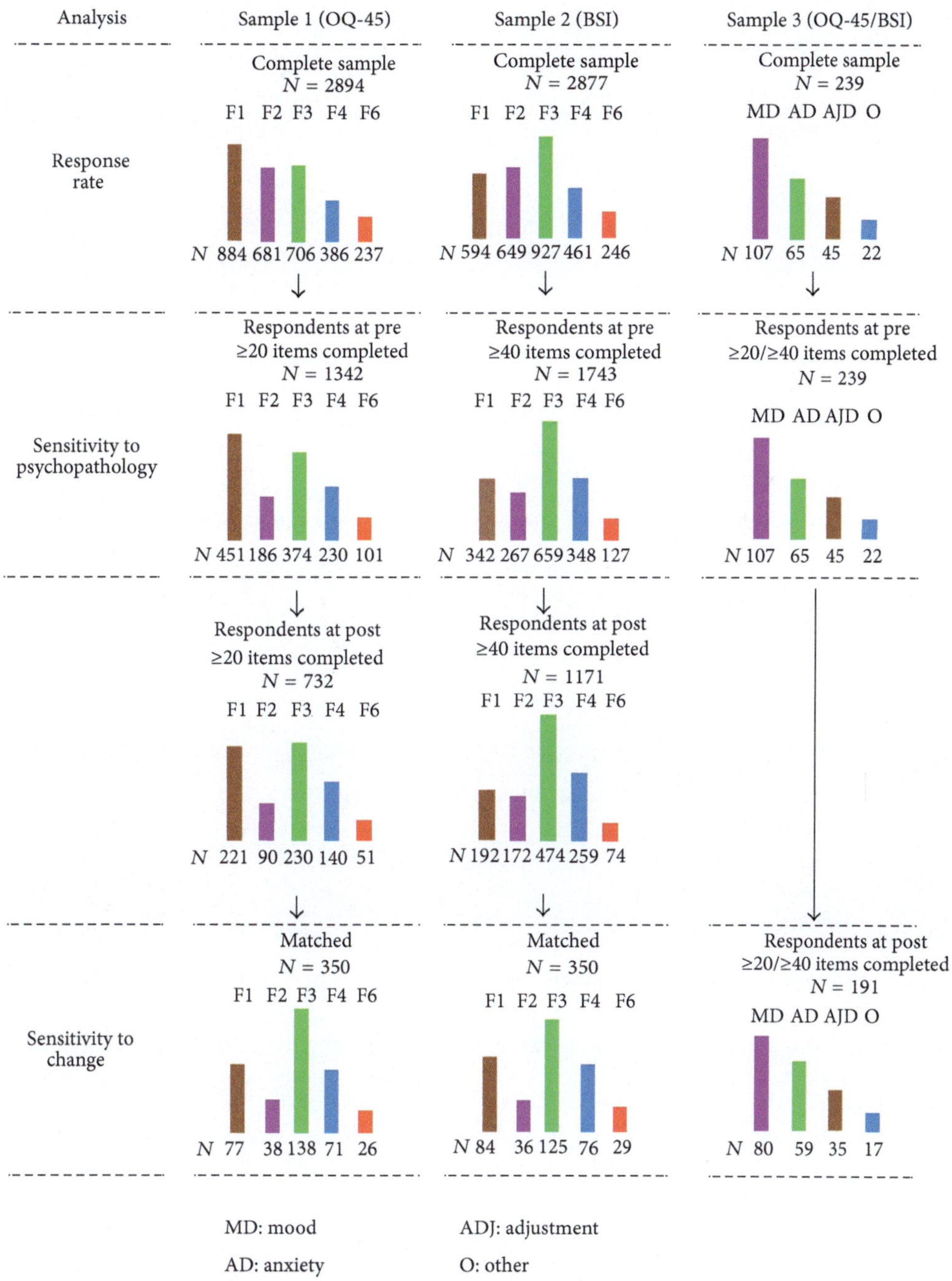

FIGURE 1: Number of cases included in the different analyses.

Besides the comparison of the proportions of cases in the principal categories of clinical significance classified by the two instruments, we also analyzed the pre-post differences using the linear mixed model; for this, the OQ-45 and BSI scores were z-transformed.

3. Results

3.1. Response Rate. The completeness of the returned questionnaires varied between the two measures. The highest number of unanswered items was found for the OQ-45 questionnaires returned by the inpatients. Questions on intimate relationships but also work-related questions were the most affected by nonresponse in sample 1. Item number 7 ("I feel unhappy in my marriage/significant relationship") was left out in 24% of the cases. A work-related item such as number 12 ("I find my work/school satisfying") had 8% missing values. Overall, the impact of incomplete responses in sample 1 was high: of the 1342 questionnaires evaluable at intake only 588 (43.8%) had been completely filled out.

Nonresponse on the BSI questionnaires returned by inpatients was not related to the content but instead to the

Table 2: Descriptive statistics and reliability (Chronbach's alpha) of the global scales.

	OQ Total Score		GSI	
	Inpatients (n_1 = 1342)	Outpatients (n_3 = 239)	Inpatients (n_2 = 1743)	Outpatients (n_3 = 239)
M (SD)	78.4 (28.9)	72.0 (19.4)	1.46 (0.79)	1.06 (0.53)
Min	0	33	0	0.26
Percentiles				
5	31	40	0.25	0.34
10	38	47	0.41	0.45
25	58	60	0.85	0.66
50	79	71	1.40	0.97
75	99	85	2.02	1.39
90	117	95	2.56	1.76
95	126	104	2.85	2.02
Max	159	143	3.79	2.78
α^*	0.95	0.91	0.97	0.95

Note: *Calculations of α are based on complete case analysis. OQ-45 from sample 1: n_1 = 588. OQ-45 from sample 3: n_3 = 198. BSI from sample 2: n_2 = 1282. BSI from sample 3: n_3 = 237.

Table 3: Statistics of the OQ-45 and the BSI/SCL-90R based on samples from Germany.

	Functional population M (SD)	Dysfunctional population Outpatients M (SD)	Dysfunctional population Inpatients M (SD)	Cut-off	Critical difference
OQ Total Score	46.2 (18.5) [20]	71.8 (21.9) [21]	79.0 (27.9) [18]*	58.8 [18]	17.8 [18]
GSI	0.31 (0.23) [22]	1.08 (0.63) [23]	1.47 (0.68) [24]†	0.60 [24]†	0.2 [25]

Note: *Pooled M and SD from the intervention and control group at admission. †Based on SCL-90R data.

position of the items. Items 1 to 10 had on average 1.5% missing values; items above number 40 reached missingness from 4% to 7.5%. Of the 1743 evaluable BSI forms at intake only 1282 (73.6%) were complete.

In the outpatient sample the incompleteness of the questionnaires was low. For the OQ-45, besides a 7% of nonresponse on item number 7, missingness varied from 0% to 3.5%. On the BSI questionnaires, missingness on the single items was always under 1%.

In the inpatient setting the response rate at both pre- and postmeasurement was about 25% for the OQ-45 in sample 1 and 40% for the BSI in sample 2. This difference has to be viewed as improvement in data monitoring over the course of the years and cannot be considered to be an indicator for better acceptance of the BSI over the OQ-45.

The response rate was dependent on the severity of psychopathology at admission and of the amount of improvement at discharge in both inpatient samples (Figure 2). Moreover, patients with schizophrenia showed the lowest response rate, with the BSI, 41% at intake and 45% at discharge. The highest rate was registered among patients having an F4 diagnosis, with 75% at intake and 65% at discharge, respectively.

In the outpatient sample the response rate at the end of the therapy did not correlate significantly with Axis I or Axis II diagnoses.

3.2. Cut-Off and Critical Difference. Table 2 shows the descriptive statistics of the scales based on data collected at the beginning of the treatment in the three samples. Table 3 reports comparative statistics from German sample 3.

The cut-off and the critical difference for the OQ Total Score were calculated using the data of the respondents from sample 1 at intake (N = 1342, M_{patient} = 78.4, SD_{patient} = 28.9, and Chronbach's α = 0.95) and data published by Lambert et al. [20] on a nonclinical sample (N = 232, $M_{\text{nonpatient}}$ = 46.2, and $SD_{\text{nonpatient}}$ = 18.5). Applying (1) and (2) led to C = 59 and $D_{95\%}$ = 18. Therefore, a patient can be classified as remitted if the following two conditions are fulfilled: (a) his OQ Total Score has decreased by at least 18 points and (b) has reached a value below 59 at the end of the treatment. If only (b) is met, then the patient is classified as improved. Both parameter values are similar to those published in Puschner et al. [18].

The calculation of the parameters for the GSI scale was based on data of the respondents from sample 2 (N = 1743, M_{patient} = 1.46, SD_{patient} = 0.79, and Chronbach's α = 0.97) and the data published in Franke [22] on a nonclinical sample (N = 600, $M_{\text{nonpatient}}$ = 0.31, and $SD_{\text{nonpatient}}$ = 0.23). The corresponding parameters of clinical significance were C = 0.57 and $D_{95\%}$ = 0.38. Schmitz et al. [24] obtained a similar cut-off value based on a sample of participants with severe impairments in which inpatient treatment was indicated.

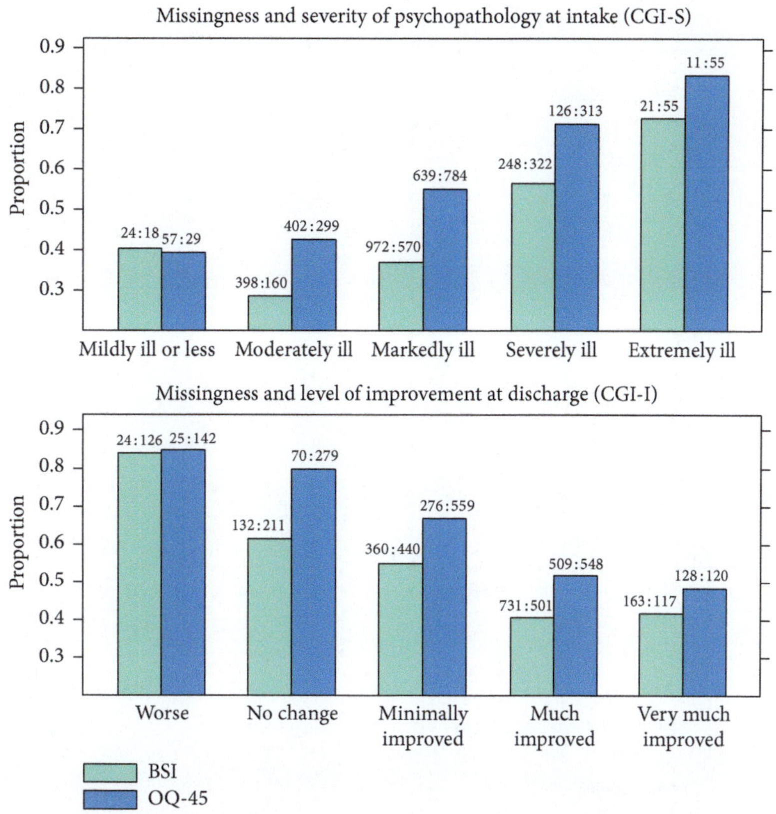

FIGURE 2: Relationship between missingness (proportion of nonresponse) and CGI ratings. The ratio between the number of respondents and the number of nonrespondents is noted on top of the bars (data from samples 1 and 2).

Lutz et al. [25] proposed a critical difference calculated with the standard deviation of the functional sample, which is consequently narrower than our value based on a commonly larger standard deviation from a clinical sample.

3.3. Sensitivity to Psychopathology. Figures 3 and 4 report the sensitivity of the global scales OQ Total Score and GSI. Figure 3 shows the profiles of different diagnosis groups on the OQ-45 scales. More than 80% of the inpatients with diagnoses F3, F4, and F6 had an OQ Total Score of at least 59 points and were therefore classified as clinical cases (caseness). Fewer than 70% of inpatients with a diagnosis F1 or F2 scored above the clinical cut-off. Considering the most important clinical disorders in an outpatient setting, that is, affective and anxiety disorders, fewer than 70% of the patients with an anxiety disorder but without a comorbid personality disorder (PD) were correctly classified as clinical cases by OQ Total Score. In contrast, sensitivity of more than 80% was attained among patients with an affective disorder, independently of additional comorbidity on the Axis II. Since the SD scale contributes the most to the Total Score scale, a high correlation of $r = 0.96$ between the two scales was present. The other two scales, that is, IR and SR, which have a minor importance in forming the Total Score, also did not vary substantially across the different type of disorders.

In contrast to the OQ-45, the BSI produced profiles with more distinctive differences between the diagnosis groups (Figure 4). Except for the patients with schizophrenia (F2), the Depression scale was the scale with the highest score for the different diagnosis groups. The largest mean on this scale was exhibited by patients with a personality disorder (F6) and not, as theoretically expected, by patients with an affective disorder (F3). Patients with schizophrenia attained the highest score on the Paranoid Ideation scale, which would be in accordance with the diagnostic criteria for this psychiatric group. However, their mean score was outperformed by that of patients with an F6 diagnosis. Overall, the highest Symptom Distress as measured by the BSI was observed on average among patients with a personality disorder in both an inpatient and an outpatient setting.

In the samples of inpatients and outpatients, the BSI with its GSI scale exhibited a higher sensitivity to psychopathology than the OQ-45 with its Total Score scale. However, the same diagnosis groups with a low average OQ Total Score, that is, F2 and F1 among the inpatients and anxiety disorders without PD among the outpatients, achieved a GSI score that was on average also lower than that of other diagnosis groups. About 25% of the respondents with an F2 diagnosis were not correctly classified as clinical cases. The caseness determined by the GSI scale was not associated with the CGI or GAF score (logistic regression: $\chi^2(2) = 0.56$, $p = 0.76$). Therefore, the substantial misclassification of patients with schizophrenia cannot be considered to be a consequence of low severity of

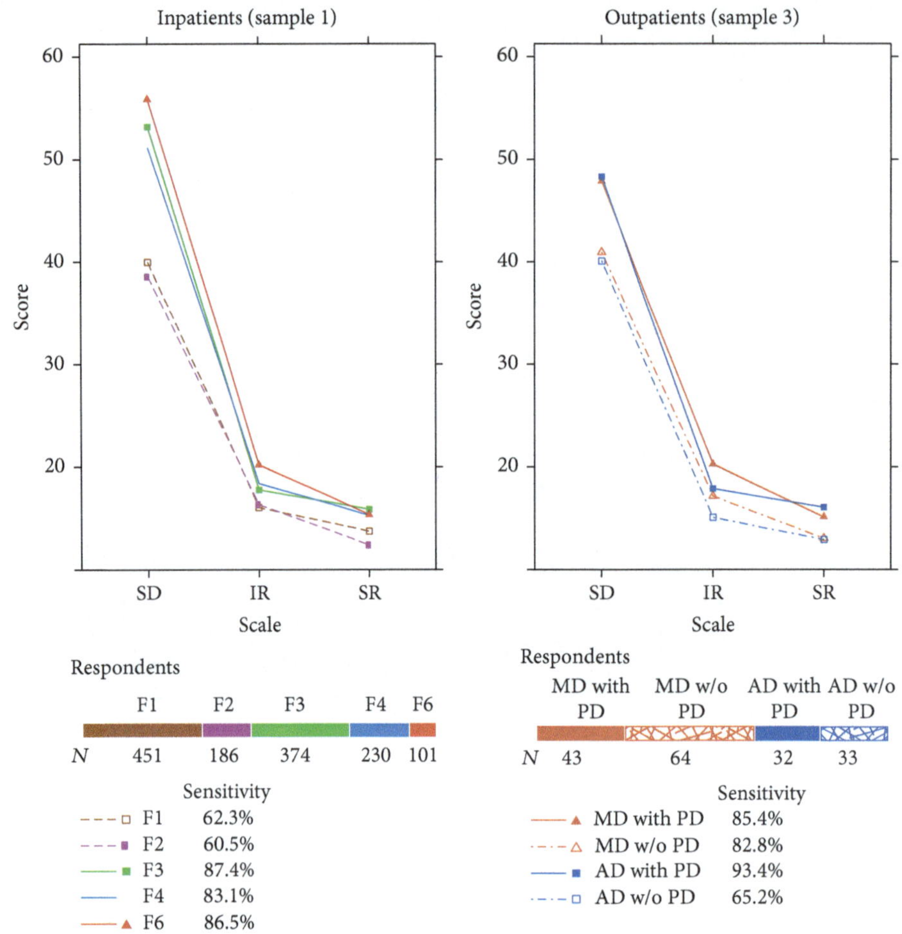

FIGURE 3: OQ-45 profiles of the respondents at intake. For sample 3 only data of patients with a principal diagnosis of mood (MD) or anxiety disorder (AD) grouped according to the presence or absence of a personality disorder (PD) are represented. Percentages represent the sensitivity to psychopathology according to the OQ Total Score.

mental illness or high psychosocial functioning of the sample analyzed.

For both instruments one would actually expect to find higher sensitivity to psychopathology with inpatients than with outpatients, but the percentages in Figures 3 and 4 do not support this expectation. The statistics in Table 2 show that respondents with 0 points on one of the questionnaires were found among the inpatients but not among the outpatients and that the 5th and the 10th percentiles in the inpatient samples were lower than the corresponding values from the outpatients. The lowest 5th percentiles of the global questionnaire scores were found for the GSI among the inpatients with substance abuse (0.15) and inpatients with schizophrenic disorders (0.11).

3.4. Sensitivity to Change. For the inpatient setting, we based our analysis of sensitivity to change on matched samples. The histograms in Figure 5 show that samples 1 and 2 were already quite similar before the matching, since they exhibited an extensive overlap of their propensity score distributions but with some density differences, however. From the smaller sample, that is, sample 1, a total of 419 patients with complete scales and covariates values were available for the matching. Of these, 350 cases could successfully be matched on a 1 : 1 ratio with cases from the larger sample 2 (the absolute standardized difference of means was smaller than 0.1 for each covariate).

Figure 6 shows the results of the clinical significance analysis. In the outpatient sample, the proportions of improved and remitted cases classified by the two measures were quite similar. In the inpatient samples, the GSI scale identified 54% improved cases compared to the 41.4% identified by the OQ Total Score. Although this difference is significant [$\chi^2(7) = 58.5$, $p < 0.001$], it does not necessarily attest a superior sensitivity to change to the BSI. This is because the GSI scale produces higher prescores than the OQ Total Score, and, therefore, patients have a higher probability of lowering their score on the GSI than on the OQ total scale during their treatment.

To balance out this difference, the scores of the two questionnaires were z-transformed and analyzed with a linear mixed model. Figure 7 shows the estimated fixed

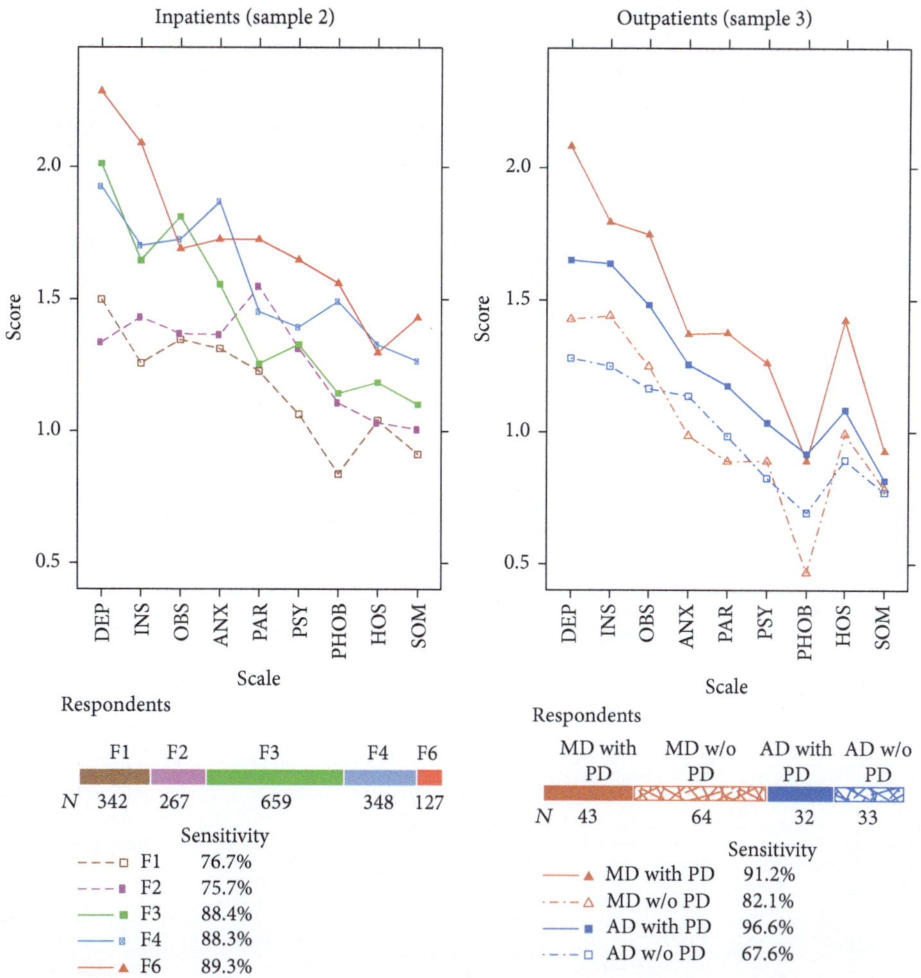

FIGURE 4: BSI profiles of the respondents at intake. For sample 3 only data of patients with a principal diagnosis of mood (MD) or anxiety disorder (AD) grouped according to the presence or absence of a personality disorder (PD) are represented. Percentages represent the sensitivity to psychopathology according to the GSI scale.

effects; they indicate that the two questionnaires recorded the same amount of change between the pre- and the postmeasurement.

4. Discussion

This study examined the applicability of the OQ-45 and the BSI for assessing the outcome quality of inpatient and outpatient treatments. Both of these self-report measures can be easily administered by a wide range of service professionals and take about 10 minutes to be filled out. Normative data and analysis results concerning their psychometric properties are available [38].

However, our analyses pointed out the following critical aspects of the performance of the two questionnaires, which have often been neglected in the literature: (1) the number of missing values that emerges in the data collection, (2) the diagnostic value of the scale profiles, and (3) the robustness of the clinical significance algorithm.

(1) Missing Data. Since Rubin's [39] seminal paper on inference with missing data, there has been a growing awareness of this problem in the scientific community. In evaluation studies, the probability of nonresponse is often correlated with the attained outcome. Our results clearly demonstrate this relationship. Respondents and nonrespondents are different in two clinically crucial aspects: nonrespondents have higher severity of mental illness and show less improvement after the treatment than respondents. Missingness is therefore a source of bias when assessing the effectiveness of a treatment, and nowadays guidelines concerning the statistical analysis of incomplete data are available [40, 41]. Different authors have pointed out that missingness as low as 10%, if not treated adequately in the statistical analysis, can lead to bias [42, 43]. In a previous analysis we were able to successfully apply multiple imputation to the outcome data of sample 3, because, first, the missing rate in the sample was relatively low (20%) and, second, the progress of the patients was additionally monitored through repeated measurements during the treatment, which generally improve the predictive power of the imputation model [27]. In contrast, with samples 1 and 2 the application of multiple imputation proved to be ineffective. On the one hand, nonresponse in these samples exceeded 50%, and according to Rubin [44] multiple

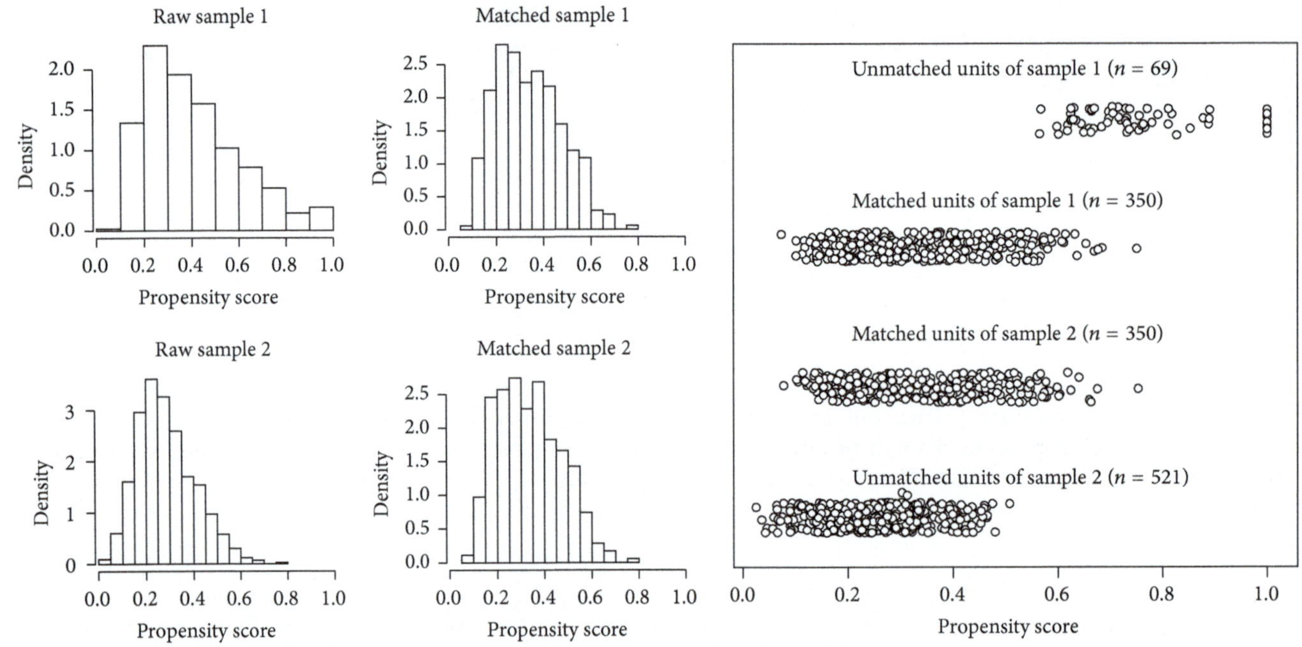

FIGURE 5: Distributions of the propensity scores of the inpatient respondents with complete covariates values. Histograms on the left show the distributions before (raw) and after (matched) the matching. The plot on the right shows the differences between matched and unmatched cases.

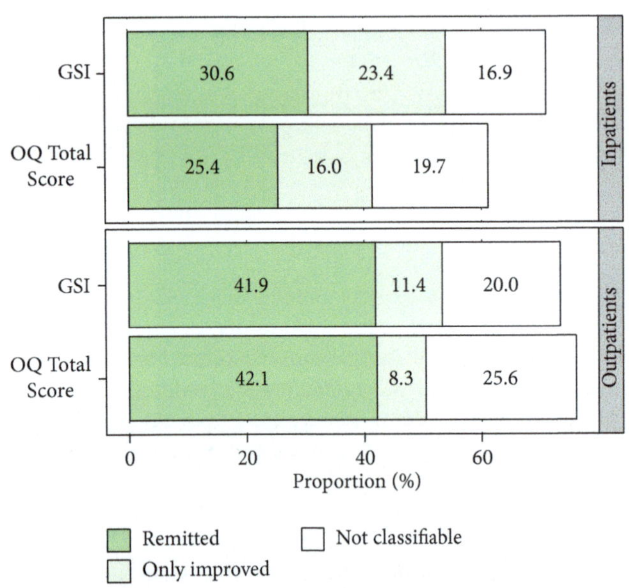

FIGURE 6: Results of the analysis of the clinical significance. Analysis of inpatient data are based on matched samples: $n_1 = n_2 = 350$. Outpatient sample: $n_3 = 191$. The category "not classifiable" refers to cases misclassified as nonclinical by the self-report measure.

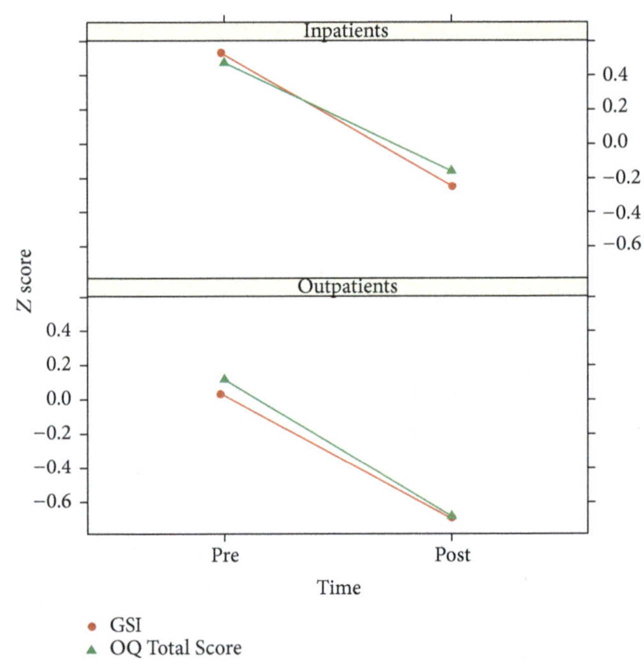

FIGURE 7: Average pre-post changes in z scores. Analysis of inpatient data are based on matched samples: $n_1 = n_2 = 350$. Outpatient sample: $n_3 = 191$.

imputation was conceived to deal with a typical fraction of missing information of 30% or less. On the other hand, the drastic reduction of the data collection to only pre-post measurements, in order to minimize administrative expense, makes it hard to obtain robust estimations of the missing data through imputation models. All in all, the high proportion of missing data discourages the use of self-report measures with the patients with severe impairments usually found in a psychiatric hospital setting in favor of clinician-administered measures.

(2) Diagnostic Value of the Profiles. Questionnaires like OQ-45 and BSI have a relatively large number of items, so that

different reliable Likert scales may be formed that allow the creation of a person's profile. Can these profiles be used, for instance, to facilitate the formulation of a psychiatric diagnosis? Our results do not support the use of these questionnaires as screening instruments to facilitate the assessment of ICD-10 diagnoses. In the construction of the OQ-45 this was never an intended purpose [45], but the nine primary symptom dimensions of the BSI suggest a possible application for screening purposes. In our sample, inpatients with personality disorders attained on average higher scores than inpatients in other diagnosis groups on six of the nine BSI scales. These patients had a higher mean score on the Depression scale than patients with an affective disorder and a higher mean score on the Paranoid Ideation scale than patients with schizophrenia. Poor diagnostic efficacy of the nine scales in assessing DSM-IV symptom disorders was also reported by Pedereen and Karterud [46]. Two different approaches have been suggested for dealing with the low discriminant validity of the BSI scales. The first is to consider the questionnaire through its GSI score as more appropriate for measuring the overall degree of psychological distress instead of the precise nature of the psychopathology [38]. From this optic, the Outcome Questionnaire with 45 items in its full version or 30 items in its short version would seem to be a more time-effective choice than BSI when measuring general level of psychological distress in a less time-consuming way. The second approach consists in improving the factorial structure of the questionnaire. To this purpose, different authors have used the bifactor structural model in recent years. This model is used to build a general distress factor and more specific components of psychopathology. Thomas [47] demonstrated that a bifactor model of the BSI items can achieve higher accuracy than an oblique simple structure in diagnosing some disorders, such as depression or generalized anxiety disorder. Brodbeck et al. [48] also proposed a bifactor solution that correlates with DSM-IV diagnoses, especially depressive disorders, anxiety disorders, and personality disorders. One of their results in line with ours is that patients with personality disorders are characterized by a high level of general distress. Overall, it seems that improving the factor structure of the BSI can lead to improved sensitivity in identifying depressive or anxiety disorders, but we doubt that it can do the same with patients with substance abuse or acute psychotic disorders. A nonnegligible part of these patients tends to score low, and their profiles resemble those of healthy persons or remitted patients. These results support the hypothesis that patients with these disorders are inclined to underestimate their own emotional and behavioral difficulties. As pointed out by Burlingame et al. [8] the disadvantages of using self-report measures with inpatients with severe and persistent mental illness "include an insufficient clinical picture as a result of the dependence on patients' ability to accurately describe their condition, which at times is doubtful because of denial, minimization of symptoms, or responder bias" (p. 448).

(3) Robustness in the Outcome Evaluation. Clinical significance, as originally proposed by Jacobson and Truax [19], is considered, beside pre-post effect sizes, to be a gold standard as a performance indicator in routine outcome monitoring [49]. This approach encompasses two steps: first, identifying the subsample of patients that reached a reliable change and then determining which among them moved outside the range of the dysfunctional population. This method presupposes a valid and consistent distinction between functionality and dysfunctionality already *at the onset of the treatment.* Therefore, the percentage of cases that can be adequately categorized depends on the sensitivity of the instrument. For self-report questionnaires measuring important mental health problems, the expected sensitivity is of at least 80% [50, 51]. Our results reveal a heterogeneous picture in this regard. For inpatients with an F3, F4, or F6 diagnosis the sensitivity to psychopathology of both instruments exceeds 80%. However, the questionnaires exhibited low values with inpatients with a principal diagnosis of substance abuse or schizophrenia. Especially within the latter group, which represents an important diagnosis group in an inpatient setting, about 25% of the respondents were misclassified as nonclinical subjects according to the GSI score. The patients with schizophrenia analyzed in this study had a mean GAF score of 32 points at admission and were hospitalized on average 36 days in a primary care hospital. Thus, the substantial misclassification cannot be explained by a lack of mental illness but instead by limitations, either of the measures used in assessing psychopathology or of the methodology used in assessing caseness. Analyses based on outpatients have reported sensitivity of above 90% for the OQ total scale [52] as well as the GSI scale [46]. Sensitivity values of at least 80% based on inpatient data were reported by Moessner et al. [53] for both global scales using data from inpatients with an F3, F4, F5, or F6 diagnosis and by Timman et al. [54] for the OQ Total Score using an inpatient sample with personality disorders. Nevertheless, our analyses do not support a generalization of this high accuracy in detecting caseness among inpatients with an F1 or F2 diagnosis. A lack of research on the generalizability of the OQ-45 was confirmed by Lambert and Hawkins [55], who admitted that much of the research "demonstrating the use of the OQ-45 has been conducted with young, educated patients" (p. 496).

Concerning the limitations of our methodology in assessing clinical significance, we see the following possibilities for improvement: (1) *construct psychological functioning scales using a bifactor model.* For both questionnaires, there are various published results demonstrating that this kind of factor analysis is able to improve the fit of the scale structure to the data [47, 48, 56]; (2) *determine the cut-off scores with the receiver operating characteristic (ROC) curve.* This method can provide more accurate cut-off scores than the weighted midpoints calculated by the Jacobson and Truax method, especially when data are not normally distributed [57]. The procedure requires raw data from both a healthy and a patient sample; however, (3) *avoid the necessity of cut-off scores between functionality and dysfunctionality by using the percentage of improvement approach.* A different outcome evaluation that could be applied as a complement to the Jacobson and Truax method consists in analysis of the relative change from the baseline severity [58]. A reduction of at least 50% of the initial symptom level can be considered as response to treatment, whereas a reduction of at least 75% is necessary to rate the outcome as remission [59].

Concerning the comparison of the two outcome instruments, the overall better accuracy of BSI in detecting clinical cases that emerged in our analyses means that patients' prescores are on average lower with the OQ-45 than with the BSI questionnaire. Patients with low scores already at the beginning obviously have on average a minor probability of further lowering their scores during the treatment, independently of the quality of the treatment. Consequently, this disparity between the two measures leads to a higher sensitivity to change for the BSI.

5. Conclusion

On the whole, the comparison of the two questionnaires, BSI and OQ-45, as instruments to be used for routine outcome assessment leads to the following statements:

(i) In an *inpatient setting* both questionnaires have basically the same *sensitivity to change*. However, the OQ-45 has a lower *sensitivity to psychopathology* than the BSI, a characteristic that also has an impact on sensitivity to change. Another drawback affecting the OQ-45 is that inpatients tend to leave out the questions on intimate relationships or work. Unfortunately, in the inpatient setting, the nonresponse rate with both self-report measures is higher than 30%, leading to potentially nonrepresentative results.

(ii) In an *outpatient setting*, the superiority of the BSI in *both types of sensitivity* is minimal. Therefore, OQ-45 can be considered as an equivalent alternative to the BSI in routine outcome monitoring, with the advantage that it is less time-consuming.

(iii) Due to the limited sensitivity to psychopathology in *both treatment settings*, it is not advisable to base clinical assessment on data collected only with these self-report questionnaires; they should be complemented with clinician-completed ratings.

Competing Interests

The authors declare that they have no competing interests.

References

[1] APA Task Force on Quality Indicators, *Quality Indicators. Defining and Measuring Quality in Psychiatric Care for Adults and Children. Report of the APA Task Force on Quality Indicators and Report of the APA Task Force on Quality Indicators for Children*, American Psychiatric Publishing, Washington, DC, USA, 2002.

[2] B. M. Ogles, M. J. Lambert, and S. A. Fields, *Essentials of Outcome Assessment*, John Wiley & Sons, New York, NY, USA, 2002.

[3] A. J. Rush, M. B. First, and D. Blacker, *Handbook of Psychiatric Measures*, American Psychiatric Publishing, Washington, DC, USA, 2008.

[4] T. Wobrock, S. Weinmann, P. Falkai, and W. Gaebel, "Quality assurance in psychiatry: quality indicators and guideline implementation," *European Archives of Psychiatry and Clinical Neuroscience*, vol. 259, no. 2, pp. S219–S226, 2009.

[5] L. R. Derogatis and N. Melisaratos, "The brief symptom inventory: an introductory report," *Psychological Medicine*, vol. 13, no. 3, pp. 595–605, 1983.

[6] L. R. Derogatis, *SCL-90-R Revised Manual*, Johns Hopkins School of Medicine, Baltimore, Md, USA, 1983.

[7] T. L. Kramer and G. R. Smith, "Behavioral health outcomes," in *Textbook of Administrative Psychiatry: New Concepts for a Changing Behavioral Health System*, J. A. Talbott and R. E. Hales, Eds., pp. 135–144, American Psychiatric Publishing, 2001.

[8] G. M. Burlingame, T. W. Dunn, S. Chen et al., "Special section on the GAF: selection of outcome assessment instruments for inpatients with severe and persistent mental illness," *Psychiatric Services*, vol. 56, no. 4, pp. 444–451, 2005.

[9] H. L. Piersma, W. M. Reaume, and J. L. Boes, "The Brief Symptom Inventory (BSI) as an outcome measure for adult psychiatric inpatients," *Journal of Clinical Psychology*, vol. 50, no. 4, pp. 555–563, 1994.

[10] M. Hoe and J. Brekke, "Testing the cross-ethnic construct validity of the brief symptom inventory," *Research on Social Work Practice*, vol. 19, no. 1, pp. 93–103, 2009.

[11] W. D. Wood, "An attempt to validate the psychoticism scale of the brief symptom inventory," *British Journal of Medical Psychology*, vol. 55, no. 4, pp. 367–373, 1982.

[12] M. E. Johnson, C. L. Chipp, C. Brems, and D. B. Neal, "Receiver operating characteristics for the brief symptom inventory depression, paranoid ideation, and psychoticism scales in a large sample of clinical inpatients," *Psychological Reports*, vol. 102, no. 3, pp. 695–705, 2008.

[13] N. J. Preston and T. J. Harrison, "The Brief Symptom Inventory and the Positive and Negative Syndrome Scale: discriminate validity between a self-reported and observational measure of psychopathology," *Comprehensive Psychiatry*, vol. 44, no. 3, pp. 220–226, 2003.

[14] M. J. Lambert, J. J. Morton, D. Hatfield et al., *Administration and Scoring Manual for the OQ-45*, American Professional Credentialing Services, Nashville, Tenn, USA, 2004.

[15] M. E. Maruish, *Essentials of Treatment Planning*, John Wiley & Sons, New York, NY, USA, 2002.

[16] L. Bufka and N. Camp, "Brief measures for screening and measuring mental health outcomes," in *Handbook of Assessment and Treatment Planning for Psychological Disorders*, M. M. Antony and D. H. Barlow, Eds., vol. 2, pp. 62–94, Guilford Press, New York, NY, USA, 2010.

[17] L. A. Doerfler, M. E. Addis, and P. W. Moran, "Evaluating mental health outcomes in an inpatient setting: convergent and divergent validity of the OQ-45 and Basis-32," *The Journal of Behavioral Health Services and Research*, vol. 29, no. 4, pp. 394–403, 2002.

[18] B. Puschner, D. Schöfer, C. Knaup, and T. Becker, "Outcome management in in-patient psychiatric care," *Acta Psychiatrica Scandinavica*, vol. 120, no. 4, pp. 308–319, 2009.

[19] N. S. Jacobson and P. Truax, "Clinical significance: a statistical approach to defining meaningful change in psychotherapy research," *Journal of Consulting and Clinical Psychology*, vol. 59, no. 1, pp. 12–19, 1991.

[20] M. J. Lambert, W. Hannöver, K. Nisslmüller, M. Richard, and H. Kordy, "Fragebogen zum Ergebnis von Psychotherapie,

[Questionnaire on the results of psychotherapy: reliability and validity of the German translation of the Outcome Questionnaire 45.2 (OQ-45.2)]," *Zeitschrift für klinische Psychologie und Psychotherapie*, vol. 31, no. 1, pp. 40–46, 2002.

[21] B. Puschner, S. Haug, S. Häfner, and H. Kordy, "Impact of treatment setting on the course of improvement. Inpatient versus outpatient psychotherapy," *Psychotherapeut*, vol. 49, no. 3, pp. 182–192, 2004.

[22] G. H. Franke, "Erste Studien zur Güte des Brief Symptom Inventory (BSI) [First studies about the psychometric quality of the brief symptom inventory (BSI)," *Zeitschrift für Medizinische Psychologie*, vol. 6, pp. 159–166, 1997.

[23] C. Geisheim, K. Hahlweg, W. Fiegenbaum, M. Frank, B. Schroeder, and I. von Witzleben, "Das Brief Symptom Inventory (BSI) als Instrument zur Qualitätssicherung in der Psychotherapie," *Diagnostica*, vol. 48, no. 1, pp. 28–36, 2002.

[24] N. Schmitz, N. Hartkamp, and G. H. Franke, "Assessing clinically significant change: application to the SCL-90-R," *Psychological Reports*, vol. 86, no. 1, pp. 263–274, 2000.

[25] W. Lutz, J. R. Böhnke, K. Köck, and A. Bittermann, "Diagnostik und psychometrische Verlaufsrückmeldungen im Rahmen eines Modellprojektes zur Qualitätssicherung in der ambulanten Psychotherapie," *Zeitschrift für Klinische Psychologie und Psychotherapie*, vol. 40, no. 4, pp. 283–297, 2011.

[26] V. Tschuschke, A. Crameri, M. Koehler et al., "The role of therapists' treatment adherence, professional experience, therapeutic alliance, and clients' severity of psychological problems: prediction of treatment outcome in eight different psychotherapy approaches. Preliminary results of a naturalistic study," *Psychotherapy Research*, vol. 25, no. 4, pp. 420–434, 2015.

[27] A. Crameri, A. von Wyl, M. Koemeda, P. Schulthess, and V. Tschuschke, "Sensitivity analysis in multiple imputation in effectiveness studies of psychotherapy," *Frontiers in Psychology*, vol. 6, no. 1042, pp. 1–11, 2015.

[28] P. Staczan, R. Schmuecker, M. Koehler et al., "Effects of sex and gender in ten types of psychotherapy," *Psychotherapy Research*, 2015.

[29] H. U. Wittchen, M. Zaudig, and T. Fydrich, *Structured Clinical Interview for DSM-IV. Axis I and II*, Hogrefe, Göttingen, Germany, 1997.

[30] J. Busner and S. D. Targum, "The clinical global impressions scale: applying a research tool in clinical practice," *Psychiatry (Edgmont)*, vol. 4, no. 7, pp. 28–37, 2007.

[31] J. Endicott, R. L. Spitzer, J. L. Fleiss, and J. Cohen, "The global assessment scale. A procedure for measuring overall severity of psychiatric disturbance," *Archives of General Psychiatry*, vol. 33, no. 6, pp. 766–771, 1976.

[32] G. H. Franke, *Brief Symptom Inventory von Derogatis (BSI)*, Hogrefe, Göttingen, Germany, 2000.

[33] P. R. Rosenbaum and D. B. Rubin, "The central role of the propensity score in observational studies for causal effects," *Biometrika*, vol. 70, no. 1, pp. 41–55, 1983.

[34] R. Kenett and S. Salini, *Modern Analysis of Customer Surveys: With Applications Using R*, John Wiley & Sons, New York, NY, USA, 2011.

[35] D. Ho, K. Imai, G. King, and E. Stuart, "Matchit: nonparametric preprocessing for parametric casual inference," *Journal of Statistical Software*, vol. 42, no. 8, pp. 1–28, 2011.

[36] E. A. Stuart, "Matching methods for causal inference: a review and a look forward," *Statistical Science*, vol. 25, no. 1, pp. 1–21, 2010.

[37] D. B. Rubin, "Using propensity scores to help design observational studies: application to the tobacco litigation," *Health Services and Outcomes Research Methodology*, vol. 2, no. 3-4, pp. 169–188, 2001.

[38] A. M. Tarescavage and Y. S. Ben-Porath, "Psychotherapeutic outcomes measures: a critical review for practitioners," *Journal of Clinical Psychology*, vol. 70, no. 9, pp. 808–830, 2014.

[39] D. B. Rubin, "Inference and missing data," *Biometrika*, vol. 63, no. 3, pp. 581–592, 1976.

[40] C. H. Mallinckrodt, Q. Lin, and M. Molenberghs, "A structured framework for assessing sensitivity to missing data assumptions in longitudinal clinical trials," *Pharmaceutical Statistics*, vol. 12, no. 1, pp. 1–6, 2013.

[41] National Research Council, *The Prevention and Treatment of Missing Data in Clinical Trials*, The National Academies Press, Washington, DC, USA, 2010.

[42] V. Kristman, M. Manno, and P. Côté, "Loss to follow-up in cohort studies: how much is too much?" *European Journal of Epidemiology*, vol. 19, no. 8, pp. 751–760, 2004.

[43] A. M. Wood, I. R. White, and S. G. Thompson, "Are missing outcome data adequately handled? A review of published randomized controlled trials in major medical journals," *Clinical Trials*, vol. 1, no. 4, pp. 368–376, 2004.

[44] D. B. Rubin, "Discussion on multiple imputation," *International Statistical Review*, vol. 71, no. 3, pp. 619–625, 2003.

[45] M. J. Lambert, *Prevention of Treatment Failure: The Use of Measuring, Monitoring, and Feedback in Clinical Practice*, American Psychological Association, Washington, DC, USA, 2010.

[46] G. Pedereen and S. Karterud, "Is SCL-90R helpful for the clinician in assessing DSM-IV symptom disorders?" *Acta Psychiatrica Scandinavica*, vol. 110, no. 3, pp. 215–224, 2004.

[47] M. L. Thomas, "Rewards of bridging the divide between measurement and clinical theory: demonstration of a bifactor model for the Brief Symptom Inventory," *Psychological Assessment*, vol. 24, no. 1, pp. 101–113, 2012.

[48] J. Brodbeck, N. Stulz, S. Itten, D. Regli, H. Znoj, and F. Caspar, "The structure of psychopathological symptoms and the associations with DSM-diagnoses in treatment seeking individuals," *Comprehensive Psychiatry*, vol. 55, no. 3, pp. 714–726, 2014.

[49] E. de Beurs, M. Barendregt, A. de Heer et al., "Comparing methods to denote treatment outcome in clinical research and benchmarking mental health care," *Clinical Psychology & Psychotherapy*, vol. 23, no. 4, pp. 308–318, 2016.

[50] J. J. M. H. Strik, A. Honig, R. Lousberg, and J. Denollet, "Sensitivity and specificity of observer and self-report questionnaires in major and minor depression following myocardial infarction," *Psychosomatics*, vol. 42, no. 5, pp. 423–428, 2001.

[51] I. Bjelland, A. A. Dahl, T. T. Haug, and D. Neckelmann, "The validity of the Hospital Anxiety and Depression Scale: an updated literature review," *Journal of Psychosomatic Research*, vol. 52, no. 2, pp. 69–77, 2002.

[52] I. Amble, T. Gude, S. Stubdal et al., "Psychometric properties of the Outcome Questionnaire-45.2: the Norwegian version in an international context," *Psychotherapy Research*, vol. 24, no. 4, pp. 504–513, 2014.

[53] M. Moessner, C. Gallas, S. Haug, and H. Kordy, "The clinical psychological diagnostic system (KPD-38): sensitivity to change and validity of a self-report instrument for outcome monitoring and quality assurance," *Clinical Psychology and Psychotherapy*, vol. 18, no. 4, pp. 331–338, 2011.

[54] R. Timman, K. de Jong, and N. de Neve-Enthoven, "Cut-off scores and clinical change indices for the dutch outcome questionnaire (OQ-45) in a large sample of normal and several psychotherapeutic populations," *Clinical Psychology & Psychotherapy*, 2015.

[55] M. J. Lambert and E. J. Hawkins, "Measuring outcome in professional practice: considerations in selecting and using brief outcome instruments," *Professional Psychology: Research and Practice*, vol. 35, no. 5, pp. 492–499, 2004.

[56] A. G. Thalmayer, "Alternative models of the Outcome Questionnaire-45," *European Journal of Psychological Assessment*, vol. 31, no. 2, pp. 120–130, 2015.

[57] M. Gönen, *Analyzing Receiver Operating Characteristic Curves with SAS*, SAS Institute, Cary, NC, USA, 2007.

[58] W. Hiller, A. C. Schindler, and M. J. Lambert, "Defining response and remission in psychotherapy research: a comparison of the RCI and the method of percent improvement," *Psychotherapy Research*, vol. 22, no. 1, pp. 1–11, 2012.

[59] M. L. Crismon, M. Trivedi, T. A. Pigott et al., "The Texas medication algorithm project: report of the Texas consensus conference panel on medication treatment of major depressive disorder," *The Journal of Clinical Psychiatry*, vol. 60, no. 3, pp. 142–156, 1999.

25

Arabic Translation and Psychometric Evaluation of the Depression Literacy Questionnaire among Adolescents

Hussain Ahmed Darraj,[1] Mohamed Salih Mahfouz,[2] Rashad Mohamed Al Sanosi,[3] Mohammed Badedi,[4] Abdullah Sabai,[4] Abdulrahman AL Refaei,[5] and Hussain Mutawm[6]

[1]*Jazan Health Affairs, Ministry of Health, Jazan 45911, Saudi Arabia*
[2]*Family and Community Medicine Department, Faculty of Medicine, Jazan University, P.O. Box 2531, Jazan 45142, Saudi Arabia*
[3]*Substance Abuse Research Centre (SARC), Jazan University, Jazan 45142, Saudi Arabia*
[4]*Public Health Administration, Jazan Health Affairs, Ministry of Health, Jazan 82723, Saudi Arabia*
[5]*Jazan General Directorate of Education, Ministry of Education, Jazan 82614, Saudi Arabia*
[6]*Departments of English, Faculty of Languages and Translation, King Khalid University, Abha 62529, Saudi Arabia*

Correspondence should be addressed to Mohamed Salih Mahfouz; mm.mahfouz@gmail.com

Academic Editor: Nicola Magnavita

Background. Depression is a serious mental health disease. Globally, it is estimated that almost 350 million people suffer from depression. It is important to assess depression literacy including knowledge and beliefs about mental disorders among adolescents. *Objective.* This study was conducted to validate the Arabic version of the Depression Literacy Questionnaire (D-Lit) among adolescents. *Methods.* A cross-sectional study was conducted among a sample size of 120 adolescents. Statistical analysis included face validation, confirmatory factor analysis, and reliability testing. A test-retest was carried out within a two-week interval. *Results.* The mean score for depression literacy among participants was 8.6 (SD = 4.48), the median was 8, and the interquartile range was 7. Preliminary construct validation analysis confirmed that factor analysis was appropriate for the Arabic version of D-Lit. The total internal consistency was measured by Cronbach's alpha coefficient and split-half test and the results were 0.78 and 0.71, respectively. The test-retest reliability measured by Pearson's correlation was 0.92 and spearman rho was equal to 0.91. *Conclusions.* Face validity, construct validity, and reliability analysis were found satisfactory for the Arabic version of D-Lit. The Arabic D-Lit was found valid and reliable to be used in the future studies.

1. Background

Depression is a serious mental health disease and generally characterized by sadness, loss of interest in activities, and decreased energy [1]. Evidence suggests that the onset of major depression predominantly manifests during adolescence stage. Furthermore, it influences a child's psychological, social, and academic functioning. Owing to that, they will be vulnerable to the risk of substance abuse and suicidal behavior [2, 3].

Depressive disorders in developing countries represent a key determinant of health-related disability. It is considered as a major source of nonfatal disease [4, 5]. Globally, it is estimated that almost 350 million people suffer from depression [6]. In the United Kingdom, it is reported that 60% of adolescents experienced depressive symptoms [7]. In the Eastern Mediterranean Region, the prevalence of mental disorders among children and adolescents was 10%–36%, which is either similar to or significantly higher than the global estimates [8]. In the neighboring country of the United Arab Emirates, just over 22% of children aged 6 to 18 years were reported to have mental health problems [9]. In Saudi Arabia, a recent study showed that the prevalence of depression among boys who are secondary school students in

Abha city was approximately 38.2% [10]. Another study was conducted in the same region and showed that the prevalence of depression was 13.9% among girl students [11].

It is important to assess mental health literacy including knowledge and beliefs about mental disorders among adolescents [12]. A high level of mental health literacy on depression leads to a better understanding and outcomes of depressive disorders. A recent definition of mental health literacy is "the capacity to understand how to enhance and maintain good mental health; understand mental disorders and their treatments; decrease stigma against those living with a mental disorder and enhance help-seeking efficacy" [13]. Lack of mental health literacy results in a delay in seeking appropriate treatment and creates difficulties communicating with health professionals [14]. Schools are a typical venue in which to embed mental health literacy because the school students are more familiar with educational activities [15, 16].

One of the useful international assessment tools for mental health literacy specific to depression is the Depression Literacy Questionnaire (D-Lit) [17]. To date, Depression Literacy Questionnaire (D-Lit) validation studies have been made in numerous languages [17, 18]. Up to our best knowledge the Depression Literacy Questionnaire (D-Lit) has not so far been validated in Arabic.

The aim of the study was to translate the English-language version of the "Questionnaire on the Depression Literacy Questionnaire (D-Lit)" into Arabic and to validate the Arabic language version among adolescents so that it could be used in Arabic-speaking populations. Face validity, internal consistency, test-retest reliability, and construct validity were assessed.

2. Materials and Methods

2.1. The Instrument. The Depression Literacy Questionnaire (D-Lit) consists of 22 items, assessing the respondents' knowledge about depression. For each statement, respondents selected what they believed to be the correct response from three possible choices (true, false, or I don't know). There is a mix of true and false items in each scale. For example, "loss of confidence and poor self-esteem may be a symptom of depression" (D-Lit; true) and "people with depression disorder often hear voices that are not there" (D-Lit; false). Respondents' answers were scored 1 point for each correct answer, and the total score was ranged from 0 to 22. The higher score indicates a higher literacy toward depression.

2.2. Study Design and Participants. This study employed a cross-sectional study design. The source population was adolescent students in Jazan city. Four schools, two intermediate and two secondary schools, for boys and girls were randomly selected. The number of study participants for each phase was determined according to the type of validation method. 30 students were recruited in phase one which was focused on face validity, while in phase two, for construct validity, the sample size was calculated depending on Gorsuch's [19]. For reliability testing, the required sample size was calculated based on Cronbach's alpha formula. Taking into consideration 10% dropout, the final required sample size was 120 participants. In test-retest phase (phase three), the sample size was based on intraclass correlation coefficient (ICC) [20]. The minimally acceptable ICC value ($r1 = 0.7$) versus an alternative ICC value reflecting the expectations ($r1 = 0.8$) was chosen. The power was 80% and the significance level was 5%. The required sample size was 40 participants [20].

2.3. Translation and Cross-Cultural Adaptation. The planned procedures for translating the D-Lit were based on the guidelines of translation and cross-cultural adaptation by Beaton et al. [21]. Translation and back translation were conducted in order to confirm accuracy and appropriateness of Depression Literacy Questionnaire (D-Lit) wording. The instrument was translated by two independent persons from English into Arabic at the same time. One of them was aware of the study's purpose and goals, and the other one was not. Both translators had discussed the differences between their translations to resolve any differences until they developed a consensus about the Arabic wording of each item. Two back translations into English were done by two independent persons. The back translation was conducted with no prior exposure to the English-language version of the questionnaire. Then, Expert Committee Review was conducted. Principal investigator, translators, Arabic language expert, social expert, and psychiatrist discussed any discrepancies found between the original D-Lit and items and the back-translated versions the questionnaire. The committee also assessed the suitability of the instrument to be used for adolescents which was found appropriate. To avoid any limitation of the applicability of this version of the scale, the final translation was in classic Arabic, which can be used in other Arab countries with different dialects. The final Arabic version of the questionnaire is shown in Appendix B.

2.4. Data Collection. Data was collected from selected schools with no missing data. In the phase one, face validation was conducted. The selected participants ($n = 30$) were asked to go through the Arabic version of the D-Lit. After reading through the instrument, students were asked if they fully understood the instrument and its meaning. Participants reported clear understanding of the translated instrument.

In the second phase, construct validation and reliability testing were conducted. The Arabic version of the D-Lit was distributed to the participants ($n = 120$). The researcher briefly explained the content and how to answer the instrument before asking the participants to complete the instrument. The participants were encouraged to ask if they had any problem with the instrument. The average time taken to complete the instrument was 15 minutes. The completed instruments were returned to the researcher. At the end of phase two, no participants had indicated problems with the Arabic version of the D-Lit.

In phase three, test-retest reliability was conducted after a two-week interval. In this phase, we were able to reach 65 participants who had been involved in phase two and the same Arabic version of the D-Lit was given to them. The aim was to test if the participants would provide the same answer as in the previous phase.

2.5. Statistical Analysis. The collected data was analyzed using SPSS version 19.0. Descriptive statistics was used to summarize the demographic information and to obtain the descriptive details of depression literacy among the participants. In order to assess the factor structure of the translated version of the D-List prior to factor analysis, the preliminary analysis which indicates the adequacy of the instrument for factor analysis was evaluated. The preliminary analysis is represented by the value of the Kaiser-Meyer-Olkin (KMO) Measure of Sampling Adequacy, Individual Measure of Sampling Adequacy (MSA), and Bartlett's test of sphericity. The KMO value is expected to exceed the acceptable limit of 0.50 [22]. Lastly, Bartlett's test of sphericity indicates the appropriateness of factor analysis for the translated instrument [23]; thus it is expected to be significant. The analysis then proceeded with an assessment of the factor structure, since confirmatory factor analysis was conducted using SPSS application.

Assessment of the factor structure includes factor loading where items that are highly loaded into each factor were examined and then compared to previous studies. To assess the reliability of the Arabic version of the D-Lit, the internal consistency and test-retest reliability of the translated instrument were measured. The internal consistency reliability of the instruments is represented by Cronbach's alpha coefficient (α). Subsequently, Pearson's correlation coefficient (R) was calculated to evaluate the test-retest reliability. The correlation coefficient was calculated for the total score of the translated instrument.

2.6. Ethical Considerations. The study proposal and instrument were approved by the faculty of Medicine Ethical Committee. Authorization was granted from the headmasters of the selected schools. During the distribution of the questionnaire, students were told that the information collected would be kept anonymous and that participation was completely voluntary. Informed consent was sought from the eligible participants following full disclosure regarding the study before data collection is done. Proxy consent for children was obtained from parents or the person responsible. The purpose of the study was explained and participants were assured that they may withdraw from the study at any time during the study.

3. Results

3.1. Study Participants Background. Table 1 shows the background characteristics of the study population. A total of 120 students from 4 intermediate and secondary schools in Jazan city were involved in the study. Almost 88.3% (106) were Saudi, and 50% (60) were males.

3.2. Arabic-Translated Version of the D-Lit Scores. In the current study, the mean score for depression literacy among the participants was 8.6 (SD = 4.48), the median equals 8, the interquartile range was 7, and the range was 16. The descriptive summary of the Arabic-translated version of the D-Lit among the participants is tabulated in Table 2.

TABLE 1: Background characteristics of the students.

Characteristic	(n)	(%)
Nationality		
Saudi	106	88.3
Non-Saudi	14	11.7
Sex		
Male	60	50
Female	60	50
Grade		
Excellent	77	73.3
Very good	20	19
Good	7	6.7
Poor	1	1
Total	120	100

TABLE 2: Arabic-translated version of the D-Lit scores.

Mean score (SD)	8.6 (SD = 4.48)	
Measurements	Frequency (n)	Percentage (%)
Below mean score	64	53.4
Above mean score	56	46.6

Based on the mean score, the participants were divided into two groups: participants who scored below the mean score and participants who scored above the mean score. The percentage of those who scored above the mean score (46.6%) is shown to be less than those who scored below the mean score (53.4%).

3.3. Reliability Testing. The overall estimate of the reliability of the Arabic-translated version of the D-Lit (Cronbach's alpha) was 0.78 and split-half was equal to 0.71. The item-to-total score correlations were between $r = 0.20$ and $r = 0.55$, with 15 items exceeding the 0.30 criterion [24] and 7 items more than 0.2. The test-retest reliability of the total score, measured by Pearson's correlation, was scored and is found to be perfect $R = 0.92$ and Spearman rho was 0.91.

3.4. Readability Testing. Gunning Fog index is 6.26 for the Arabic version of D-Lit which indicates the number of years of formal education that a person requires in order to easily understand the questions in the D-Lit scale on the first reading.

3.5. Factor Analysis. The preliminary analysis for factor analysis of the Arabic-translated version of the D-Lit showed a satisfactory result. The determinant was >0.00001. The value of the KMO measure of sampling adequacy was 0.63, while Bartlett's test for sphericity was found highly significant ($p < 0.001$). The factor loading of the translated instrument is shown in Table 3. It confirms that all the items of the scale have been explained by a single factor (component 1). Multiple components have been emerged to indicate the possibility of other specific dimensions of this scale, but we are going to ignore it because our objective is to confirm

TABLE 3: Results of factor analysis.

N	Item to total score correlation	Factor loading	Communalities
Q1	0.220	0.354	0.540
Q2	0.399	0.442	0.826
Q3	0.550	0.772	0.906
Q4	0.237	0.287	0.558
Q5	0.455	0.534	0.904
Q6	0.234	0.273	0.724
Q7	0.283	0.275	0.810
Q8	0.315	0.383	0.693
Q9	0.313	0.438	0.547
Q10	0.234	0.286	0.696
Q11	0.474	0.704	0.846
Q12	0.381	0.401	0.829
Q13	0.253	0.277	0.298
Q14	0.206	0.254	0.841
Q15	0.421	0.671	0.831
Q16	0.212	0.224	0.636
Q17	0.314	0.393	0.897
Q18	0.212	0.240	0.784
Q19	0.377	0.389	0.715
Q20	0.336	0.522	0.499
Q21	0.388	0.440	0.771
Q22	0.365	0.419	0.717

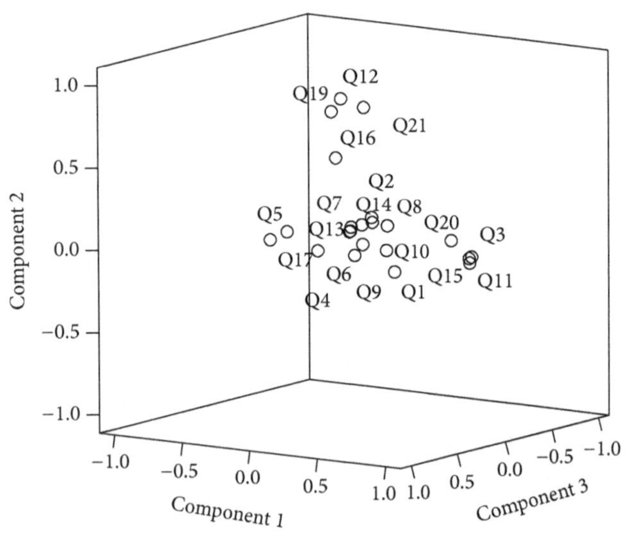

FIGURE 1: Component plot in rotated space.

the existing factor in the original scale. The screen plot also clearly suggested that the dimensions underlay the items of the scale (Figure 1).

As shown in Table 3, a component 1 extracted factor explained 100% of the variance in the items of the scale. Thus, factor rotation was not needed. All communality values were above 0.30, as recommended by Tabachnick and Fidell, 2001 [25].

4. Discussion

This study represents the first attempt to examine the reliability and the validity of an Arabic version of the 22-item Depression Literacy Questionnaire (D-Lit). The results provide solid support for the scale's reliability and validity among adolescent school students. Reliability was demonstrated through adequate estimates of internal consistency; Cronbach's alpha was estimated at 0.78, which exceeds the minimum criterion of 0.70 [26]. This internal consistency estimate is consistent with findings from other studies of D-Lit measures, which reported alpha of 0.7 in a sample of adults [17] and alphas of 0.88 and 0.92, respectively, in Greek and Italian versions of the D-Lit [18]. The test-retest reliability of the total score, measured by Pearson's correlation was found to be perfect ($R = 0.92$). Spearman rho was found to be 0.91, which was the same as the reliability for the English, Greek, and Italian versions of the D-Lit (alpha = 0.71, alpha = 0.80, and alpha = 0.78, resp.) [17, 18].

The corrected item-to-total correlations for 15 items exceeded the 0.30 criterion [24] and 7 items more than 0.2 suggesting the homogeneity of the measure and that each item was measuring a unique construct. This finding was not reported in the original English version of the D-Lit.

The findings of the factor analysis provide further support for the construct validity of the Arabic D-Lit. All items have been explained by a single factor which indicates that the Arabic version of the D-Lit is valid to measure depression literacy as one scale.

Gunning Fog index is 6.26 for the Arabic version of D-Lit which indicates the number of years of formal education a person requires to easily understand the questions in the D-Lit scale on the first reading. On the other hand, we have measured the Gunning Fog index for the original English version which was found to be 14.49. This further confirms that Arabic D-Lit is appropriate for the level of adolescent students.

5. Limitations

Around half $n = 65$ of participants dropped during the second phase of the study and hence did not fill the same questionnaire, compared to participants in the first time test $n = 120$; this dropout was due to midterm exams but still it was a statistically appropriate sample for test-retest as the minimal sample size was calculated to be 40 participants.

6. Conclusion

The results of the analysis of the psychometric properties of the Arabic version of the D-Lit in adolescent school students yield promising evidence that the 22-item D-Lit has acceptable reliability and validity. The findings also indicate that the D-Lit is potentially useful for assessing depression literacy that precedes the development and designing of depression

Table 4: D-Lit.

3	2	1	الرجاء اختيار الاجابة المناسبة (صح، خطأ، لا أعلم) لكل من الأسئلة التالية:	*N*
لا أعلم	خطأ	صح	الأشخاص الذين يعانون من الاكتئاب غالبا ما يتكلمون بطريقة مشوشة وغير مترابطة.	1
لا أعلم	خطأ	صح	المصابون بالاكتئاب قد يشعرون بالذنب عندما لا يكونوا على خطأ.	2
لا أعلم	خطأ	صح	السلوك المتهور والطائش هو عرض من أعراض الاكتئاب.	3
لا أعلم	خطأ	صح	فقدان الثقة وضعف الثقة بالنفس قد يكونا من أعراض الاكتئاب.	4
لا أعلم	خطأ	صح	عدم المشي على التصدعات في الرصيف قد تكون علامة على الاكتئاب.	5
لا أعلم	خطأ	صح	الأشخاص الذين يعانون من الاكتئاب-كثيرا ما يسمعون أصواتا غير موجودة.	6
لا أعلم	خطأ	صح	النوم الكثير أو القليل جدا قد يكون علامة على الاكتئاب.	7
لا أعلم	خطأ	صح	الإفراط في تناول الطعام أو فقدان الرغبة في الغذاء قد يكون علامة على الاكتئاب.	8
لا أعلم	خطأ	صح	الاكتئاب لا يؤثر على ذاكرتك وتركيزك.	9
لا أعلم	خطأ	صح	وجود شخصيات متعدده ومختلفة في الإنسان قد تكون علامة على الاكتئاب.	10
لا أعلم	خطأ	صح	الاشخاص قد يتحركون ببطء أكثر أو يصبحون منفعلون نتيجة لاكتئابهم.	11
لا أعلم	خطأ	صح	المعالج النفسي السريري يمكن أن يصف أدوية مضادات الاكتئاب.	12
لا أعلم	خطأ	صح	الاكتئاب المتوسط يعطل حياة الشخص بقدر التصلب المتعدد أو الصمم.	13
لا أعلم	خطأ	صح	معظم الناس الذين يعانون من الاكتئاب يحتاجون إلى التنويم في المستشفى.	14
لا أعلم	خطأ	صح	العديد من الناس المشهورين قد عانوا من الاكتئاب.	15
لا أعلم	خطأ	صح	العديد من طرق علاج الاكتئاب هي أكثر فعالية من أدوية مضادات الاكتئاب.	16
لا أعلم	خطأ	صح	المشورة هي فعّالة مثل العلاج السلوكي المعرفي للاكتئاب.	17
لا أعلم	خطأ	صح	العلاج السلوكي المعرفي هو فعّال كما مضادات الاكتئاب في حالات الاكتئاب الخفيفة الى المتوسطة.	18
لا أعلم	خطأ	صح	من المرجح أن تكون الفيتامينات هي أكثر فائدة لعلاج الاكتئاب من بين جميع العلاجات البديلة ونمط الحياة.	19
لا أعلم	خطأ	صح	الناس الذين يعانون من الاكتئاب يجب عليهم التوقف عن تناول مضادات الاكتئاب بمجرد أن يشعروا بالتحسن.	20
لا أعلم	خطأ	صح	مضادات الاكتئاب تسبب الادمان.	21
لا أعلم	خطأ	صح	مفعول الأدوية المضادة للاكتئاب عادة ما يظهر فوراً.	22

literacy educational programs for adolescent school students and to monitor the effectiveness of these interventions to produce the desired change, which is important for combating depression stigma and improving help-seeking behavior.

Appendix

A. Depression Literacy Questionnaire Items (D-Lit)

Answer each item with one of three options – true, false or don't know.

(1) People with depression often speak in a rambling and disjointed way.

—

(2) People with depression may feel guilty when they are not at fault.

—

(3) Reckless and foolhardy behavior is a common sign of depression.

—

(4) Loss of confidence and poor self-esteem may be a symptom of depression.

—

(5) Not stepping on cracks in the footpath may be a sign of depression.

—

(6) People with depression often hear voices that are not there.

—

(7) Sleeping too much or too little may be a sign of depression.

—

(8) Eating too much or losing intereslt in food may be a sign of depression.

—

(9) Depression does not affect your memory and concentration.

—

(10) Having several distinct personalities may be a sign of depression.

—

(11) People may move more slowly or become agitated as a result of their depression.

—

(12) Clinical psychologists can prescribe antidepressants.

—

(13) Moderate depression disrupts a person's life as much as multiple sclerosis or deafness.

—

(14) Most people with depression need to be hospitalized.

—

(15) Many famous people have suffered from depression.

—

(16) Many treatments for depression are more effective than antidepressants.

—

(17) Counseling is as effective as cognitive behavioral therapy for depression.

—

(18) Cognitive behavioral therapy is as effective as antidepressants for mild to moderate depression.

—

(19) Of all the alternative and lifestyle treatments for depression, vitamins are likely to be the most helpful.

—

(20) People with depression should stop taking antidepressants as soon as they feel better.

—

(21) Antidepressants are addictive.

—

(22) Antidepressant medications usually work straight away.

—

B. Arabic Version of the D-Lit

See Table 4.

Competing Interests

The authors have no competing interests to declare.

Authors' Contributions

Hussain Ahmed Darraj prepared the research proposal; Hussain Ahmed Darraj, Mohamed Salih Mahfouz, and Mohammed Badedi designed this research paper; Hussain Ahmed Darraj and Mohamed Salih Mahfouz performed data analysis; Hussain Ahmed Darraj, Mohamed Salih Mahfouz, Mohammed Badedi, and Abdullah Sabai wrote the paper. Mohamed Salih Mahfouz, Rashad Mohamed Al Sanosi, Abdulrahman AL Refaei, and Hussain Mutawm provided significant input on the paper. All authors read and approved the final paper.

Acknowledgments

The authors would like to thank Dr. Nabil Joseph Awadalla for his valuable comments and suggestions in the early work. Also, the authors thank the staff from Jazan University for their efforts in supervising the data collection phase. The authors appreciate the efforts of the Education Directorate in Jazan Region, administrative staff, and teachers for coordination and help with data collection. Also, the authors would like to thank Professor Kathy Griffiths for the permission to use the Depression Literacy Questionnaire.

References

[1] World Health Organization, *The World Health Report 2001: Mental Health: New Understanding, New Hope*, World Health Organization, Geneva, Switzerland, 2001.

[2] C. Hammen and B. E. Compas, "Unmasking unmasked depression in children and adolescents: the problem of comorbidity," *Clinical Psychology Review*, vol. 14, no. 6, pp. 585–603, 1994.

[3] B. Birmaher, N. D. Ryan, D. E. Williamson et al., "Childhood and adolescent depression: a review of the past 10 years. Part I," *Journal of the American Academy of Child & Adolescent Psychiatry*, vol. 35, no. 11, pp. 1427–1439, 1996.

[4] N. Sartorius, "The economic and social burden of depression," *Journal of Clinical Psychiatry*, vol. 62, no. 15, pp. 8–11, 2001.

[5] G. Miller, "The unseen: mental illness's global toll," *Science*, vol. 311, no. 5760, pp. 458–461, 2006.

[6] Mental disorders fact sheet no. 396, October 2015, http://www.who.int/mediacentre/factsheets/fs396/en.

[7] R. Harrington and A. Clark, "Prevention and early intervention for depression in adolescence and early adult life," *European Archives of Psychiatry and Clinical Neuroscience*, vol. 248, no. 1, pp. 32–45, 1998.

[8] WHO, *Maternal, Child and Adolescent Mental Health: Challenges and Strategic Directions 2010–2015*, World Health Organization Regional Office for the Eastern Mediterranean. Regional Committee for the EM/RC57 Fifty-Seventh Session Original: Arabic Agenda Item 4, 2010.

[9] V. Eapen, M. E. Jakka, and M. T. Abou-Saleh, "Children with psychiatric disorders: the Al Ain community psychiatric survey," *Canadian Journal of Psychiatry*, vol. 48, no. 6, pp. 402–407, 2003.

[10] K. S. Al-Gelban, "Depression, anxiety and stress among Saudi adolescent school boys," *Journal of The Royal Society for the Promotion of Health*, vol. 127, no. 1, pp. 33–37, 2007.

[11] K. S. Al Gelban, "Prevalence of psychological symptoms in Saudi Secondary School girls in Abha, Saudi Arabia," *Annals of Saudi Medicine*, vol. 29, no. 4, pp. 275–279, 2009.

[12] A. F. Jorm, A. E. Korten, P. A. Jacomb, H. Christensen, B. Rodgers, and P. Pollitt, "'Mental health literacy': a survey of the public's ability to recognise mental disorders and their beliefs about the effectiveness of treatment," *Medical Journal of Australia*, vol. 166, no. 4, pp. 182–186, 1997.

[13] Y. Wei, J. A. Hayden, S. Kutcher, A. Zygmunt, and P. McGrath, "The effectiveness of school mental health literacy programs to address knowledge, attitudes and help seeking among youth," *Early Intervention in Psychiatry*, vol. 7, no. 2, pp. 109–121, 2013.

[14] I. Rootman and D. Gordon-El Bihbety, *A Vision for a Health Literate Canada: Report of the Expert Panel on Health Literacy*, 2008.

[15] M. S. Atkins, K. E. Hoagwood, K. Kutash, and E. Seidman, "Toward the integration of education and mental health in schools," *Administration and Policy in Mental Health and Mental Health Services Research*, vol. 37, no. 1-2, pp. 40–47, 2010.

[16] J. Wyn, H. Cahill, R. Holdsworth, L. Rowling, and S. Carson, "MindMatters, a whole-school approach promoting mental health and wellbeing," *Australian and New Zealand Journal of Psychiatry*, vol. 34, no. 4, pp. 594–601, 2000.

[17] A. Gulliver, K. M. Griffiths, H. Christensen et al., "Internet-based interventions to promote mental health help-seeking in elite athletes: an exploratory randomized controlled trial," *Journal of Medical Internet Research*, vol. 14, no. 3, p. e69, 2012.

[18] L. A. Kiropoulos, K. M. Griffiths, and G. Blashki, "Effects of a multilingual information website intervention on the levels of depression literacy and depression-related stigma in Greek-born and Italian-born immigrants living in Australia: a randomized controlled trial," *Journal of Medical Internet Research*, vol. 13, no. 2, 2011.

[19] R. L. Gorsuch, *Factor Analysis*, Erlbaum, Hillsdale, Mich, USA, 1983.

[20] S. D. Walter, M. Eliasziw, and A. Donner, "Sample size and optimal designs for reliability studies," *Statistics in Medicine*, vol. 17, no. 1, pp. 101–110, 1998.

[21] D. E. Beaton, C. Bombardier, F. Guillemin, and M. B. Ferraz, "Guidelines for the process of cross-cultural adaptation of self-report measures," *Spine*, vol. 25, no. 24, pp. 3186–3191, 2000.

[22] H. F. Kaiser, "An index of factorial simplicity," *Psychometrika*, vol. 39, no. 1, pp. 31–36, 1974.

[23] A. Field, *Discovering Statistics Using SPSS*, Sage, Thousand Oaks, Calif, USA, 2009.

[24] B. C. Cronk, *How to Use SPSS: A Step-by-Step Guide to Analysis and Interpretation*, Pyrczak, Glendale, Calif, USA, 2004.

[25] B. G. Tabachnick and L. S. Fidell, *Using Multivariate Statistics*, 2001.

[26] J. Nunnally and I. Bernstein, "Statistical foundations," in *Psychometric Theory*, pp. 31–208, McGraw-Hill, New York, NY, USA, 3rd edition, 1994.

26

Clinical Profile and Comorbidity of Obsessive-Compulsive Disorder among Children and Adolescents: A Cross-Sectional Observation in Bangladesh

Md. Hafizur Rahman Chowdhury, Mohammad S. I. Mullick, and S. M. Yasir Arafat

Department of Psychiatry, Bangabandhu Sheikh Mujib Medical University, Dhaka, Bangladesh

Correspondence should be addressed to S. M. Yasir Arafat; arafatdmc62@gmail.com

Academic Editor: Veit Roessner

Obsessive compulsive disorder (OCD) is a common disorder characterised by persistent and unwanted intrusive thoughts, images, and urges and repetitive behaviours or mental acts and can cause pervasive impairments. In Bangladesh, the prevalence of OCD among children is 2% which is higher than in previous reporting. This study was aimed at looking into the type, frequency, and severity of symptoms of OCD and comorbidity among children and adolescents. A consecutive 60 OCD cases from a child mental health service with age range of 5–18 years were recruited and divided into below and above 12 years of age group. The assessment was carried out using standardized Bangla version of Development and Wellbeing Assessment and Children's Yale-Brown Obsessive Compulsive Scale was administered. Of the obsession, contamination was the highest followed by doubt, and of the compulsion, washing/cleaning was the highest followed by checking, repeating, and ordering rituals. More than half of the subjects had severe OCD and comorbidity was present in 58% subjects. Specific phobia, social phobia, major depressive disorder, and tic disorder were more prevalent. These symptoms and comorbidity profile can serve the baseline data for a country like Bangladesh and further large scale study would better generalize the study results.

1. Introduction

Obsessive-compulsive disorder (OCD) is a relatively common disorder with a lifetime prevalence of 1–3% in children and adolescents, characterised by persistent and unwanted intrusive thoughts, images, and urges (obsessions) and repetitive behaviours or mental acts (compulsions), and typically runs a chronic, wax, and wane course and can cause pervasive impairments in social, academic, and familial functioning [1–6]. Males and females are equally commonly affected from adolescence onwards, but males predominate in prepubertal OCD [7]. The presentation of obsessions and compulsions is heterogeneous in children and adolescents and most of these differences are related to the developmental limitations of younger children compared to adults, and so on [1, 3, 6]. Moreover, OCD is a highly comorbid disorder in childhood with up to 80% of affected children meeting diagnostic criteria for another mental health disorder, most commonly another anxiety disorder, depressive disorder, attention deficit disorder, oppositional defiant disorder (ODD), conduct disorder (CD), or tic disorder, and as many as 50–60% of youth experiencing two or more other mental disorders during their lifetime [3, 6, 8, 9]. A community based epidemiological survey reported that prevalence of OCD among children in Bangladesh is 2% and that is in line with the other cultures [10]. It is evident that the pattern of presentation of obsessive-compulsive disorder between children and adolescent might be different and researchers' clinical observation is that the pattern of presentation of obsessions and compulsions among children and adolescents may be different in Bangladesh due to different cultural and religious background. So, it was aimed to find out the type and frequency of the symptoms of OCD among children and adolescents and to delineate the comorbidity of OCD in children and adolescents in Bangladesh.

2. Methods

2.1. Ethical Consideration. The researchers were duly concerned about the ethical issues related to the study. Formal ethical clearance was taken from the Institutional Review Board (IRB) of the Bangabandhu Sheikh Mujib Medical University (BSMMU) for conducting the study. Confidentiality of the person and the information was maintained; observed and unauthorized persons did not have any access to the data. Informed written consent was taken from the subjects as well as from the legal guardians after informing the nature and purpose of the study, the procedure of study, the right to refuse, and acceptance and withdrawal from participating in the study and the participants did not gain financial benefit from this study. The present study posed a very low risk to the participants, as procedures such as medical treatments, invasive diagnostics, or procedures causing psychological, spiritual, or social harm were not included.

2.2. Design, Subjects, and Instruments. This was a cross-sectional observational study carried out in the Child and Adolescent Outpatient Services of the Department of Psychiatry, BSMMU, Dhaka. Data were collected with the help of convenient sampling during the period of January 2009 to December 2009 from a total of 60 consecutive patients with OCD between 5 and 18 years of age. All children up to 18 years diagnosed as OCD by a psychiatrist were included into the study. Data were collected with the researchers themselves having sound psychopathological background. The cases were divided into two groups: children up to 11 years and adolescents from 12–18 years. For assessment of OCD and comorbidity, structured instrument for assessment of child psychopathology, standardized and validated Bangla parent version of Development and Wellbeing Assessment (DAWABA), was administered [10]. In addition, Self DAWABA was used for the adolescent cases. DAWABA generated ICD-10 DCR [11] diagnoses were assigned for the cases where only Axis one diagnosis was considered. For assessment of symptom pattern and severity of OCD, Children's Yale-Brown Obsessive-Compulsive Scale (CY-BOCS) [12] was used. This scale has five sections: instruction, obsessions checklists, severity items for obsessions, compulsions checklist, and severity items in compulsion. The CY-BOCS comprises 10 severity items, five for the obsessions and five for the compulsions. The severity items assess five aspects pertaining to obsessions and compulsions: frequency, interference, distress, resistance, and control. The 10 severity items are rated on a five-point scale with responses: none, mild, moderate, severe, and extreme for the frequency; interference and distress items are rated as always resists and completely yields to the resistance; and control items are rated as complete control, much control, moderate control, little control, and no control. This scale was translated in Bangla through translation-back translation and committee translation procedure and standardized and validated by the researchers. The translated Bangla version of this scale was used for assessment of pattern and severity of OCD among children and adolescents. Sociodemographic characteristics were assessed by a questionnaire designed for the study. All collected data were cleaned by checking and rechecking for omissions, inconsistencies, and improbabilities. Data were edited, coded, and entered into the computer. After managing data properly, it was analyzed in Statistical Package for Social Science (SPSS) version 12.

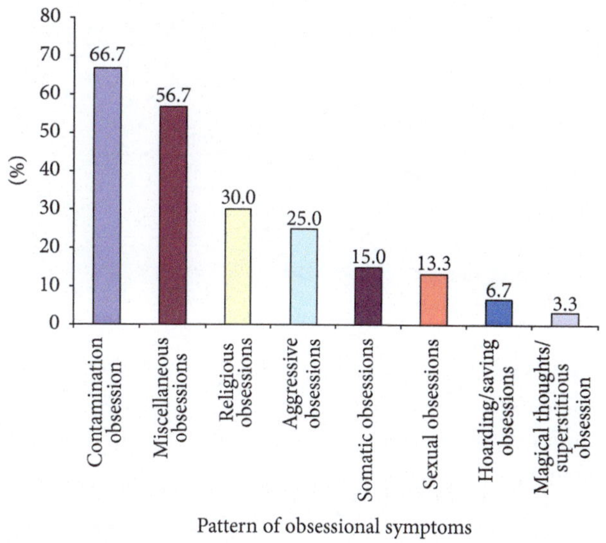

FIGURE 1: Pattern of obsessive symptoms among 8–18-year-old respondents ($n = 60$).

3. Results

All the 60 respondents were students; 21 were children and 39 were adolescents and 43 (71.7%) were boys and 17 (28.3%) were girls. Their age ranged from 8 to 18 years with the mean of 13.9 ± 3.44 years. Majority of cases came from urban areas (81.7%) with middle income group (57.7%). Forty-five percent of cases had first-degree family history of psychiatric disorder and the highest percentage had OCD (63%) followed by mood disorder (15%) and anxiety disorders (15%).

It was found that the highest percentage of patients had contamination obsession (66.7%) followed by miscellaneous obsessions (56.7%) that mainly included pathological doubt and religious obsession (30%) (Figure 1). Proportion of aggressive obsessions (25.6%), religious obsessions (36%), and miscellaneous obsessions (64%) were found to be higher among the adolescents group whereas contamination obsessions (71%) were found to be high among the children group.

Regarding compulsive symptoms, the highest percentage of patients had washing/cleaning compulsion (65%) followed by checking compulsion (50%) (Figure 2).

Axis one comorbidity was present among 51.7% of cases with OCD. The highest percentage had specific phobia (10%) followed by major depressive disorder (10%) (Table 1).

Table 2 shows characteristics feature of obsession according to Children's Yale-Brown Obsessive Scale with the mean score of time spent on obsession and obsession-free interval; and interference from obsessions was higher among the adolescents than that of children. Mean obsession score was significantly higher in the adolescents than the children, which was statistically significant and obtained from unpaired Student's t-test (Table 2).

Table 1: Pattern of comorbidity among 8–18-year-old respondents.

Pattern of comorbidity	Age in years <12 (n = 21)		≥12 (n = 39)		Total (n = 60)	
	Number	%	Number	%	Number	%
Generalized anxiety disorder	0	.0	2	5.1	2	3.3
Specific phobia	6	28.6	0	.0	6	10.0
Tic disorder	5	23.8	0	.0	5	8.3
Conduct disorder	0	.0	2	5.1	2	3.3
Oppositional defiant disorder	2	9.5	2	5.1	4	6.7
Hyperkinetic disorder	4	23.8	0	.0	4	9.0
Major depressive disorder	0	.0	6	15.4	6	10.0
Social phobia	1	4.8	5	12.8	6	10.0
Autism spectrum disorder	1	4.8	1	2.6	2	3.3
Comorbidity						
OCD only	8	38.1	21	53.8	29	48.3
Comorbidity	13	61.9	18	46.2	31	51.7

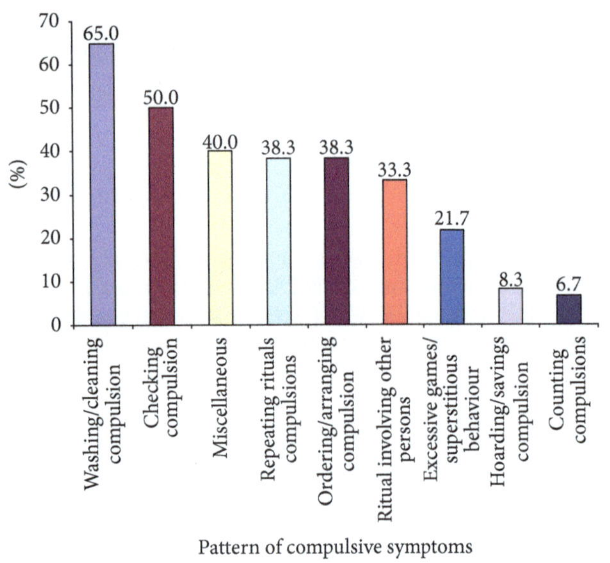

Figure 2: Pattern of compulsive symptoms among 8–18-year-old respondents (n = 60).

Characteristics feature of compulsion according to Children's Yale-Brown Obsessive Scale is shown in Table 3.

Percent distribution of severity of OCD among the respondents according to CY-BOCS revealed that more than half of the patients had severe OCD (53.3%) followed by 36.7% who had extreme OCD, 6.7% who had moderate OCD, and only 3.3% who had mild OCD. The proportion of extreme OCD was found to be high among the adolescents (48.7%) whereas severe OCD was higher among the children (71.4%). The mean score for OCD was 26.81 ± 5.2 for the children and 30.46 ± 5.9 for the adolescents and mean difference was statistically significant ($p < 0.05$).

Table 4 shows relationship between morbidity and selected sociodemographic characteristics of the patients. Analysis found that the OCD with comorbidity was found to be high among the younger patients (61.9%) whereas OCD only was found among the adolescents (53.8%).

4. Discussion

This study aimed at looking into the type, frequency, and severity of symptoms of OCD and comorbidity among children and adolescents in Bangladesh and, to the authors' best knowledge, it is the first study to reveal the finding in geographic area as well as the culture.

In the present study, it was found that 45% of patients had 1st-degree family history of psychiatric illness obtained by history. The overall pattern of family history indicated that highest percentage had OCD (63%) followed by mood disorder (15%) and also other anxiety disorders (15%) followed by psychosis (7.4%). However, the proportions of OCD (75%) and mood disorder (16.7%) were found to be high among children whereas, among adolescents, highest percentage had OCD (53.3%) followed by other anxiety disorders. This result gives further evidence that suggests a biological basis for OCD and genetic studies that find higher concordance rates of OCD in first-degree family members and twins than in general population [1–5, 13]. Considering the caregivers' perception about the child's disease, 88.3% believed that it was mental illness, which indicates good awareness among parents of OCD patients, but we should also keep in mind that most of the parents came from good educational and economic background. According to CY-BOCS, the pattern indicates that the highest percentage of patients had contamination obsession (66.7%) followed by miscellaneous obsessions (56.7%) (which mainly includes pathological doubt) and religious obsessions (30%) and these findings are consistent with the findings of other similar types of representative studies [1, 2, 14, 15]. Mean obsession score was significantly higher in the adolescents than the children, which can be explained by cognitive developmental stages. The CY-BOCS pattern of compulsion indicates that

TABLE 2: Characteristics feature of obsession according to Children's Yale-Brown Obsessive Scale.

Characteristics	Age in years <12 ($n = 21$) Number	%	≥12 ($n = 39$) Number	%	Total ($n = 60$) Number	%	p value
Time spent on obsession							
Mild	2	9.5	2	5.1	4	6.7	
Moderate	9	42.9	10	25.6	19	31.7	
Severe	10	47.6	15	38.5	25	41.7	
Extreme	0	.0	12	30.8	12	20.0	
Mean ± SD score	2.38 ± 0.7		2.95 ± 0.9		2.75 ± 0.9		0.013
Obsession-free interval							
Long	1	4.8	3	7.7	4	6.7	
Moderately long	16	76.2	14	35.9	30	50.0	
Short	3	14.3	17	43.6	20	33.3	
Extremely short	1	4.8	5	12.8	6	10.0	
Mean ± SD score	2.19 ± 0.6		2.62 ± 0.8		2.47 ± 0.8		0.040
Interference from obsessions							
Long	1	4.8	3	7.7	4	6.7	
Moderately long	10	47.6	7	17.9	17	28.3	
Short	10	47.6	10	25.6	20	33.3	
Extremely short	0	.0	19	48.7	19	31.7	
Mean ± SD score	2.43 ± 0.6		3.15 ± 1.0		2.90 ± 0.9		0.003
Distress of obsessions							
Long	1	4.8	2	5.1	3	5.0	
Moderately long	4	19.0	3	7.7	7	11.7	
Short	12	57.1	12	30.8	24	40.0	
Extremely short	4	19.0	22	56.4	26	43.3	
Mean ± SD score	2.90 ± 0.8		3.38 ± 0.8		3.22 ± 0.8		0.035
Resistance							
Much resistance	1	4.8	1	2.6	2	3.3	
Some resistance	1	4.8	3	7.7	4	6.7	
Often yields	17	81.0	23	59.0	40	66.7	
Completely yields	2	9.5	12	30.8	14	23.3	
Mean ± SD score	2.95 ± 0.6		3.18 ± 0.7		3.10 ± 0.7		0.204
Control over obsessions							
Much control	1	4.8	0	.0	1	1.7	
Moderate control	1	4.8	3	7.7	4	6.7	
Little control	17	81.0	23	59.0	40	66.7	
No control	2	9.5	13	33.3	15	25.0	
Mean ± SD score	2.95 ± 0.6		3.26 ± 0.6		3.15 ± 0.6		0.063
Total obsession score	13.62 ± 2.8		15.92 ± 3.1		15.12 ± 3.2		0.006

p value reached from unpaired Student's t-test.

the highest percentage of patients had washing/cleaning compulsion followed by checking compulsion and miscellaneous compulsion, and the findings are in agreement with other findings [14, 15]. Present study revealed that the comorbidity was present among 51.7% of children and adolescent OCD patients, which is in between the widely variable range of other studies [3, 5, 6, 13, 16, 17]. However, comorbidity was higher among children (61.9%) than the adolescents (46.2%) but the difference was not statistically significant, reached from Chi square test. This finding (more early onset OCD is associated with more comorbidity) is also consistent with other studies' findings [18]. The pattern of comorbidity also indicated that the highest percentage had specific phobia followed by major depressive disorder, social phobia, tic disorder, oppositional defiant disorder, hyperkinetic disorder, generalized anxiety disorder, conduct disorder, mental retardation, and autism spectrum disorder. This finding is partly comparable to other findings except absence of alcohol

TABLE 3: Characteristics feature of compulsion according to Children's Yale-Brown Compulsive Scale.

Characteristics	Age in years				Total (n = 60)		p value
	<12 (n = 21)		≥12 (n = 39)				
	Number	%	Number	%	Number	%	
Time spent on compulsion							
Mild	1	4.8	2	5.1	3	5.0	
Moderate	9	42.9	16	41.0	25	41.7	
Severe	11	52.4	13	33.3	24	40.0	
Extreme	0	.0	8	20.5	8	13.3	
Mean ± SD score	2.48 ± 0.6		2.69 ± 0.9		2.62 ± 0.8		0.312
Compulsion-free interval							
Long	1	4.8	2	5.1	3	5.0	
Moderately long	15	71.4	21	53.8	36	60.0	
Short	5	23.8	13	33.3	18	30.0	
Extremely short	0	.0	3	7.7	3	5.0	
Mean ± SD score	2.19 ± 0.5		2.44 ± 0.7		2.35 ± 0.7		0.171
Interference from compulsions							
Long	1	4.8	2	5.1	3	5.0	
Moderately long	11	52.4	12	30.8	23	38.3	
Short	9	42.9	19	48.7	28	46.7	
Extremely short	0	.0	6	15.4	6	10.0	
Mean ± SD score	2.38 ± 0.6		2.74 ± 0.8		2.62 ± 0.7		0.069
Distress of compulsions							
Long	1	4.8	2	5.1	3	5.0	
Moderately long	5	23.8	6	15.4	11	18.3	
Short	13	61.9	15	38.5	28	46.7	
Extremely short	2	9.5	16	41.0	18	30.0	
Mean ± SD score	2.76 ± 0.7		3.15 ± 0.9		3.02 ± 0.8		0.082
Resistance							
1	1	4.8	1	2.6	2	3.3	
2	4	19.0	8	20.5	12	20.0	
3	14	66.7	22	56.4	36	60.0	
Completely yields	2	9.5	8	20.5	10	16.7	
Mean ± SD score	2.81 ± 0.7		2.95 ± 0.7		2.90 ± 0.7		0.471
Control over compulsion							
Much control	1	4.8	1	2.6	2	3.3	
Moderate control	5	23.8	8	20.5	13	21.7	
Little control	13	61.9	20	51.3	33	55.0	
No control	2	9.5	10	25.6	12	20.0	
Mean ± SD score	2.76 ± 0.7		3.00 ± 0.8		2.92 ± 0.7		0.240
Total obsession score	13.19 ± 2.8		14.54 ± 3.4		14.07 ± 3.2		0.121

p value reached from unpaired Student's t-test.

and drug related disorders and eating disorder, which can be explained by Bangladeshi sociocultural background [19, 20]. Comorbidity pattern also showed two specific patterns for children and adolescent groups. The proportions of major depressive disorder (15.4%) followed by social phobia (12.8%), generalized anxiety disorder (5.1%), and conduct disorder (5.1%) were higher among the adolescents whereas specific phobia (28.6%), tic disorder (23.8%), hyperkinetic disorder (19%), mental retardation (4.8%), and autism spectrum disorder were higher among the children. This finding is somewhat consistent with other studies' findings [3, 5, 6, 13, 21].

5. Conclusion

Though generalization of the study finding may be difficult because of small sample size, single centre exposer, and

TABLE 4: Relationship between morbidity and selected sociodemographic characteristics.

Characteristics	Number	Morbidity: OCD only Number	OCD only %	Comorbidity Number	Comorbidity %	p value
Age in years						
<12	21	8	38.1	13	61.9	0.244
≥12	39	21	53.8	18	46.2	
Sex						
Male	43	24	55.8	19	44.2	0.065
Female	17	5	29.4	12	70.6	
Residence						
Urban	49	25	51.0	24	49.0	0.379
Rural	11	4	36.4	7	63.6	
Religion						
Muslim	54	25	46.3	29	53.7	0.344
Non-Muslim	6	4	66.7	2	33.3	
Level of education						
Primary	17	6	35.3	11	64.7	0.204
Secondary and above	43	23	53.5	20	46.5	
Father's level of education						
Below graduate	19	10	52.6	9	47.4	0.650
Graduate and above	41	19	46.3	22	53.7	
Monthly family income (Tk.)						
Up to US $280	31	15	48.4	16	51.6	0.993
> US $280	29	14	48.3	15	51.7	

p value reached from Chi square test.

tertiary care level coverage, it is the first study to explore the issue; and findings of the study will help our health professionals to address the symptom pattern of OCD, its severity, and comorbid conditions among child and adolescent patients in Bangladesh. It will increase the space and will help creating an information baseline to carry out further study in this field in future. Further, large-scale, multicentre study can be conducted to explore OCD symptoms with severity adequately and necessary policies can be formulated based on the study result.

Abbreviations

OCD: Obsessive-compulsive disorder
IRB: Institutional Review Board
BSMMU: Bangabandhu Sheikh Mujib Medical University
DAWBA: Development and Wellbeing Assessment
DCR: Diagnostic criteria for research
CY-BOCS: Children's Yale-Brown Obsessive-Compulsive Scale
SPSS: Statistical Package for Social Science.

Disclosure

This study was a self-funded study.

Competing Interests

The authors declare having no conflict of interests.

Authors' Contributions

MHR Chowdhury and MSI Mullick contributed the conception, design, and the acquisition of data. MHR Chowdhury, MSI Mullick, and SMY Arafat contributed the drafting and the critical revision of the manuscript. SMY Arafat contributed the final approval of the manuscript.

References

[1] B. J. Sadock, V. A. Sadock, and P. Ruiz, *Synopsis of Psychiatry*, 11th edition, 2015.

[2] P. Cowen, P. Harrison, and T. Burns, *Shorter Oxford Textbook of PSHIATRY*, Oxford University Press, 6th edition, 2012.

[3] C. Tanidir, H. Adaletli, H. Gunes et al., "Impact of gender, age at onset, and lifetime tic disorders on the clinical presentation and comorbidity pattern of obsessive-compulsive disorder in children and adolescents," *Journal of Child and Adolescent Psychopharmacology*, vol. 25, no. 5, pp. 425–431, 2015.

[4] G. Krebs and I. Heyman, "Obsessive-compulsive disorder in children and adolescents," *Archives of Disease in Childhood*, vol. 100, no. 5, pp. 495–499, 2015.

[5] E. H. Decloedt and D. J. Stein, "Current trends in drug treatment of obsessive-compulsive disorder," *Journal of Neuropsychiatric Disease and Treatment*, vol. 6, pp. 233–242, 2010.

[6] A. K. Langley, A. B. Lewin, R. L. Bergman, J. C. Lee, and J. Piacentini, "Correlates of comorbid anxiety and externalizing disorders in childhood obsessive compulsive disorder," *European Child & Adolescent Psychiatry*, vol. 19, no. 8, pp. 637–645, 2010.

[7] S. E. Swedo, J. L. Rapoport, H. Leonard, M. Lenane, and D. Cheslow, "Obsessive-compulsive disorder in children and adolescents. Clinical phenomenology of 70 consecutive cases," *Archives of General Psychiatry*, vol. 46, no. 4, pp. 335–341, 1989.

[8] I. Heyman, E. Fombonne, H. Simmons, T. Ford, H. Meltzer, and R. Goodman, "Prevalence of obsessive-compulsive disorder in the British nationwide survey of child mental health," *British Journal of Psychiatry*, vol. 179, pp. 324–329, 2001.

[9] A. H. Zohar, "The epidemiology of obsessive-compulsive disorder in children and adolescents," *Child and Adolescent Psychiatric Clinics of North America*, vol. 8, no. 3, pp. 445–460, 1999.

[10] M. S. I. Mullick and R. Goodman, "The prevalence of psychiatric disorders among 5–10 year olds in rural, urban and slum areas in Bangladesh," *Social Psychiatry and Psychiatric Epidemiology*, vol. 40, no. 8, pp. 663–671, 2005.

[11] World Health Organization, *The ICD-10 Classification of Mental and Behavioural Disorders: Diagnostic Criteria for Research*, World Health Organization, Geneva, Switzerland, 1993.

[12] D. McKay, J. Piacentini, S. Greisberg et al., "The Children's Yale-Brown obsessive-compulsive scale: item structure in an outpatient setting," *Psychological Assessment*, vol. 15, no. 4, pp. 578–581, 2003.

[13] A. B. Lewin, S. Chang, J. McCracken, M. McQueen, and J. Piacentini, "Comparison of clinical features among youth with tic disorders, obsessive-compulsive disorder (OCD), and both conditions," *Psychiatry Research*, vol. 178, no. 2, pp. 317–322, 2010.

[14] A. M. Albano, L. S. Knox, and D. H. Barlow, *Clinical Handbook of Anxiety Disorders in Children and Adolescents*, Jason Aranson, New Jersey, NJ, USA, 1995.

[15] J. D. Stein and E. Hollander, Eds., *Textbook of Anxiety Disorders*, American Psychiatric, Washington, DC, USA, 2002.

[16] M. Allsopp and C. Verduyn, "A follow-up of adolescents with obsessive-compulsive disorder," *British Journal of Psychiatry*, vol. 154, pp. 829–834, 1989.

[17] H. L. Leonard, S. E. Swedo, M. C. Lenane et al., "A 2- to 7-year follow-up study of 54 obsessive-compulsive children and adolescents," *Archives of General Psychiatry*, vol. 50, no. 6, pp. 429–439, 1993.

[18] C. Wewetzer, T. Jans, B. Müller et al., "Long-term outcome and prognosis of obsessive-compulsive disorder with onset in childhood or adolescence," *European Child and Adolescent Psychiatry*, vol. 10, no. 1, pp. 37–46, 2001.

[19] D. Semple, R. Smyth, J. Burns, R. Darjee, and A. Mcintosh, *Oxford Handbook of Psychiatry*, Oxford University Press, Oxford, UK, 1st edition, 2005.

[20] J. Toro, M. Cervera, E. Osejo, and M. Salamero, "Obsessive-compulsive disorder in childhood and adolescence: A Clinical Study," *Journal of Child Psychology and Psychiatry*, vol. 33, no. 6, pp. 1025–1037, 1992.

[21] B. Juliana and C. Maria, "Impact of age at onset and duration of illness on the expression of co-morbidities in OCD," *The Journal of Clinical Psychiatry*, vol. 65, no. 1, pp. 22–27, 2004.

27

Psychometric Validation of the Bangla Version of the Patient-Doctor Relationship Questionnaire

S. M. Yasir Arafat

Department of Public Health, ASA University Bangladesh, ASA Tower, 23/3 Bir Uttam ANM Nuruzzaman Sarak, Shyamoli, Dhaka 1207, Bangladesh

Correspondence should be addressed to S. M. Yasir Arafat; arafatdmc62@gmail.com

Academic Editor: Ulrich Schweiger

Background. The patient-doctor relationship is an important issue in health care as it is linked to patient satisfaction, treatment adherence, and treatment outcome. The PDRQ-9 is brief instrument which has an excellent overall internal consistency to measure it. *Objective.* It was aimed at developing a culturally adapted and validated Bangla version of Patient-Doctor Relationship Questionnaire (PDRQ-9). *Method.* Data were collected during the period of May 2015 to July 2015 from 50 patients by interviewing with the final Bangla version of PDRQ-9 obtained by ideal translation-back translation procedure with nonprobability purposive consecutive sampling and analyzed by Statistical Package of Social Science (SPSS) 16.0 and Microsoft Excel 2007 version software. *Result.* The internal consistency of Bangla PDRQ-9 was measured by Cronbach's α which was 0.97. Only one factor was extracted from varimax rotation factor analysis with high commonalities between the items. *Conclusion.* Bangla version of PDRQ-9 is valid, accepted, and widely applicable in clinical practice, research, public health, and primary health care in Bangladesh.

1. Introduction

The patient-doctor relationship (PDR) is an important concept in health care [1]. Throughout the history of medicine, patients and doctors have scrutinized and debated their relationship, which is undoubtedly one of the most difficult among interpersonal relations, for a variety of reasons [2]. It has been linked to patient satisfaction, treatment adherence, and treatment outcome. In primary care, "knowing the patient is at least as important as knowing the disease," and physicians with a warm and friendly style are more effective than physicians with a more formal style [3]. It was found that patients search out a Primary Care Practitioner (PCP) who matches their own representation of an ideal and validate their choice in a dynamic communicative process [4]. Patient satisfaction is a concept that reflects the patient's perception regarding the care quality and treatment received. Generally evaluated by self-report, several questionnaires focused on decision making, access, and use of the different health services or on the treatment satisfaction [5]. The measurement instruments of the patient-doctor relationship make it possible to quantify the patient's opinion regarding communication, satisfaction, and accessibility in the dealing with the doctor and the treatment followed [5]. Substantial efforts have been made to develop instruments and to assess the PDR from the patient's point of view. A systematic review found 19 instruments with a variety of dimensions and used diverse conceptual models for the PDR and recommended the use of the Patient-Doctor Relationship Questionnaire (PRDQ-9) as a brief (9 items) questionnaire with excellent overall internal consistency [1]. Bengali is one of the sixth most widely spoken languages in the world with nearly 300 million users. In 2050 estimated Bengali speaking population will be nearly 400 million [6]. At present there is no culturally adapted scale to measure the patient doctor relationship in Bangla. So, it was aimed at developing a culturally adapted and validated Bangla version of Patient-Doctor Relationship Questionnaire (PDRQ-9) for use in assessing the relationship between the physician and the patient as PDRQ-9 is brief short easily applicable tool.

2. Materials and Methods

2.1. Ethical Consideration. The researcher was duly concerned about the ethical issues relate to the study. Formal ethical clearance was taken from the ethical review committee of the ASA University Bangladesh for conducting the study and formal permission was taken from the questionnaire developing author, Christina M. Van der Feltz-Cornelis. Confidentiality of the person and the information was maintained and observed and unauthorized persons did not have any access to the data. Informed written consent was taken from the subject informing the nature and purpose of the study, the procedure of study, and the right to refuse, accept, and withdraw to participate in the study and the participants did not gain financial benefit from this study. The present study posed a very low risk to the participants, as procedures such as medical treatments, invasive diagnostics, or procedures causing psychological, spiritual, or social harm were not included.

2.2. Instrument Development. The adaptation to Bengali was performed according to the state-of-the-art procedure of forward-backward translation of English PDRQ-9 by 1 medical doctor and 1 psychologist; both of them are native speakers of the Bangla and are fluent in English. The 2 Bangla versions were compared, and an updated Bangla forward version was compiled. This version was translated back into English by a professional translator with experience in medical translation and by 1 medical doctor who had not been involved in the forward translation. The back-translated versions were then compiled and compared by the researcher. These versions were submitted to the University expert committee. Thus, an optimized Bangla version was generated and with that optimized Bangla version pretesting was done and supposed changes were made accordingly. Thus, the final Bangla version of PDRQ-9 was developed [7].

2.3. Design and Subjects. The current study was a part of Master of Public Health (M.P.H.) thesis under the department of Public Health, ASA University Bangladesh. The descriptive, cross-sectional study was conducted at Psychiatry Out-Patient Department (OPD) of Dhaka Medical College Hospital (DMCH) and data were collected during the period of May 2015 to July 2015 from 50 patients with the final Bangla version of PDRQ-9 with nonprobability purposive consecutive sampling. The interview was performed by the researcher himself through face-to-face interview technique. The participants who were above the age of 14 years, were willing to participate in the study, and can read Bangla were included in the study. Participants not willing to participate and who made first visit to the respective physicians were excluded. Sample size was estimated on basis of more than 5 : 1 ratio of participants to item as variable recommendations available considering rules of thumb regarding the minimum ratio of participants to variables 2 : 1 or extracted factors 20 : 1 [8]. The questionnaire encompasses nine statements and the respondents were requested to indicate the appropriateness of each statement as a description of how they feel about their doctor in different aspects. After managing data properly it was analyzed in SPSS 16 version and Microsoft Excel Software 2007 version.

3. Result

3.1. Demographic Characteristics of Respondents. In this PDRQ-9 Bangla validation study age, gender, educational status, occupation, religion, marital status, net family income, residence, family type, number of family members, and duration of follow-up were considered as demographic variables. Age of the respondents was found as mean ± SD (range): 35.6 ± 10.71 (14–66) years; 62% were male and 38% were female; 64% live in town, 16% in mini town, and 20% in village; 72% were married, 16% unmarried, 8% widow, and 4% divorced; 52% had nuclear family and 48% belonged to joint family environment.

Mean PDRQ-9 score of individual item ranged from 3.02 ± 1.11 to 3.30 ± 1.11. The highest score was 3.30 ± 1.11 for item-6 "Agreeness on the nature of symptoms." The lowest score was 3.02 ± 1.11 for item-9 "Accessibility" (Table 1).

3.2. Reliability of PDRQ-9 Bangla. Cronbach's Alpha (α) value was 0.97. (When interpreting Cronbach's Alpha (α), it ranges from 0 to 1. A value of $\geq$0.70 reflects good reliability.)

Interitem correlation matrix showed a value of significant correlation (Table 2). (When interpreting correlation, it ranges from 0 to 1. A value of $\geq$0.50 reflects the items are significantly correlated.)

3.3. Validity of Bangla Version of PDRQ-9. Face validity, content validity, and *criterion validity* was systematically assessed and maintained during the development of the research instrument and at the time of interview by the interview response. Construct validity was assessed, done by Exploratory Factor Analysis, the principal component with varimax rotation and internal consistency. KMO and Bartlett's test of sphericity was applied to the fitness of data for factor analysis and the KMO and Bartlett's Test of sampling adequacy was 0.9 where a value of $\geq$0.5 of KMO is considered as a good sampling adequacy.

3.4. Construct Validity. Construct validity was assessed by factor analysis. It showed high commonalities between the items before and after extraction ranging from 0.79 to 0.85. The varimax rotation showed only one component was extracted (Table 3).

4. Discussion

Psychometrics has a very important role in public health, psychiatry, primary health care, and many other fields even in health promotional strategy for measuring the attitude. Relationship between patient and physician has been discussed from the origin of medicine. PDRQ-9 was developed by Van Der Feltz-Cornelis et al. in 2004, a Patient-Doctor Relationship Questionnaire (PDRQ-9) in primary care based on Alexander and Luborsky developed the Helping Alliance

TABLE 1: Distribution of item characteristics of PDRQ-9 Bangla ($N = 50$).

Item number	PDRQ-9 item	Mean ± SD	Corrected item-total correlation
1	My physician helps me	3.06 ± 1.03	0.88
2	My physician has enough time for me	3.20 ± 1.17	0.89
3	I trust my physician	3.22 ± 1.09	0.87
4	My physician understands me	3.14 ± 1.22	0.88
5	My physician is dedicated to help me	3.10 ± 1.07	0.88
6	My physician and I agree on the nature of my medical symptoms	3.30 ± 1.11	0.86
7	I can talk to my physician	3.22 ± 1.18	0.92
8	I feel content with my physician's treatment	3.24 ± 1.22	0.87
9	I find my physician easily accessible	3.02 ± 1.11	0.90

TABLE 2: Interitem correlation of PDRQ-9 Bangla.

	Interitem correlation matrix							
q1								
q2	.79							
q3	.85	.77						
q4	.76	.82	.70					
q5	.89	.80	.88	.73				
q6	.72	.81	.70	.92	.69			
q7	.85	.87	.87	.80	.83	.80		
q8	.79	.77	.80	.86	.79	.83	.81	
q9	.82	.86	.79	.83	.81	.81	.86	.76

TABLE 3: Factor Analysis-Principal Component Analysis with distribution of varimax rotation of PDRQ-9 Bangla.

Rotated component matrix	
Items	Component 1
q1	.91
q2	.91
q3	.90
q4	.90
q5	.90
q6	.89
q7	.94
q8	.90
q9	.92

Questionnaire (HAQ), and Van der Linden validated Dutch version [4]. Spanish version was validated in 2009 by Adán et al., validation of the Turkish Patient-Doctor Relationship Questionnaire (PDRQ- Turkish) was done by Mergen et al. in 2012, and Zenger et al. validated the German version of PDRQ-9 in 2014 [1, 5, 9]. It was aimed at adapting the PDRQ-9 in Bangla.

Internal consistency of PDRQ-9 Bangla was found to be 0.97 (Cronbach's Alpha) which suggests significant reliability and aligns with PDRQ-9 German (0.95), PDRQ-9 Dutch (0.94), Spanish (0.92), and Turkish (0.91) validation study [1, 4, 5, 9]. The corrected item-total correlation was ≥0.87 (Table 2) which was highly significant and aligns with others as it was ≥0.94 in PDRQ-9 German validation study [1]. Factor analysis of PDRQ-9 Bangla was revealed as a single factor scale and the solution could not be rotated in the varimax rotation (Table 3) as PDRQ-9 German was unidimensional scale and PDRQ-9 Dutch, PDRQ Spanish were validated as single factor scale after removal of second factor with the help of the factor analysis without significant alteration of scale property, reliability, and validity ultimately [1, 4, 5].

5. Conclusion

The results from this evaluation indicate good psychometric properties of the PDRQ-9 Bangla. This Bangla validated scale will be helpful to assess the relationship between physician and patients in clinical practice, research, public health, and primary health care in Bangladesh. Though it is the first validated scale in Bangla for measuring the patient-doctor relationship and a very good scale to measure the relationship in a very short time in clinical practice, public heath, health research, and primary health care, with this minimum sample, generalization of the study result may be difficult. Data were collected from the patients visiting a hospital of a city, but those from hospitals or institutions of other regions and heterogeneous groups were not included. This instrument bears only the patients' direction of the relationship; doctors' direction was not to be evaluated. Larger studies involving more heterogeneous patients may help to provide a more complete picture of impact of patient-doctor relationship in Bangladesh.

Disclosure

This study was presented at 8th International Conference on Psychiatry (ICP-2015), Dhaka, 2015.

Conflict of Interests

The author has no conflict of interests to declare.

Authors' Contribution

The author has the sole contribution in every step of the study.

Acknowledgments

The author thanks Dr. Nasrin Sultana, the academic supervisor of the research, Professor Dr. MA Bari, Professor of Public Health, ASA University, Professor M. A. Hafez, Professor of Statistics (BUHS), and S. M. Hafiz Al Asad for helping in different parts of this research. The author thanks Professor Dr. Christina M. Van Der Feltz-Cornelis for permitting validating the scale.

References

[1] M. Zenger, R. Schaefert, C. van der Feltz-Cornelis, E. Brähler, and W. Häuser, "Validation of the patient-doctor-relationship questionnaire (PDRQ-9) in a representative cross-sectional German population survey," *PLoS ONE*, vol. 9, no. 3, Article ID e91964, 2014.

[2] M. Koutsosimou, K. Adamidis, A. Liakos, and V. Mavreas, "The development of an instrument for the assessment of doctor-patient relationship (dopraq-16)," *Journal of Psychology & Psychotherapy*, vol. 3, no. 3, article 118, 2013.

[3] R. M. Eveleigh, E. Muskens, H. Van Ravesteijn, I. Van Dijk, E. Van Rijswijk, and P. Lucassen, "An overview of 19 instruments assessing the doctor-patient relationship: different models or concepts are used," *Journal of Clinical Epidemiology*, vol. 65, no. 1, pp. 10–15, 2012.

[4] C. M. Van Der Feltz-Cornelis, P. Van Oppen, H. W. J. Van Marwijk, E. De Beurs, and R. Van Dyck, "A patient-doctor relationship questionnaire (PDRQ-9) in primary care: development and psychometric evaluation," *General Hospital Psychiatry*, vol. 26, no. 2, pp. 115–120, 2004.

[5] J. C. M. Adán, B. Moreno-Jiménez, R. R. Carvajal, M. G. Herrer, and P. R. López, "Psychometric validation of the spanish version of the patient-doctor relationship questionnaire (PDRQ)," *Actas Espanolas de Psiquiatria*, vol. 37, no. 2, pp. 94–100, 2009.

[6] S. R. Chowdhury, *Adaptation, Linguistic & Clinimetric Validation of the Bangla Version of the Brief Psychiatric Rating Scale (BPRS-18) for Bangladesh Index*, Bangabandhu Sheikh Mujib Medical University (BSMMU), Dhaka, Bangladesh, 2014.

[7] D. E. Beaton, C. Bombardier, F. Guillemin, and M. B. Ferraz, "Guidelines for the process of cross-cultural adaptation of self-report measures," *Spine*, vol. 25, no. 24, pp. 3186–3191, 2000.

[8] M. J. Ridd, G. Lewis, T. J. Peters, and C. Salisbury, "Patient-doctor depth-of-relationship scale: development and validation," *Annals of Family Medicine*, vol. 9, no. 6, pp. 538–545, 2011.

[9] H. Mergen, C. van der Feltz-Cornelis, N. Karoglu, B. E. Mergen, and K. Ongel, "Validity of the Turkish patient-doctor relationship questionnaire (PDRQ-Turkish) in comparison with the Europe instrument in a family medicine center," *HealthMED Journal*, vol. 6, pp. 1763–1770, 2012.

Dyslipidaemia and Medical Outcome (Health Related Quality of Life) in Patients with Schizophrenia Taking Antipsychotics in Enugu, Nigeria

Emmanuel Omamurhomu Olose,[1] John Edet,[2] Monday Nwite Igwe,[3] Donald Chidozie Chukwujekwu,[4] Miriam Chinyere Aguocha,[5] and Richard Uwakwe[6]

[1]*Department of Psychiatry, University of Calabar, Calabar, Nigeria*
[2]*Department of Clinical Services, Federal Neuropsychiatric Hospital, Calabar, Nigeria*
[3]*Department of Psychiatry, Ebonyi State University, Abakaliki, Nigeria*
[4]*Department of Psychiatry, University of Port Harcourt, Port Harcourt, Nigeria*
[5]*Department of Psychiatry, Imo State University, Orlu, Nigeria*
[6]*Department of Psychiatry, Nnamdi Azikiwe University, Awka, Nigeria*

Correspondence should be addressed to Emmanuel Omamurhomu Olose; oloseoe@yahoo.com

Academic Editor: Veit Roessner

Aim. Determine association between use (and type) of antipsychotics and dyslipidaemia in newly diagnosed schizophrenia patients attending Federal Neuropsychiatric Hospital, Enugu. *Methods.* From sixty antipsychotic naive patients with schizophrenia and sixty first-degree relatives matched for gender and age, fasting blood lipid profiles were measured at baseline and after twelve weeks. Medical Outcome Study Short Form General Health Survey was administered to patients on both occasions. Fasting lipid profile changes of both groups were compared. *Results.* Mean endpoint of total cholesterol (TC), low density lipoprotein (LD), and triglycerides (TG) in mmol/l for cases was significantly higher than initial values (TC 4.5 versus 4.3, $t = 4.3$, $p < 0.0001$), (LDL 2.8 versus 2.6, $t = 14.3$, $p < 0.0001$), and (TG 1.3 versus 1.0, $t = 12.1$, $p < 0.0001$). Mean endpoint of high density lipoprotein (HDL) in mmol/l for cases was significantly lower than initial values (1.1 versus 1.2, $t = 12.1$, $p < 0.0001$). Prevalence of dyslipidaemia for cases was 13%. Mean endpoint of TC, LDL, TG, and HDL in mmol/l for controls was not significantly different from initial values (TC 4.30 versus 4.27, $t = 1.09$, $p = 0.279$), (LDL 2.49 versus 2.46, $t = 1.28$, $p = 0.205$), (TG 0.96 versus 0.94, $t = 1.27$, $p = 0.207$), and (HDL 1.37 versus 1.38, $t = 1.61$, $p = 0.113$). Subjects on atypical antipsychotics had higher risk for dyslipidaemia. *Conclusion.* Use of antipsychotics was significantly associated with dyslipidaemia.

1. Introduction

Dyslipidaemia and lipid metabolism have attracted attention of researchers in recent times. For patients with mental disorders, the observation that the disease itself and its treatment may be associated with metabolic problems adds another layer of complexity. Abnormal lipid levels have been unequivocally associated with increased risk for cardiovascular events such as myocardial infarction and stroke in the general population [1]. They also contribute additional risk factors to patients with diabetes mellitus and coronary heart disease [2]. Patients with schizophrenia have a life expectancy 20% shorter than that of the general population [3]; approximately 2/3 of the excess mortality is due to comorbid medical illness [4]. The rate of cardiovascular mortality in patients with schizophrenia is twice that seen in the general population. Antipsychotic treatment is associated with various degrees of weight gain and dyslipidaemia [5], which may possibly contribute to excess mortality in patients with schizophrenia.

Dyslipidaemia was defined as an abnormality of any of the lipid profile components, that is, elevated total cholesterol

(TC) $\geq$ 5.2 mmol/l, low density lipoprotein cholesterol $\leq$ 3.4 mmol/l, triglycerides (TG) $\geq$ 1.7 mmol/l, and high density lipoprotein (HDL) < 1.04 mmol/l.

Patients with schizophrenia are at an increased risk of dyslipidaemia in part due to poor diet and sedentary life style [6], antipsychotic treatment is also associated with various degrees of dyslipidaemia. Elevated blood lipids particularly triglycerides are associated with some typical antipsychotics, shortly after their introduction phenothiazines were found to elevate serum triglycerides and total cholesterol levels [7]. Clozapine and olanzapine have been shown to cause significant hypertriglyceridaemia compared with typical antipsychotics. The atypicals vary in their propensity to cause weight gain; the difference in weight gain associated with these agents reflects their order of risk for insulin resistance and dyslipidaemia [8].

Given that the majority of patients with schizophrenia face chronic, even life-long treatment with APDs, the risks of metabolic symptom such as dyslipidaemia are major considerations for individuals on APD maintenance treatment.

In Nigeria studies on antipsychotic associated dyslipidaemia are scanty and the few studies are mainly cross sectional. There is a need for more longitudinal prospective studies. The present study was designed to determine the prevalence of dyslipidaemia as well as association between the use of antipsychotic drugs and dyslipidaemia in newly diagnosed patients with schizophrenia.

2. Aims and Objectives

The general aim of the study was to determine the relationship between the use of antipsychotic drugs and dyslipidaemia in newly diagnosed patients with schizophrenia attending the Federal Neuropsychiatric Hospital, Enugu.

The specific objectives of the study were the following:

(1) To determine the association between use (and type) of antipsychotic and dyslipidaemia in newly diagnosed patients with schizophrenia attending the Federal Neuropsychiatric Hospital, Enugu.

(2) To compare the patients' fasting lipid profile with those of first-degree relations not using antipsychotic medication.

(3) To determine the prevalence of dyslipidaemia in patients with schizophrenia using antipsychotic medications.

(4) To determine the medical outcome (health related quality of life both mental and physical) in patients with schizophrenia attending the Federal Neuropsychiatric Hospital, Enugu.

3. Methodology

3.1. Setting of the Study. This was a prospective study carried out at the Federal Neuropsychiatric Hospital, Enugu. The Federal Neuropsychiatric Hospital, Enugu, is the only Federal government owned psychiatric hospital in the south east geopolitical zone of Nigeria. The hospital also receives patients from Delta, Rivers, Kogi, and Benue states. On the average the hospital attends to about one thousand five hundred patients monthly out of whom about 320 are new patients.

3.2. Ethical Issues. All patients and their next of kin gave signed informed consent to participate in the study which commenced after approval was obtained from the ethics committee of the Federal Neuropsychiatric Hospital, Enugu. Ethical clearance was obtained on the 19th day of December 2013. Refusal of a patient to participate or continue in the study at any point did not affect the quality of care received from the hospital. Those found to have lipid profiles of clinical significance were discussed with the consultants/doctors in charge with a view to having the patients referred for further assessment and management. The researchers bore the cost for payment of lipid profiles analysis.

3.3. Sample Size. A minimum required sample size was calculated using the computer software (Java Stat) for comparative control study. This gave a minimum sample size of 57 for each group of participants to be studied. For the purpose of this study the sample size was inflated by 20% for each group to make more robust the findings that would be generated. Thus a total of 136 participants were recruited for the study consisting of 68 patients with schizophrenia and 68 first-degree relations (controls) to eliminate genetics as a confounding factor.

3.4. Eligibility Criteria

3.4.1. Inclusion Criteria [Patients]

(1) Participants meeting ICD-10 diagnostic criteria for schizophrenia attending hospital for the first time.

(2) Participants who are antipsychotic naive.

(3) Age, $\geq$ 18 years.

(4) Must have a first-degree relation ready to take part in the project.

(5) Must give informed consent.

3.4.2. Inclusion Criteria [Controls]

(1) First-degree relations [siblings] matched for gender and age $\pm$5 years.

(2) Age $\geq$ 18 years.

(3) Must give informed consent.

3.4.3. Exclusion Criteria [Patients and Controls]

(1) Medical conditions related to dyslipidemia (e.g., obesity, i.e., body mass index [BMI] greater than 30 at entry point, diabetes mellitus) as well as abnormal lipid profile at the point of entry.

(2) Taking medications related to dyslipidemia (e.g., oral contraceptives, thiazides, and steroids).

(3) Those who refuse to give consent.

3.5. Instruments

3.5.1. Sociodemographic Interview Schedule. This was designed by the author to obtain basic information about the participant's health and biodata. General medical diagnosis, medication in use including duration of use as well as any illness common in the family was documented. The antipsychotics as well as the dosages prescribed were noted.

3.5.2. M-CIDI (Munich Version of the Composite International Diagnostic Interview). M-CIDI was produced for the World Health Organization (WHO) and the United States (US) Alcohol Drug Abuse and Mental Health Administration by the US National Institute of Mental Health. It is used for the assessment of mental disorders and to provide diagnoses according to ICD10 and DSM IV. The CIDI package comes in modules. In this study only the schizophrenia module was used. The M-CIDI has been used previously in this environment by Olose et al. [9].

3.5.3. Medical Outcome Study Short Form General Health Survey (SF-12). SF-12 was developed by Stewart et al. [10]. The SF-12 Health Survey is a 12-item subset of the SF-36 that measures the same eight domains of health. It is a brief, reliable measure of overall health status of the respondent. The instrument can either be self-administered or given by a trained interviewer in person or by telephone to persons aged 14 and older. It takes about 2 to 3 minutes to complete. The categories/domains of health which the instrument measures are: Physical functioning, Role physical, Bodily pain, General health, Vitality, Social functioning, Role-emotional and mental health. These domains are scaled on 2 and 5-point Likert scale. The SF-12 Health Survey is published in both standard (4-week) and acute (1-week) recall versions for self-administration as well as scripts for personal interviews. The SF-12 physical and mental health summary measures are referred to as PCS-12 and MCS-12, respectively. The standard 4-week recall period was adapted for the SF36 and SF-12 to maintain comparability with the long -form Medical outcome Study (MOS) measures from which it was derived. The test-retest reliability of the PCS-12 summary measures was 0.890 in the US and 0.864 in the UK. Coefficients of 0.760 in US and 0.774 in UK were observed for the MCS-12. Fourteen validity tests involving physical criteria ranged from 0.43 to 0.93 (median = 0.6 7).

The literature has shown that concurrent validity for both the short form 12 and the short form 20 is the same in psychometric properties. The SF-20 has been validated in Nigeria [11]. In the present study the SF-12 was used to determine the overall health related status/outcome of patients.

3.5.4. Method of Lipid Profile Estimation. The method of Trinder [12] was used for the estimation of total cholesterol.

Triglyceride values were estimated by the method of Barham and Trinder [13]. LDL cholesterol was calculated by the Friedewald equation [14]: LDL = TC − TG/2.2 − HD.

3.5.5. Participant Selection and Sampling Technique

Patients. All patients with schizophrenia coming to the emergency clinic were first of all identified. Those coming for the first time were then specifically identified to determine their eligibility for inclusion. Participants that met the inclusion criteria were then traced with the assistance of medical record staff to the various service points of the hospital that is the emergency ward, inpatient ward and the outpatient department. Consecutive attendees with schizophrenia presenting for the first time were approached for recruitment.

Controls. For all the selected participants, efforts were made to get a first-degree biological relative, to eliminate genetics as a confounding factor after matching for gender and age (±5 years).

3.6. Procedure. Data collection took place from December 2013 to June 2014. The first step was to identify patients diagnosed as having schizophrenia by the doctor on duty at the emergency room.

When the participants (patients) had been identified and selected explanation of the study and how he/she was selected were proffered. Informed consent was then obtained; this was followed by administration of M-CIDI to confirm the diagnosis of schizophrenia in the patients. After patients were identified, a first-degree relative (matched for gender and age ±5 years) for whom no diagnosis of schizophrenia had been made from history and who took no antipsychotic agent was identified if they met the inclusion criteria. Sociodemographic data of age, educational status, occupation, and family history of cardiovascular disease or diabetes mellitus was then obtained. The Medical Outcome Study Short Form General Health Survey (SF-12) was also administered to all the patients. A single venous blood sample was obtained for fasting lipid profile analysis. All blood samples were processed by the same Federal Neuropsychiatric Hospital laboratory Scientist. The same procedure was carried out for the controls. At the end of 12 weeks, all the outcome measures were repeated for the patients and the control groups. At the second assessment one hundred and twenty subjects remained in the study that is sixty cases and sixty controls. Sixteen subjects dropped out of the study. Patients were categorized according to the antipsychotics (typical or atypical) that they used in the previous 12 weeks before the second assessment. As a naturalistic study the attending doctor determined the prescription of antipsychotics. Any drugs used in the preceding twelve weeks were recorded.

3.7. Statistical Analysis. Data was analyzed using the personal computer version of the Statistical Package for the Social Sciences (SPSS- PC version 20). The subjects were classified according to their lipid profile status, use of antipsychotics, and sociodemographic variables. All the antipsychotics used by the index cases were converted to their CPZ equivalent doses. Noncontinuous variables were compared using Chi-square test while the *t*-test was used for continuous variables such as age and lipid levels.

Table 1: Sociodemographic profile.

Variable	Frequency Study $N = 60$ (%)	Control $N = 60$ (%)	Statistic	p value
Gender				
Male	27 (45)	27 (45%)	$x^2 = 0.00$	1.0
Female	33 (55)	33 (55%)		
Age group				
18–22	16 (26.7)	12 (19.9)		
23–27	19 (31.6)	23 (38.4)		
28–32	16 (26.7)	16 (26.7)	$t = 0.063$	0.950
33–37	6 (10)	6 (10.0)		
38–42	3 (5)	3 (5)		
Mean age	27.00 (5.38)	27.03 (5.80)		
Marital status				
Single	50 (83.3)	39 (65)	$x^2 = 5.263$	0.0218
Married	10 (16.7)	21 (35)		
Education				
Yes	59 (98.3)	60 (100)	$x^2 = 1.008$	0.3153
No	1 (1.7)	0		
Occupation				
Employed	8 (13.3)	32 (53.3)		
Unemployed	37 (61.7)	12 (20.0)	$x^2 = 27.19$	0.0001
Student	15 (25.0)	16 (26.7)		

For the individual antipsychotics the mean baseline fasting blood lipids values were compared with the respective mean endpoint values by using t-test. All tests were two-tailed with significance level set at 0.05%.

4. Results

4.1. Sociodemographic Profile of Study (Patients) and Controls. See Table 1.

4.1.1. Antipsychotic Usage and Dosage. The cases were prescribed either typical or atypical antipsychotic drugs. Among the cases who used typical antipsychotic drugs, 39 (83%) were prescribed haloperidol, 5 (10.6%) were prescribed chlorpromazine while only 3 (6.4%) cases took trifluoperazine.

Among the 13 (21.6%) cases placed on atypical antipsychotics 9 (69%) were prescribed olanzapine and 4 (31%) took risperidone.

The mean dosage per day in milligram for cases using typical antipsychotics was 340 mg/day for those prescribed chlorpromazine and 18.46 mg/day for those prescribed haloperidol while those on trifluoperazine were prescribed 16.67 mg/day. The mean chlorpromazine equivalent dosage was 615.33 and 333.40 for those on haloperidol and trifluoperazine, respectively.

For cases prescribed atypical antipsychotics the mean daily dosage was 18.33 mg/day with a range of 15 to 20 mg for cases placed on olanzapine, six cases took 20 mg olanzapine daily while three took 15 mg of olanzapine daily. While those on risperidone received a mean daily dosage of 3.75 mg/day with a range of 3 to 4 mg, 3 cases received 4 mg/day and one received 3 mg/day. The chlorpromazine equivalent dosage for patients on olanzapine and risperidone was 366.6 and 375, respectively.

4.1.2. Association between the Use of Antipsychotics and Dyslipidaemia. The mean endpoint of total cholesterol (TC) for cases was significantly higher than the baseline (4.50 mmol/l versus 4.34 mmol/l, = 4.317, $p < 0.001$).

The mean endpoint of total cholesterol (TC) for controls was not significantly different from baseline (4.27 mmol/l versus 4.30 mmol/l, = 1.093, $p = 0.279$).

The mean endpoint of triglyceride (TG) for cases was significantly higher than the baseline (1.28 mmol/l versus 1.05 mmol/l, = 4.371, $p < 0.0001$).

The mean endpoint of TG for controls was not significantly different from baseline (0.96 mmol/l versus 0.94, = 1.276, $p = 0.207$).

The mean endpoint of high density lipoproteins (HDL) for cases was significantly lower than baseline (1.11 versus 1.23, = 12.164, $p < 0.0001$).

The mean endpoint of HDL for controls was not significantly different from baseline (1.37 versus 1.38, = 1.61, $p =$ 0.113).

The mean endpoint of low density lipoprotein (LDL) for cases was significantly higher than baseline (2.78 versus 2.64, = 4.000, $p < 0.0001$).

TABLE 2: Individual antipsychotics and change in lipid profile.

Variable	Mean baseline (SD)	Mean end point (SD)	Mean change	t-test	df	p
Haloperidol						
TC (mmol/L)	4.35 (.42)	4.44 (.43)	0.09	2.172	39	0.036
TG (mmol/L)	1.07 (.25)	1.25 (.30)	0.18	13.314	39	0.0001
HDL (mmol/L)	1.23 (.12)	1.15 (.12)	0.08	15.632	39	0.0001
LDL (mmol/L)	2.63 (.37)	2.72 (.39)	0.09	2.182	39	0.035
Chlorpromazine						
TC (mmol/L)	4.30 (.45)	4.35 (.65)	0.05	0.405	4	0.706
TG (mmol/L)	1.11 (.26)	1.45 (.05)	0.34	4.687	4	0.009
HDL (mmol/L)	1.34 (.16)	1.04 (.00)	0.30	7.511	4	0.002
LDL (mmol/L)	2.43 (.37)	2.57 (.56)	0.14	1.057	4	0.350
Trifluoperazine						
TC (mmol/L)	4.14 (.67)	4.12 (.58)	0.02	.300	2	0.792
TG (mmol/L)	1.02 (.31)	1.25 (.39)	0.23	5.111	2	0.036
HDL (mmol/L)	1.20 (.05)	1.07 (.04)	0.13	4.298	2	0.650
LDL (mmol/L)	2.46 (.49)	2.46 (.04)	0.00	0.000	2	1.000
Olanzapine						
TC (mmol/L)	4.45 (.26)	5.01 (.26)	0.56	18.068	8	0.001
TG (mmol/L)	1.00 (.15)	1.40 (.19)	0.40	18.711	8	0.001
HDL (mmol/L)	1.22 (.04)	1.04 (.04)	0.18	17.097	8	0.001
LDL (mmol/L)	2.83 (.23)	3.23 (.39)	0.40	4.724	8	0.001
Risperidone						
TC (mmol/L)	4.29 (.39)	4.49 (.40)	0.20	11.286	3	0.001
TG (mmol/L)	.99 (.17)	1.14 (.22)	0.15	4.469	3	0.021
HDL (mmol/L)	1.16 (.05)	1.08 (.05)	0.08	0.200	3	0.008
LDL (mmol/L)	2.74 (.39)	2.87 (.30)	0.13	2.532	2	0.085

TC = total cholesterol, TG = triglycerides, HDL = high density lipoprotein, LDL = low density lipoproteins, change = change in lipid profile (mmol/L).

The mean endpoint of LDL for controls was not significantly different from baseline (2.49 mmol/l versus 2.46 mmol/l, = 1.280, $p = 0.205$).

Eight (13.3%) of the cases ($n = 60$) developed dyslipidaemia whereas the lipid profiles of the controls remained within normal limits.

4.1.3. Association between the Class or Type of Antipsychotic and Dyslipidaemia. Among the thirteen (21.66%) cases that received atypical antipsychotics, 3 (23.08%) developed dyslipidaemia. From the 47 (78.34%) that received typical antipsychotics 5 (10.64%) developed dyslipidaemia ($x^2 = 1$, p value = 0.356).

The relative risk (risk ratio) for the development of dyslipidaemia in atypical versus typical antipsychotics was 1.16 (95% CI = 0.85–1.60) There was an increased risk of dyslipidaemia with atypical antipsychotics compared to typical antipsychotic therapy OR = 2.52, 95% CI = 0.51 to 12.35.

4.1.4. Individual Antipsychotics and Change in Lipid Profile. Among the cases that received typical antipsychotics 2 (40%) on chlorpromazine ($n = 5$) developed dyslipidaemia. Chlorpromazine's main effect was on the triglyceride fraction which was markedly raised (mean change = 0.34 mmol/l) and the HDL fraction which was markedly lowered (mean change = 0.30 mmol/l). The mean change in TC and LDL was an increase of 0.05 mmol/l and 0.14 mmol/l, respectively (Table 2).

Three (7.69%) cases on haloperidol ($n = 39$) developed dyslipidaemia. The mean increase for TC, TG, and LDL was 0.09 mmol/l, 0.18 mmol/l, and 0.09 mmol/l, respectively; the mean decrease for HDL was 0.08 mmol/l.

None of the cases on trifluoperazine ($n = 3$) developed dyslipidaemia. There was no mean change in the LDL fraction. The mean increase for TC and TG was 0.02 mmol/l and 0.23 mmol/l, respectively. The mean decrease in HDL was 0.13 mmol/l (Table 2). Among the patients on atypical antipsychotics olanzapine caused the most significant increase in serum TC, LDL, and TG (0.56 mmol/l, 0.40 mmol/l, and 0.40 mmol/l, resp.) and decrease in HDL (0.18 mmol/l) (Table 2).

Three (33.33%) patients on olanzapine ($n = 9$) developed dyslipidaemia. None of the patients on risperidone ($n = 4$) developed dyslipidaemia, and they had a mean increase in serum TC, LDL, and TG of 0.16 mmol/l, 0.14 mmol/l, and 0.23 mmol/l, respectively. The mean decrease in HDL was 0.12 mmol/l (Table 2).

4.1.5. Short Form 12 Medical Outcome of Patients. The Short Form 12 PCS baseline mean value for patients was 52.84 (SD = 5.54) with a range of 31.70 to 59.20. The endpoint PCS12 mean value was 52.07 (SD = 5.39) with a range of 34.20 to

58.0. There was no significant difference between the mean baseline and endpoint PCS of cases (t = .858 p = 0.394). The mean baseline short form 12 MCS components for cases was 34.60 (SD = 9.753) with a range of 13 to 55. The mean endpoint short form 12 MCS component was 51.50 SD = 4.70 with a range of 37.30 to 58.50. There was a significant difference between the mean baseline and endpoint MCS (t = 168, df = 59, p = 0.0001).

For patients placed on typical antipsychotics, the mean baseline SF 12 PCS component was 52.67 (SD = 6.02) with a range of 31.70 to 59.20. The mean endpoint PCS component was 51.58 (SD = 5.50) with a range of 34.20 to 58.0. There was no significant difference between the baseline and endpoint PCS scores (t = 0.768, p = 0.446). For typical antipsychotics, the mean baseline short form 12 MCS component was 34.72 (SD = 10.59) with a range of 34.20 to 58. The endpoint mean SF 12 MCS was 51.55 (SD = 4.73) with a range of 37.30 to 58.10. Endpoint MCS score was significantly higher than baseline (t = 12.942, df = 46, p value < 0.0001).

For patients placed on atypical antipsychotics the mean baseline SF-12 PCS component was 53.43 SD = 3.40, range 47.20 to 59.20. The mean endpoint PCS component was 53.0 SD = 4.61 range 42.60 to 57.90. There was no significant difference between baseline and endpoint PCS scores (t = 0.508, p = 0.621). The mean baseline MCS was 34.18 SD = 6.20 with a range of 26.80 to 44.70. The mean endpoint MCS was 51.32 SD = 4.96 with a range of 41.20 to 58.50. Endpoint MCS score was significantly higher compared to baseline (t = 7.892, p < 0.0001).

5. Discussion

5.1. Association between the Use of Antipsychotics and Dyslipidaemia. The present study found significant changes in lipid profile (an increase in TC, TG, LDL and decrease in HDL levels) at the end of 12 weeks among cases but no significant change among the controls. This finding is similar to that of an American study by Wirshing et al. [15] which compared the effects of atypical antipsychotics clozapine, risperidone, quetiapine, and olanzapine and typical antipsychotics haloperidol and fluphenazine on glucose and lipid profile. Two hundred and fifteen patients were reviewed from two and half years before and after initiation of antipsychotic treatment. Covariates including patients other medications were controlled for in the analysis. All the groups had significant increases in lipid profiles.

The findings in the present study are also similar to the findings in the Iranian study carried out at the cardiovascular research Centre Isfahan University of Medical Sciences by Hamidreeza et al. [16]. The objective of the Iranian study was to compare the effects of atypical and typical antipsychotics on lipid profiles. One hundred and twenty-eight patients with schizophrenia were enrolled in the study and were divided into two groups. There was no significant difference in age, gender, duration of illness, period of drug consumption and age at onset of illness in the two groups. It was found that the level of lipid profile increased in both typical and atypical users.

The findings in the present study are similar to that of a Nigerian study [17] which compared the effects of clozapine and risperidone on lipid profiles. At the end of six weeks there was a significant increase in serum TC, LDL, TG and a significant decrease in HDL in both treatment groups compared to controls.

Meyer and Koro [18] reviewed the literature since 1970 documenting the effects of antipsychotic agents on serum lipids; both typical and atypical antipsychotics were associated with lipid dysregulation. This finding is in line with the present study.

However, Smith et al. [19] conducted a comparative study of atypical antipsychotics including clozapine, risperidone, and olanzapine and typical antipsychotics and reported that most mean fasting lipid levels were within normal range and were not significantly different across the four treatment groups.

This difference in results obtained in the Smith study compared to the present study may be accounted for by the fact that in the present study only antipsychotics naive patients were enrolled, whereas in the study by Smith et al., patients with chronic schizophrenia who have been on long term therapy with antipsychotics were recruited. It has been shown that patients with schizophrenia treated for years with antipsychotic medication may develop tolerance to the effects of antipsychotics on lipid levels, so measurements of postprandial levels in addition to fasting levels may be helpful in identifying metabolic effects among such patients [17].

In the present study, 8 (13%) cases developed an abnormal lipid profile. This level is much higher than that obtained by Meyer and Koro [18] which was 7%. This difference may be accounted for by the fact that, in the Meyer and Koro study cases of dyslipidaemia were mainly defined as those who had received treatment for dyslipidaemia which may have omitted those with dyslipidaemia that did not receive treatment. In addition the study was also retrospective in nature. It has been shown that retrospective studies lack accuracy when compared to prospective studies [20].

In a study by Meyer and Koro [18], a prevalence of dyslipidemia of 23% was reported. The higher prevalence of dyslipidaemia compared to the present study may be explained by the fact that in that study mainly atypical antipsychotics were used whereas in the present study only 18% of the cases were placed on atypicals and the majority of the patients were on haloperidol. Meyer and Koro [18] in a review of the literature from 1970 to 2004 found that high potency conventional antipsychotics (e.g., haloperidol) appear to be associated with lower risk of dyslipidaemia compared to atypicals such as clozapine and olanzapine.

In a study by Lawani et al. [21] on the prevalence of metabolic syndrome in schizophrenic patients on antipsychotics in a Nigerian hospital a prevalence of 56% dyslipidaemia was obtained. The high level of dyslipidaemia seen in that study compared to the present study may be due to the duration of treatment which was 1–39 years with a mean duration of 6.09 years. The duration of use of antipsychotics is a determinant for the development of lipid abnormalities among patients with schizophrenia [18]. Also in the present study patients were screened for dyslipidaemia and some of its associated risk factors; patients with dyslipidaemia were omitted at baseline, whereas the Lawani et al. study was a cross sectional study without screening for metabolic risk factors.

The exclusion of patients with dyslipidaemia and obesity at baseline (onset of study) ensures that any dyslipidaemia noticed at the end of the study period is a likely reflection of the effect of the prescribed antipsychotic medication on the patients lipid profile. Although not sufficient to establish causality, this eliminates the likelihood for the occurrence of a type II error in this study. This is one of the strengths of this study unlike the situation in the study by Lawani et al. [21] mentioned above.

Different studies give different prevalence levels of dyslipidaemia and this probably may be accounted for by the different definitions of dyslipidemia in the studies as well as differences in ethnicity, sample size, drug used in the various studies, and duration of follow-up.

5.2. Association between the Class of or Type of Antipsychotic and Dyslipidemia. Although, in the present study, a greater percentage of cases receiving atypical antipsychotics (23.07%) developed dyslipidemia in comparison to 10.64% of those receiving typical antipsychotics, the association is not statistically significant. It seems that the effect of antipsychotics on lipid profiles depends on the individual antipsychotics and is not a class effect. The lack of class effect is highly consistent with the Joint Consensus Statement [22] issued by the American Diabetes Association, the American Psychiatric Association, the American Association of Clinical Endocrinologists and the North American Association for the study of obesity. This consensus statement issued in 2004 classified clozapine and olanzapine as being associated with an increased risk of worsening lipid profiles, whereas aripiprazole and ziprasidone were not associated with an increased risk for detrimental serum lipid changes. The statement noted that there were conflicting data about the effects of quetiapine and risperidone on lipids.

Furthermore, Lidenmeyer et al. [23] found significant increases in mean total cholesterol after treatment with olanzapine and clozapine but there was no elevation with haloperidol or risperidone, thus even though risperidone is an atypical antipsychotic it showed minimal effects on cholesterol levels.

In the present study, lipid profile increased in both typical and atypical antipsychotic users. This result is similar to a previous Iranian study by Hamidreeza et al. [16] which showed an increase in lipid profile in both the typical and atypical drug users. In that study the typical group had significantly higher mean TC and LDL levels than the atypical group, which could probably be explained by the fact that in the typical group 81.3% of the patients used phenothiazines, whereas in the present study in the typical group majority (82%) used haloperidol. Butyrophenones (Haloperidol) are associated with less chances of significant increase in visceral obesity which may be an important factor for development of insulin resistance and the metabolic syndrome [23]. These two conditions are associated with dyslipidemia which may probably explain the difference in study outcome of the Hamidreeza et al. study showing higher lipid profile levels in the typical antipsychotic group.

Among the atypical antipsychotics, olanzapine had a greater effect on lipid levels in the present study. The effects of olanzapine and risperidone exposure were evaluated in a large health care data base (the UK General Practice Research Database) [UK GPRD] [17]. Olanzapine was associated with a 3 fold risk in the odds of developing hyperlipidaemia compared with typical antipsychotics. Risperidone was not associated with increased odds of developing hyperlipidaemia compared with no antipsychotic or typical antipsychotic exposure. The UK GPRD result is consistent with the present study. In the present study the elevation of triglyceride was 14% with risperidone; other researchers have reported levels of 20% [24].

Meyer and Koro [18] in a retrospective study demonstrated that risperidone did not have any significant effect on serum cholesterol but caused concurrent increases in triglyceride levels. Meyer and Koro study also demonstrated a significant increase in levels of both triglycerides and cholesterol in olanzapine treated patients. These findings are in line with the present study.

Several other studies have confirmed the significant effect of olanzapine on the rise in serum lipids that is triglycerides [25], total cholesterol [25], LDL cholesterol [26], and HDL decline [27]. These are similar to the findings in the present study.

Among the typical antipsychotics used in the present study, chlorpromazine produced the greatest change in lipid profiles. There was a significant rise in total cholesterol and triglycerides as well as a significant reduction of HDL which has been demonstrated in previous studies [28, 29].

In the present study, haloperidol had the least effect on lipid profiles which is in line with the study by Krakowski et al. [30] that showed minimal change in all metabolic parameters with haloperidol after 3 months of treatment.

5.3. Medical Outcome Survey 12-Item Short Form Health Survey (SF-12) for Patients. The SF-12 scores have been normalised to yield a mean of 50 and a standard deviation of ten in the United States with higher scores indicating better functioning.

The physical component summary (PCS) baseline mean value of 52.84 (SD 5.54) did not differ significantly from the endpoint value 52.07 (SD 5.39). Thus, the effect of antipsychotics did not significantly affect the PCS component, though a few patients scored less after 12 weeks of medication probably due to side effects of medication whereas some improved.

The baseline mean (mental component summary) MCS component for patients (34.60 SD 9.75) differed significantly from the mean endpoint MCS component which was 51.50 (SD 4.54). Thus the endpoint MCS component for patients was significantly higher than baseline probably reflecting the effect of antipsychotics on symptom improvement leading to an improvement in the patient's health related quality of life.

The mean endpoint PCS for typical antipsychotic was 51.58; for atypical it was 52.8. The mean endpoint MCS for typical was 51.87, for atypical it was 51.42. Thus, it can be seen that the use of antipsychotics was associated with an improvement in the health related quality of life as measured by SF-12; it improved equally in those on both typical and atypical antipsychotics.

Patient's health related quality of life (HRQOL) may be affected directly by the treatments used to manage them. While antipsychotic medications have a positive effect due to symptom improvement, the side effect of antipsychotics such as weight gain and obesity would be expected to negatively affect functional status and overall quality of life. The deleterious side effects of antipsychotic medications, such as obesity negatively affecting functional status were not seen in this study probably because of the short duration. The final SF 12 values in the present study were much higher than in a study by George et al. [31]. The study by George et al. evaluated the health related quality of life (HRQOL) among patients treated with lurasidone. Stable but symptomatic out patients were switched from their current antipsychotics in a six week open label trial. Mental and physical component summary scores (MCS and PCS) were assessed using SF-12. Change in HRQOL from baseline to endpoint were compared using ANCOVA. Improvements in SF-12 MCS scores were observed (in the study by George et al.) for all patients and those switched from quetiapine or aripiprazole and the SF-12 PCS scores remained comparable to baseline in all patient groups. The higher SF 12 seen in the present study compared to the George et al. study may be due to the fact that George et al. used patients with a mean age of forty three who had been ill for some time and had probably developed negative symptoms. Additionally, the present study result may possibly reflect better prognosis of schizophrenia in developing countries [32].

Additional Points

Limitations. (1) The duration of follow-up was short. (2) This study did not control for important confounding factors such as diet, smoking, alcohol consumption, and levels of physical activity; therefore one cannot draw direct causal inferences. (3) This is a hospital based study and findings may not be generalized to the general population. In spite of these limitations, the findings from this study can serve as an important reference point for future epidemiological studies. *Strengths.* (1) Use of drug naive patients as prior use of antipsychotics may mask metabolic effects. (2) It used biological relations as comparison to eliminate genetics as a confounding factor. (3) It has the prospective longitudinal design. (4) This is a naturalistic study so the use and dosages of antipsychotics were determined by the attending doctors.

Disclosure

This study is funded entirely by the authors alone.

Competing Interests

The authors declare that there is no conflict of interests regarding the publication of this paper.

Authors' Contributions

Emmanuel Omamurhomu Olose, John Edet, Donald Chidozie Chukwujekwu, Monday Nwite Igwe, and Miriam Chinyere Aguocha designed the study while Emmanuel Omamurhomu Olose wrote the protocol for the study. Emmanuel Omamurhomu Olose, John Edet, Monday Nwite Igwe, Donald Chidozie Chukwujekwu, and Richard Uwakwe did the literature search and Miriam Chinyere Aguocha did the data analysis. Emmanuel Omamurhomu Olose wrote the initial draft of the study, Donald Chidozie Chukwujekwu drew the tables, and all the authors read and made corrections for the final draft of this manuscript.

References

[1] W. B. Kannel, W. P. Castelli, T. Gordon, and P. M. McNamara, "Serum cholesterol, lipoproteins, and the risk of coronary heart disease: The Framingham Study," *Annals of Internal Medicine*, vol. 74, no. 1, pp. 1–12, 1971.

[2] O. O. Ogunkeye and I. S. Ighogboja, "Increase in total serum triglyceride and phospholipid in kwashiorkor," *Annals of Tropical Paediatrics*, vol. 12, no. 4, pp. 463–466, 1992.

[3] S. C. Newman and R. C. Bland, "Mortality in a cohort of patients with schizophrenia: a record linkage study," *Canadian Journal of Psychiatry*, vol. 36, no. 4, pp. 239–245, 1991.

[4] S. Brown, "Excess mortality of schizophrenia. A meta-analysis," *British Journal of Psychiatry*, vol. 171, pp. 502–508, 1997.

[5] J. W. Newcomer, "Second generation antipsychotics and metabolic effects a comprehensive literature," *CNS Drugs*, vol. 19, supplement, pp. 1–93, 2005.

[6] D. Casey, "Dyslipedemia and atypical antipsychotic drugs," *Journal of Clinical Psychiatry*, vol. 65, supplement 18, pp. 29–35, 2004.

[7] M. Clark, K. Dubowski, and J. Colmore, "The effect of chlorpromazine on serum cholesterol in chronic schizophrenic patients," *Clinical Pharmacology & Therapeutics*, vol. 11, no. 6, pp. 883–889, 1970.

[8] D. W. Haupt and J. W. Newcomer, "Hyperglycemia and antipsychotic medications," *Journal of Clinical Psychiatry*, vol. 62, supplement 27, pp. 15–26, 2001.

[9] O. E. Olose, R. Uwakwe, M. Oche et al., "Hyperglycaemia and Weight gain among schizophrenia patients treated with antipsychotic in Enugu Nigeria," *Nigerian Journal of Psychiatry*, vol. 10, no. 1, 2012.

[10] A. L. Stewart, R. D. Hays, and J. E. Ware, "The MOS short-form general health survey: reliability and validity in a patient population," *Medical Care*, vol. 26, no. 7, pp. 724–735, 1988.

[11] A. Onighaiye M, *The impact of the length of time in the university. Ego self esteem and stress manifestation in students [thesis]*, University of Lagos, Lagos, Nigeria, 1996.

[12] P. Trinder, "Determination of blood glucose using 4-amino phenazone as oxygen acceptor," *Journal of Clinical Pathology*, vol. 22, no. 2, article no. 246, 1969.

[13] D. Barham and P. Trinder, "An improved colour reagent for the determination of blood glucose by the oxidase system," *The Analyst*, vol. 97, no. 1151, pp. 142–145, 1972.

[14] W. T. Friedwald, R. I. Levy, and D. S. Fredickson, "Estimation of the concentration of low-density lipoprotein cholesterol in plasma, without use of the preparative ultracentrifuge," *Clinical Chemistry*, vol. 18, no. 6, pp. 499–502, 1972.

[15] D. A. Wirshing, J. A. Boyd, L. R. Meng, J. S. Ballon, S. R. Marder, and W. C. Wirshing, "The effects of novel antipsychotics on glucose and lipid levels," *Journal of Clinical Psychiatry*, vol. 63, no. 10, pp. 856–865, 2002.

[16] R. Hamidreeza, K. Azam, A. Hamid et al., "Lipid profile in antipsychotic users. A comparative study. ARVA," *Atheroscler*, vol. 9, no. 3, pp. 198–202, 2013.

[17] O. B. Idonije, O. O. Festus, U. Akpamu, O. Okhiai, O. I. Inbhogbe, and G. B. S. Iyalomhe, "A comparative study of the effects of clozapine and risperidone monotherapy on lipid profile in Nigerian patients with schizophrenia," *International Journal of Pharmacology*, vol. 8, no. 3, pp. 169–176, 2012.

[18] J. M. Meyer and C. E. Koro, "The effects of antipsychotic therapy on serum lipids: a comprehensive review," *Schizophrenia Research*, vol. 70, no. 1, pp. 1–17, 2004.

[19] R. C. Smith, J. P. Lidenmeyer, N. Bark et al., "Clozapine, Risperidone, Olanzapine and Conventional Antipsychotics drug effect on glucose lipid and leptin in schizophrenia patients," *International Journal Neuro Psychopharmacol*, vol. 8, no. 2, pp. 183–194, 2005.

[20] C. Bushe and B. Leonard, "Association between atypical antipsychotic agents and type 2 diabetes: review of prospective clinical data," *British Journal of Psychiatry*, vol. 184, no. 47, pp. s87–s93, 2004.

[21] A. O. Lawani, B. O. James, O. Marakinyo et al., "Prevalence of metabolic syndrome in schizophrenic on antipsychotics in a Nigerian Psychiatric Hospital," *Nigerian Journal Psychiatric*, vol. 7, no. 2, 2009.

[22] American Diabetes Association, American Psychiatric Association, American Association of Clinical Endocrinologists, and North American Association for the Study of Obesity, "Consensus development conference on antipsychotic drugs and obesity and diabetes," *Diabetes Care*, vol. 27, no. 2, pp. 596–601, 2004.

[23] J.-P. Lindenmayer, P. Czobor, J. Volavka et al., "Changes in glucose and cholesterol levels in patients with schizophrenia treated with typical or atypical antipsychotics," *The American Journal of Psychiatry*, vol. 160, no. 2, pp. 290–296, 2003.

[24] H. S. Khalili, S. Dashti-Khavidaki, H. Okhovatpour, and P. Ghaeli, "Effects of risperidone on lipid profile," *Annals of Pharmacotherapy*, vol. 41, no. 5, pp. 899–900, 2007.

[25] A. Must, J. Spadano, E. H. Coakley, A. E. Field, G. Colditz, and W. H. Dietz, "The disease burden associated with overweight and obesity," *JAMA*, vol. 282, no. 16, pp. 1523–1529, 1999.

[26] J. Ishigoka, M. Nuraski, S. Miur et al., "The olanzapine early phase II study Group efficacy and safety of olanzapine, an atypical antipsychotic in patients with schizophrenia results of open label multicentre study in Japan Psychiatry," *Journal of Clinical Neuroscience*, vol. 55, no. 4, pp. 353–363, 2001.

[27] G. Simpson, P. Weiden, T. Pigott, S. Romano, and C. Siu, "Ziprasidone vs olanzapine in schizophrenia: 6-month continuation study," *European Neuropsychopharmacology*, vol. 12, supplement 3, p. 311, 2002.

[28] J. M. Meyer, "Effect of atypical anti-psychotics on weight and serum lipid levels," *Journal of Clinical Psychiatry*, vol. 62, supplement 27, pp. 27–34, 2001.

[29] J. Muench and A. M. Hamer, "Adverse effects of antipsychotic medications," *American Family Physician*, vol. 81, no. 5, pp. 617–622, 2010.

[30] M. Krakowski, P. Czobor, and L. Citrome, "Weight gain, metabolic parameters, and the impact of race in aggressive inpatients randomized to double-blind clozapine, olanzapine or haloperidol," *Schizophrenia Research*, vol. 110, no. 1-3, pp. 95–102, 2009.

[31] A. George, H. Mariam, L. Anthony et al., "Health related quality of life among patients treated with lurasidone from a switch trial in patients with schizophrenia," *BMC Psychiatry*, vol. 14, article 53, 2014.

[32] G. Harrison, K. Hopper, T. Craig et al., "Recovery from psychotic illness: a 15- and 25-year international follow-up study," *British Journal of Psychiatry*, vol. 178, pp. 506–517, 2001.

Canadian Physicians' Attitudes towards Accessing Mental Health Resources

Tariq M. Hassan,[1] M. Selim Asmer,[2] Nadeem Mazhar,[2] Tariq Munshi,[2] Tanya Tran,[3] and Dianne L. Groll[2]

[1] *Providence Care Mental Health Services, 752 King Street West, Kingston, ON, Canada K7L 4X3*
[2] *Department of Psychiatry, Queen's University at Kingston, ON, Canada*
[3] *Queen's University at Kingston, ON, Canada*

Correspondence should be addressed to Tariq M. Hassan; hassant@providencecare.ca

Academic Editor: Nicola Magnavita

Despite their rigorous training, studies have shown that physicians experience higher rates of mental illness, substance abuse, and suicide compared to the general population. An online questionnaire was sent to a random sample of physicians across Canada to assess physicians' knowledge of the incidence of mental illness among physicians and their attitudes towards disclosure and treatment in a hypothetical situation where one developed a mental illness. We received 139 responses reflecting mostly primary care physicians and nonsurgical specialists. The majority of respondents underestimated the incidence of mental illness in physicians. The most important factors influencing respondent's will to disclose their illness included career implications, professional integrity, and social stigma. Preference for selecting mental health treatment services, as either outpatients or inpatients, was mostly influenced by quality of care and confidentiality, with lower importance of convenience and social stigma. Results from this study suggest that the attitudes of physicians towards becoming mentally ill are complex and may be affected by the individual's previous diagnosis of mental illness and the presence of a family member with a history of mental illness. Other factors include the individual's medical specialty and level of experience. As mental illness is common among physicians, one must be conscious of these when offering treatment options.

1. Introduction

In 2008, the WHO reported mental illnesses as the leading cause of disability in the US and Canada [1]. The incidence of mental illness among Canadians has been estimated at approximately 18.6% per year and has been shown to affect those of all genders, occupations, and sociocultural backgrounds [2, 3]. All considered, the impact of mental illness on the Canadian economy has totaled about $20.7 billion in 2012, and this number is expected to increase by 1.9% each year [4]. Many recent studies have shown that approaching this problem is not as simple as one would expect. Barriers to seeking care for mental illness in Canada include not only a lack of resources, but also stigma which makes patients reluctant to seek help [5].

In discussing the burden of mental illness among Canadians, the mental health needs of physicians are often overlooked. Due to recent changes in the healthcare landscape, physicians have an increasingly demanding task of excelling in clinical, academic, and managerial roles [6]. However, despite their rigorous training, studies have shown that physicians experience higher rates of mental illness, substance abuse, and suicide compared to the general population [7]. In one study, physicians were found to be at almost 6 times higher risk for suicide than the general population [8]. This increasingly evident problem has led the American Medical Association (AMA) to coin the term impaired physician as "one unable to fulfill professional or personal responsibilities because of psychiatric illness, alcoholism, or drug dependency" [9]. In addition to psychiatric illnesses, physicians have also been shown to suffer from *professional burnout*, a psychological "syndrome characterized by a loss of enthusiasm for work (emotional exhaustion), feelings of cynicism (depersonalization), and a low sense of personal accomplishment" [10]. In a recent study of US physicians, almost half reported at least one symptom of burnout [10]. Although not in itself a mental illness, burnout may "reduce the effectiveness and overall positive energy a physician may have on a daily basis" and has been shown to have a relationship with increased rates of physical illness, depression, and substance use [11–13]. Aside from its personal impact, decreased physician wellness has been linked to decreased quality of healthcare and poorer patient outcomes [14].

Physicians' attitudes towards illness and coping begin early in medical training. Medical students were found to be more likely to underestimate their risk for mental illness [15]. Another contributor was found to be students' lack of personal experience with mentally ill patients, which would make them uncertain or hesitant about recognizing signs of mental illness or knowing how to seek help. Within a culture where weakness is not tolerated and doctors are seen as being "invulnerable" to illness, young medical trainees felt that their distress was overlooked and that they were discouraged from seeking help [16]. This seems to be further fortified in postgraduate training, where surveyed residents continue to experience stigma, with fears of jeopardizing their training status by seeking help for illnesses [17]. This attitude tends to worsen as one enters practice, as taking care of oneself tends to be "low on a physician's list of priorities" [18], and a third of physicians do not have a family physician themselves [19].

Only a handful of studies have begun to look at the prevalence of mental health concerns among Canadian physicians. Data from the 2007-2008 Canadian Physician Study revealed nearly a fifth to quarter of physicians admitting to symptoms of depression and anhedonia. This seemed to be higher in females and family physicians. Contributing factors identified included stress and poor work-life balance. Most strikingly, more than a quarter of Canadian physicians reported "mental health concerns that made it difficult for them to handle their workload in the past month" [20].

Only recently have we begun to gain insight into the burden of mental health concerns among Canadian physicians. However, little is known about what proportion of these individuals seek help. Learning more about what keeps physicians from accessing mental health services is our goal for this study. Until recently, there has been little interest in exploring the factors that present barriers for physicians to seek mental healthcare in particular. For example, a recent study revealed that among a group of physicians in the UK, over 75% of participants cited stigma as a factor influencing them to withhold disclosure of their mental illness to a professional [21].

Although very limited data exists for some physician populations outside of Canada, our literature review revealed no published literature reflecting Canadian physicians' attitudes towards becoming mentally ill or having a mental illness.

The goal of the current study was to explore barriers impacting access to mental healthcare for Canadian physicians. In the hypothetical situation that one developed a mental illness, our questionnaire explored where one would seek advice and which factors would affect a physician's decision to select a specific outpatient or inpatient treatment facility. Furthermore, we hypothesized that there would be differences among these attitudes based on whether the physician had previously experienced a mental illness and had witnessed a family member suffer from a mental illness and/or their medical specialty and years of experience.

2. Methods

This is a random sample, cross-sectional study. Eligible participants included all physicians registered to practice in Canada. Residents and medical students were excluded. A random sample of 6000 physicians (approximately 10% of physicians listed) were selected from Scott's Canadian Medical Directory [22] and sent a letter of information regarding the study with a link to an online survey. A secure, online questionnaire using Fluid Surveys was used. Both English and French versions were deployed, and there was an option to change the language either at the beginning or in the middle of the survey. There was also a link to receive a paper survey with a prepaid envelope. The paper survey was identical to the online version in structure and content of questions. No identifying information was collected from subjects, and the authors had no way of correlating survey responses with individual subjects.

All subjects were eligible to enter a draw to win one of several $50 gift cards. To enter the draw, the subjects entered their name and address into a secure form. This data was used to identify the location of subjects, although this information was not linked to the original questionnaire. A letter with a link to a survey was sent to subjects and responses were collected from January 15 to April 30, 2015.

2.1. Ethical Consideration. Prior to commencement, ethical approval was granted from the Queen's University Health Sciences and Affiliated Teaching Hospitals Research Ethics Board.

2.2. Statistical Analysis. All survey responses were entered directly into the Fluid Survey site and then downloaded into an excel file where they were checked for completeness and then analyzed using SPSS (IBM Corp) v22. Descriptive variables such as frequency counts, percentages, means, and standard deviations were used to describe the study participants. A series of two-sample chi-square tests (χ^2) were conducted to examine differences in responses based on identifying information (i.e., years of experience and specialty type).

3. Results

3.1. Sample Characteristics. Of the 6000 questionnaires deployed, we received 137 responses (2.12% response rate). 92% of surveys were completed in English, and 8% were completed in French. Demographic information is summarized in Table 1. Respondents were mostly from Ontario (36%)

Table 1: Demographics of survey respondents.

	N	%
Language		
English	118	92.2
French	10	7.8
Missing	—	—
Location		
Ontario	46	35.9
Quebec	24	18.8
British Columbia	10	7.8
Alberta	10	7.8
Nova Scotia	7	5.5
New Brunswick	2	1.6
Newfoundland and Labrador	2	1.6
Saskatchewan	2	1.6
Prince Edward Island	1	0.8
Missing	24	18.8
Practicing years		
Less than 5	27	21.1
5 to 20	41	32.0
Greater than 20	59	46.5
Missing	1	0.8
Specialization		
Nonsurgical specialist	59	46.1
Primary care	54	42.2
Surgical specialist	9	7.0
Full-time research/admin	5	3.9
Missing	1	0.8
Personal history of mental illness		
No	85	66.4
Yes	43	33.6
Missing	—	—
Family history of mental illness		
No	43	33.6
Yes	85	66.4
Missing	—	—

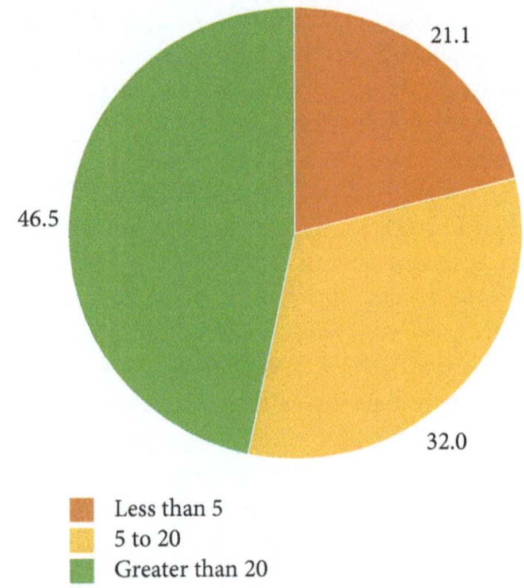

Figure 1: Canadian physicians divided by range of years they have been practicing. Data values represent frequencies in percentages ($N = 128$).

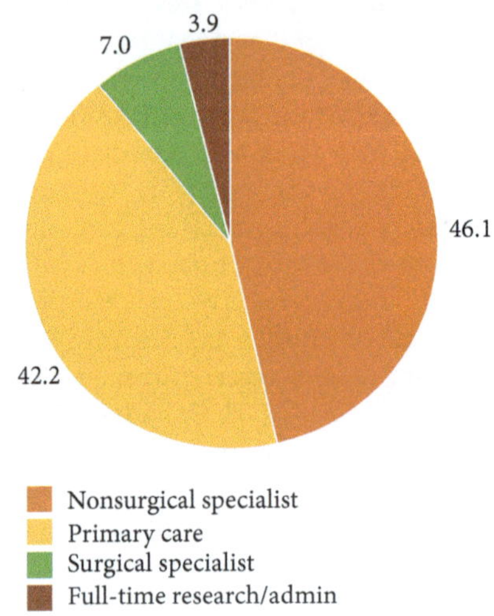

Figure 2: Canadian physicians divided by specialization. Data values represent frequencies in percentages ($N = 127$).

and Quebec (19%), with lesser representations from all other Canadian provinces. Location information was missing for 18% of respondents, as they had not filled out their address for the draw. The greatest proportion of respondents were physicians with over 20 years of medical experience (46.5%), with a smaller proportion of physicians with 5–20 years of experience (32.0%) and 21.1% with less than 5 years of experience (Figure 1). Most respondents were characterized as being nonsurgical specialists (45.6%) and primary care physicians (41.9%) (Figure 2). The proportion of respondents reporting having had a personal history of mental illness was 31.6%. The proportion of respondents having had a family history of mental illness was 62.5% (Figure 3).

3.2. Estimates of Incidence of Mental Illness among Physicians. Most respondents estimated the incidence of mental illness among physicians to be "about the same" as the general population (60.9%) (Figure 4). This estimate was significantly associated with family history of mental illness: χ^2 (N = 137) = 9.67, p = 0.008, and Cramer's V = 0.28, with respondents who had a family history being more likely to respond as "about the same" or "higher" than the general population. Respondents with no family history of mental illness (23.8%) were more likely to incorrectly estimate the incidence as being lower than in the general population.

3.3. Disclosure of Mental Illness. The majority of participants (58.8%) preferred to disclose their mental illness to a family member, while much lower proportions of participants preferred to disclose their mental illness to their family physician (12.5%) or other healthcare professionals (9.6%). There was no correlation with varying levels of experience or past history of personal mental illness or family mental illness.

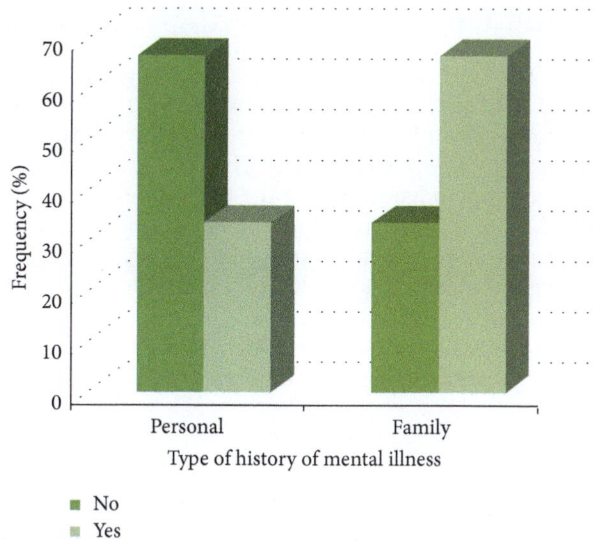

Figure 3: Frequency of Canadian physicians with or without personal and family history of mental illness (N = 128).

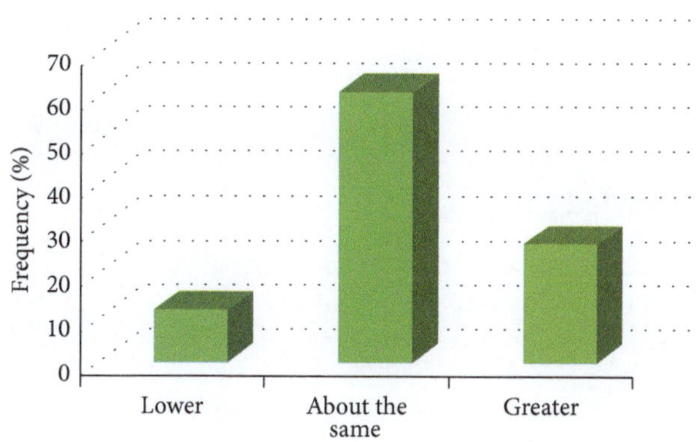

Figure 4: Canadian physicians divided by their estimation of the incidence of mental illness amongst physicians relative to the general population (N = 127).

3.4. Seeking Advice for Management of Illness. Respondents were asked how they would seek advice in the hypothetical scenario where they would develop a mental illness affecting their functioning. As a first choice, respondents indicated a noticeably stronger preference towards formal outpatient advice (e.g., a referral through a family physician) (69.5%) compared to informal outpatient advice (e.g., advice from a friend or colleague) (18%). Self-medication (5.5%) or no treatment (3.1%) was least preferred (Table 2). There was no significant correlation with years of experience or personal and/or family history of mental illness.

3.5. Preferences with regard to Obtaining Treatment. Respondents were asked to select which factors would affect where they would seek outpatient care. The most important factors were quality of care (53.7%), followed by confidentiality (30.9%) (Table 3). Convenience and social stigma were least important, having been selected by 11.0% and 0.7% of respondents, respectively. Differences in years of experience

Table 2: Top picks for outpatient services.

Factor	Primary	Secondary	Tertiary
Formal	69.5	21.1	8.6
Informal	18	62.5	9.4
Self-medication	5.5	4.7	20.3
No treatment	3.1	2.3	21.1
Other	3.9	9.4	40.6

Table 3: Most important factors influencing top pick for outpatient treatment.

Factor	Frequency (%)
Quality of care	56.3
Confidentiality	32
Convenience	10.9
Social stigma	0.8

Table 4: Top picks for inpatient services.

Factor	Primary	Secondary	Tertiary
Local government facility	30.5	9.4	12.5
Out-of-area government facility	21.1	34.4	27.3
Local private facility	16.4	34.4	41.4
Out-of-area private facility	32	21.9	18.8

Table 5: Most important factor influencing top pick for inpatient treatment.

Factor	Frequency (%)
Quality of care	43.8
Confidentiality	45.3
Convenience	6.3
Social stigma	4.7

or personal or family history of mental illness were not associated with different responses.

If inpatient treatment was to become necessary, no statistical differences were found regarding which facility type (government or private) or location (i.e., local or out-of-area facilities) respondents would choose (Table 4). There was no significant difference in response associated with different participant demographics. As with outpatient services, quality of care and confidentiality were the most important factors influencing facility selection (43.8% and 45.3%, resp.) (Table 5). Convenience and social stigma were the least important factors affecting facility selection (6.3% and 4.7%, resp.).

4. Discussion

4.1. Representativeness of the Study Sample. This is the first nationwide study in Canada exploring the attitudes of physicians towards becoming mentally ill and their preferences towards disclosing their mental illness, seeking treatment advice, and choosing a treatment facility. The response rate for this study was much lower for our survey was smaller than previous studies we have published [21, 23]. A strength of our study was that respondents reflected a variety of specialty types, mostly nonsurgical specialists and primary care physicians, which account for the biggest proportion of physicians in Canada. Surgical specialists were significantly underrepresented, possibly due to busier lifestyles and less free time to complete the survey. However, this data does not adequately represent Canadian physicians due to the low response rate and small sample size. The data suffered from undercoverage and nonresponse biases. The overrepresentation of physicians with a previous history of mental illness, as well as with family history of mental illness, indicated a source of voluntary response bias.

4.2. Understanding the Impact of Mental Illness. Over the past two decades, we have developed a greater understanding of physician mental illness, including its incidence, causes, and complications. One of the first questions in the survey explored knowledge of the prevalence of mental illness among physicians. Most participants indicated that the prevalence was the same as the general population, when in fact it is known to be higher. This indicates a need for physicians to be more educated during their training about how mental illness can affect them. More and more medical schools are promoting "wellness" and "resilience" as part of their medical school curricula, but these efforts are still in their infancy and are focused mostly on primary prevention. While these efforts are very effective in helping to improve rates of depression, anxiety, and burnout, there is currently little emphasis on secondary prevention and seeking help once a serious mental illness may be suspected [24, 25].

4.3. Seeking Advice: Has Stigma Improved? When selecting which factors would affect their decision to disclose their mental illness and to seek help, social stigma was consistently one of the least selected factors. This is reassuring in the sense that it indicates that physicians understand the importance of formal mental healthcare in the treatment of psychiatric conditions and that they are not invulnerable. This is in stark contrast to previous studies in which physicians would much rather self-medicate than risk having their mental illness documented in their medical record [26]. Our results may suggest an overall trend towards decreasing stigma towards mental illness in today's doctors.

4.4. Quality of Care Is Most Important. The two most important factors identified in this study that influenced physicians' decision to select a treatment center, whether as inpatient or outpatient, were quality of care and confidentiality. This is consistent with our previous study of psychiatrists in Canada. As we move towards more centers using electronic patient records, physicians may be concerned about the confidentiality of their medical records. This may indicate a need for more education or modifications to existing physician healthcare programs to highlight both quality of care and confidentiality as part of their care services.

5. Conclusion

The results of our study indicate the decreasing importance of stigma in physicians' thinking regarding their own mental health concerns and the importance of quality of care and confidentiality in physicians seeking help. It remains important to continue advocating for the importance of mental health during medical training and educating physicians about the burden of mental illness in the physician population. Ongoing research is needed to further understand the factors that affect physicians' choices to seek treatment for their mental illness, as well as the effectiveness of education in affecting mental illness rates among physicians.

Disclosure

This paper was presented as a Poster Presentation at the American Psychiatric Association meeting in Toronto, ON, on May 16, 2015. It was presented as a symposium at the Canadian Psychiatric Association Meeting in Vancouver, BC, on October 1, 2015.

Competing Interests

The authors declare that they have no competing interests.

Acknowledgments

This study was supported by a financial grant from the Queen's University Department of Psychiatry.

References

[1] WHO, *The Global Burden of Disease: 2004 Update*, WHO, Geneva, Switzerland, 2008.

[2] Public Health Agency of Canada, "Chapter 1: mental illnesses in Canada: an overview," in *A Report on Mental Illnesses in Canada*, 2012, http://www.phac-aspc.gc.ca/publicat/miic-mmac/chap_1-eng.php.

[3] D. R. Offord, M. H. Boyle, D. Campbell et al., "One-year prevalence of psychiatric disorder in Ontarians 15 to 64 years of age," *Canadian Journal of Psychiatry*, vol. 41, no. 9, pp. 559–563, 1996.

[4] The Conference Board of Canada, *Mental Illness Imposes High Costs on the Canadian Economy*, The Conference Board of Canada, 2012.

[5] L. W. Roberts and B. S. Bandstra, "Addressing stigma to strengthen psychiatric education," *Academic Psychiatry*, vol. 36, no. 5, pp. 347–350, 2012.

[6] M. N. Miller and K. R. McGowen, "The painful truth: physicians are not invincible," *Southern Medical Journal*, vol. 93, no. 10, pp. 966–973, 2000.

[7] A. Wilson, A. Rosen, P. Randal et al., "Psychiatrically impaired medical practitioners: an overview with special reference to impaired psychiatrists," *Australasian Psychiatry*, vol. 17, no. 1, pp. 6–10, 2009.

[8] K. Hawton, A. Clements, S. Simkin, and A. Malmberg, "Doctors who kill themselves: a study of the methods used for suicide," *QJM*, vol. 93, no. 6, pp. 351–357, 2000.

[9] E. V. M. L. Boisaubin and R. E. Levine, "Identifying and assisting the impaired physician," *The American Journal of the Medical Sciences*, vol. 322, no. 1, pp. 31–36, 2001.

[10] T. D. Shanafelt, S. Boone, L. Tan et al., "Burnout and satisfaction with work-life balance among US physicians relative to the general US population," *Archives of Internal Medicine*, vol. 172, no. 18, pp. 1377–1385, 2012.

[11] A. Iacovides, K. N. Fountoulakis, S. Kaprinis, and G. Kaprinis, "The relationship between job stress, burnout and clinical depression," *Journal of Affective Disorders*, vol. 75, no. 3, pp. 209–221, 2003.

[12] G. R. Holt, "Physician burnout: a serious concern for the medical profession," *Southern Medical Journal*, vol. 106, no. 5, p. 297, 2013.

[13] T. Honkonen, K. Ahola, M. Pertovaara et al., "The association between burnout and physical illness in the general population—results from the Finnish Health 2000 Study," *Journal of Psychosomatic Research*, vol. 61, no. 1, pp. 59–66, 2006.

[14] J. E. Wallace, J. B. Lemaire, and W. A. Ghali, "Physician wellness: a missing quality indicator," *The Lancet*, vol. 374, no. 9702, pp. 1714–1721, 2009.

[15] M. E. Whitcomb, "Helping physicians in training to care for themselves," *Academic Medicine*, vol. 79, no. 9, pp. 815–816, 2004.

[16] F. E. Fox, N. J. Doran, K. J. Rodham, G. J. Taylor, M. F. Harris, and M. O'Connor, "Junior doctors' experiences of personal illness: a qualitative study," *Medical Education*, vol. 45, no. 12, pp. 1251–1261, 2011.

[17] C. Moutier, M. Cornette, J. Lehrmann et al., "When residents need health care: stigma of the patient role," *Academic Psychiatry*, vol. 33, no. 6, pp. 431–441, 2009.

[18] L. Gundersen, "Physician burnout," *Annals of Internal Medicine*, vol. 135, no. 2, pp. 145–148, 2001.

[19] C. P. Gross, L. A. Mead, D. E. Ford, and M. J. Klag, "Physician, heal thyself? Regular source of care and use of preventive health services among physicians," *Archives of Internal Medicine*, vol. 160, no. 21, pp. 3209–3214, 2000.

[20] M. T. Compton and E. Frank, "Mental health concerns among Canadian physicians: results from the 2007-2008 Canadian Physician Health Study," *Comprehensive Psychiatry*, vol. 52, no. 5, pp. 542–547, 2011.

[21] T. M. Hassan, S. O. Ahmed, A. C. White, and N. Galbraith, "A postal survey of doctors' attitudes to becoming mentally ill," *Clinical Medicine*, vol. 9, no. 4, pp. 327–332, 2009.

[22] MDSelect, *Canadian Medical Directory 2015*, Scott's Directories, Toronto, Canada, 61st edition, 2015.

[23] T. M. Hassan, S. Sikander, N. Mazhar, T. Munshi, N. Galbraith, and D. Groll, "Canadian psychiatrists' attitudes to becoming mentally ill," *British Journal of Medical Practitioners*, vol. 6, no. 2, article 619, 2013.

[24] S. J. Slavin, D. L. Schindler, and J. T. Chibnall, "Medical student mental health 3.0: improving student wellness through curricular changes," *Academic Medicine*, vol. 89, no. 4, pp. 573–577, 2014.

[25] B. C. Drolet and S. Rodgers, "A comprehensive medical student wellness program—design and implementation at Vanderbilt School of Medicine," *Academic Medicine*, vol. 85, no. 1, pp. 103–110, 2010.

[26] C. Lehmann, "Psychiatrists not immune to effects of stigma," *Psychiatric News*, vol. 36, no. 14, p. 11, 2001.

Permissions

All chapters in this book were first published in Psychiatry , by Hindawi Publishing Corporation; hereby published with permission under the Creative Commons Attribution License or equivalent. Every chapter published in this book has been scrutinized by our experts. Their significance has been extensively debated. The topics covered herein carry significant findings which will fuel the growth of the discipline. They may even be implemented as practical applications or may be referred to as a beginning point for another development.

The contributors of this book come from diverse backgrounds, making this book a truly international effort. This book will bring forth new frontiers with its revolutionizing research information and detailed analysis of the nascent developments around the world.

We would like to thank all the contributing authors for lending their expertise to make the book truly unique. They have played a crucial role in the development of this book. Without their invaluable contributions this book wouldn't have been possible. They have made vital efforts to compile up to date information on the varied aspects of this subject to make this book a valuable addition to the collection of many professionals and students.

This book was conceptualized with the vision of imparting up-to-date information and advanced data in this field. To ensure the same, a matchless editorial board was set up. Every individual on the board went through rigorous rounds of assessment to prove their worth. After which they invested a large part of their time researching and compiling the most relevant data for our readers.

The editorial board has been involved in producing this book since its inception. They have spent rigorous hours researching and exploring the diverse topics which have resulted in the successful publishing of this book. They have passed on their knowledge of decades through this book. To expedite this challenging task, the publisher supported the team at every step. A small team of assistant editors was also appointed to further simplify the editing procedure and attain best results for the readers.

Apart from the editorial board, the designing team has also invested a significant amount of their time in understanding the subject and creating the most relevant covers. They scrutinized every image to scout for the most suitable representation of the subject and create an appropriate cover for the book.

The publishing team has been an ardent support to the editorial, designing and production team. Their endless efforts to recruit the best for this project, has resulted in the accomplishment of this book. They are a veteran in the field of academics and their pool of knowledge is as vast as their experience in printing. Their expertise and guidance has proved useful at every step. Their uncompromising quality standards have made this book an exceptional effort. Their encouragement from time to time has been an inspiration for everyone.

The publisher and the editorial board hope that this book will prove to be a valuable piece of knowledge for researchers, students, practitioners and scholars across the globe.

List of Contributors

Rolf Wynn
Department of Clinical Medicine, Faculty of Health Sciences, UiT The Arctic University of Norway, 9037 Tromsø, Norway
Department of Psychogeriatric Services, Division of Mental Health and Addictions, University Hospital of North Norway, 9291 Tromsø, Norway

Paolo Cassano, Cristina Cusin, David Mischoulon, Angela Pisoni, Trina Chang, Albert Yeung, Dawn F. Ionescu, Samuel R. Petrie, Andrew A. Nierenberg and Maurizio Fava
Depression Clinical & Research Program, Massachusetts General Hospital, Boston, MA 02114, USA

Dan V. Iosifescu
Depression Clinical & Research Program, Massachusetts General Hospital, Boston, MA 02114, USA
Wellman Center for Photomedicine, Massachusetts General Hospital, Boston, MA 02114, USA

Michael R. Hamblin
Wellman Center for Photomedicine, Massachusetts General Hospital, Boston, MA 02114, USA

Luis De Taboada
LiteCure LLC,Newark, DE 19702, USA

Masahito Fushimi
Akita Prefectural Mental Health andWelfare Center, 2-1-51 Nakadori, Akita City, Akita Prefecture 010-0001, Japan
Akita Occupational Health Promotion Center, 6-6 Senshukubota-machi, Akita City, Akita Prefecture 010-0874, Japan

A. D. Faye, S. Gawande, R. Tadke, V. C. Kirpekar and S. H. Bhave
Department of Psychiatry, NKP Salve Institute of Medical Sciences and Lata Mangeshkar Hospital, Digdoh Hills, Hingna Road, Nagpur, Maharashtra 440019, India

A. P. Pakhare
Department of Community and Family Medicine, All India Institute of Medical Sciences, Bhopal 462020, India

B. Tayade
Department of Chest Medicine, NKP Salve Institute of Medical Sciences and Lata Mangeshkar Hospital, Digdoh Hills

Tolesa Fanta, Dawit Assefa and Mekbit Getachew
Amanuel Mental Specialized Hospital, Addis Ababa, Ethiopia

Telake Azale
Department of Psychiatry, Faculty of Medicine and Health Science, University of Gondar, Gondar, Ethiopia

Klas Lanthén
Skåne University Hospital, Södra Förstadsgatan 101, 214 28 Malmö, Sweden

Mikael Rask
Department of Health and Caring Sciences, Linnaeus University, Lückligs Plats, 351 95 Växjö, Sweden

Charlotta Sunnqvist
Department of Care Science, Faculty for Health and Society, Malmö University, JanWaldenströms Gata 25, 205 06 Malmö, Sweden

Adam Simning and Yeates Conwell
Department of Psychiatry, University of Rochester, 300 Crittenden Boulevard, Rochester, NY 14642, USA

Edwin van Wijngaarden
Department of Public Health Sciences, University of Rochester, 265 Crittenden Boulevard, Rochester, NY 14642, USA

Getasew Legas Molla
Debre Tabor Hospital, Debre Tabor, Ethiopia

Haregwoin Mulat Sebhat
Psychiatry Department, University of Gondar, P.O. Box 196, Gondar, Ethiopia

Zebiba Nasir Hussen
Amanuel Mental Specialized Hospital, P.O. Box 1971, Addis Ababa, Ethiopia

Amsalu Belete Mekonen
College of Health Sciences, Debre Tabor University, P.O. Box 272, Debre Tabor, Ethiopia

Wubalem Fekadu Mersha and Tesfa Mekonen Yimer
College of Medicine and Health Sciences,Wolaita Sodo University, P.O. Box 138,Wolaita Sodo, Ethiopia

Lauren R. Godier, Jessica C. Scaife and Rebecca J. Park
Oxford Brain-Body Research into Eating Disorders, Department of Psychiatry, University of Oxford, Oxford OX3 7JX, UK

Sven Braeutigam
Oxford Brain-Body Research into Eating Disorders, Department of Psychiatry, University of Oxford, Oxford OX3 7JX, UK
Oxford Centre for Human Brain Activity, Department of Psychiatry, University of Oxford, Oxford OX3 7JX, UK

Ysbrand J. Pijl and Diederik E. Tenback
GGz Centraal Psychiatric Center, Innova, 3818 EWAmersfoort, Netherlands

Janique G. Jessurun
GGz Centraal Psychiatric Center, Innova, 3818 EWAmersfoort, Netherlands
Division of Pharmacoepidemiology & Clinical Pharmacology, Utrecht Institute for Pharmaceutical Sciences, Faculty of Science, Utrecht University, 3584 CG Utrecht, Netherlands

Peter N. van Harten
GGz Centraal Psychiatric Center, Innova, 3818 EWAmersfoort, Netherlands
Department of Psychiatry and Neuropsychology, Maastricht University, 6211 LK Maastricht, Netherlands

Toine C. G. Egberts and Ingeborg Wilting
Division of Pharmacoepidemiology & Clinical Pharmacology, Utrecht Institute for Pharmaceutical Sciences, Faculty of Science
Utrecht University, 3584 CG Utrecht, Netherlands
Department of Clinical Pharmacy, University Medical Center Utrecht, 3584 CX Utrecht, Netherlands

Binoy Krishna Tarafder
Department of Medicine, Faridpur Medical College, Faridpur, Bangladesh

Mohammad Ashik Imran Khan
Pulmonology, Bangabandhu Sheikh Mujib Medical University, Bangladesh

Md. Tanvir Islam
Internal Medicine, Bangabandhu Sheikh Mujib Medical University, Bangladesh

Sheikh Abdullah Al Mahmud
Pediatrics, Sheikh Sayera Khatun Medical College, Gopalganj, Bangladesh

Md. Humayun Kabir Sarker and Imtiaz Faruq
Sheikh Sayera Khatun Medical College, Gopalgang, Bangladesh

Md. Titu Miah
Medicine, Dhaka Medical College Hospital, Dhaka, Bangladesh

S. M. Yasir Arafat
Department of Psychiatry, Bangabandhu Sheikh Mujib Medical University, Bangladesh

Kionna Oliveira Bernardes Santos
PhysicalTherapy Department, Federal University of Bahia (UFBA), Avenida Reitor Miguel Calmon s/n, Vale do Canela, 40.110-100 Salvador, BA, Brazil

Fernando Martins Carvalho
Department of Preventive and Social Medicine, Federal University of Bahia (UFBA), Avenida Reitor Miguel Calmon s/n, Vale do Canela, 40.110-100 Salvador, BA, Brazil

Tânia Maria de Araújo
Health Department, State University of Feira de Santana (UEFS), Avenida Transnordestina, s/n Novo Horizonte, 44036-900 Feira de Santana, BA, Brazil

Leila R. Kalankesh
Tabriz Health Services Management Research Center, Tabriz, Iran
School of Management and Medical Informatics, Tabriz University of Medical Sciences, Tabriz, Iran

Nazila Moftian and Zahra Nasiry
School of Management and Medical Informatics, Tabriz University of Medical Sciences, Tabriz, Iran

Mostafa Farahbakhsh
Tabriz Research Center of Psychiatry and Behavioral Sciences, Tabriz University of Medical Sciences, Tabriz, Iran

Rebecca A. Fein
Laboratory Informatics Institute, Smyrna, GA, USA
National Alliance of Research Associates Programs (NARAP), Hartford, CT, USA

Anish Khalil, Haran Innocent, Zainab Mansoor and Shehrbano Rizvi
Shifa College of Medicine, Shifa Tameer-e-Millat University, Islamabad, Pakistan

Muhammad Faheem
Oncology Department, Nuclear Medicine, Oncology and Radiotherapy Institute [NORI], Islamabad, Pakistan

Ammad Fahim
Department of Research, Shifa International Hospital, Islamabad, Pakistan

Hizra Farrukh
Rawalpindi Medical College, Islamabad, Pakistan

Mehdi Sayyah
Education Development Center, Ahvaz Jundishapur University of Medical Sciences, Ahvaz, Iran

Kaveh Eslami and Leila Kouti
School of Pharmacy, Ahvaz Jundishapur University of Medical Sciences, Ahvaz 61357-15794, Iran

Shabnam AlaiShehni
Student Research Committee, Ahvaz Jundishapur University of Medical Sciences, Ahvaz, Iran

Kindie Mekuria
Woldia Hospital,Woldia, Ethiopia

Haregwoin Mulat
Psychiatry Department, University of Gondar, Gondar, Ethiopia

Habtamu Derajew
Amanuel Mental Specialized Hospital, Addis Ababa, Ethiopia

Tesfa Mekonen, Wubalem Fekadu
Psychiatry Department, Bahir Dar University, Bahir Dar, Ethiopia

Amsalu Belete, Getasew Legas, and Simegnew Kibret
College of Medicine and Health Sciences, Debre Tabor University, Debre Tabor, Ethiopia

Solomon Yimer
Psychiatry Department, Dilla University, Dilla, Ethiopia

Melak Menberu
College of Health Sciences, Mizan-Tepi University, Mizan-Tepi, Ethiopia

Asmamaw Getnet
Finote Selam Hospital, Finote Selam, Ethiopia

Jennifer Downey
Department of Psychiatry, New York State Psychiatric Institute and Columbia University College of Physicians and Surgeons,
New York, NY 10032, USA

Richard C. Friedman
Department of Psychiatry, Weill Cornell Medical School, New York, NY 10021, USA

Elizabeth Haase
Department of Psychiatry, Carson Tahoe Health System, Carson City, NV 89701, USA

David Goldenberg
Department of Psychiatry,Weill Cornell Medical College, New York, NY 10021, USA

Robinette Bell
Department of Psychiatry, University of Colorado School of Medicine, Aurora, CO 80045, USA

Sidney Edsall
Behavioral Health and Recovery Services, San Mateo County Psychiatric Department, San Mateo, CA 94403, USA

Siranesh Tesfaye
Department of Psychiatry, Felege Hiwot Referral Hospital, Bahir Dar, Ethiopia

Nigussie Debencho
Department of Pharmacology, Amanuel Mental Specialized Hospital, Addis Ababa, Ethiopia

Teresa Kisi
Department of Epidemiology and Biostatistics, Institute of Public Health, College of Medicine and Health Science, University of Gondar, Gondar, Ethiopia

Minale Tareke
Bahir Dar University, College of Medicine and Health Science, Bahir Dar, Ethiopia

Misael Benti
Psychiatry Department, Gimbi General Hospital, Oromia, Ethiopia

Jemal Ebrahim and Asres Bedaso
School of Nursing and Midwifery, College of Medicine and Health Sciences, Hawassa University, Hawassa, Ethiopia

Tadesse Awoke
Department of Biostatistics and Epidemiology, College of Medicine and Health Sciences, University of Gondar, Gondar, Ethiopia

Zegeye Yohannis
Research and Training Directorate, Amanuel Specialized Mental Hospital, Addis Ababa, Ethiopia

H. Poissant
Department of Education and Pedagogy, UQAM, Montreal, QC, Canada H2L 2C4

L. Rapin
Department of Linguistics, UQAM, Montreal, QC, Canada H2L 2C4

S. Chenail and A. Mendrek
Department of Psychology, Bishop's University, Sherbrooke, QC, Canada J1M 1Z7

Cathrin Martin
Department of Neuroscience, Uppsala University, Uppsala, Sweden

Cecilia Rastad
Department of Neuroscience, Uppsala University, Uppsala, Sweden
Center for Clinical Research Dalarna (CKF), Falun, Sweden

Lennart Wetterberg,
Department of Clinical Neuroscience, Karolinska Institute, St. Göran, Stockholm, Sweden

Edmialem Gezahegn
Psychiatric Clinic, University of Gondar Hospital, Gondar, Ethiopia

Melkie Edris
Departmpent of Human Nutrition, Institute of Public Health, University of Gondar, Gondar, Ethiopia

Berihun Assefa Dachew
Department of Epidemiology and Biostatistics, Institute of Public Health, University of Gondar, Gondar, Ethiopia

P. Fusar-Poli, I. Bonoldi, R. Patel, V. Bhavsar, S. Tognin, S. Badger and M. Calem
Institute of Psychiatry Psychology and Neuroscience (IoPPN), King's College London, London SE5 8AF, UK
OASIS Service, South London and Maudsley NHS Foundation Trust, London SE11, UK

M. Cappucciati, G. Rutigliano and M. Rocchetti
Institute of Psychiatry Psychology and Neuroscience (IoPPN), King's College London, London SE5 8AF, UK

T. Y. Lee, K. Lim and J. S. Kwon
Department of Psychiatry, Seoul National University College of Medicine, Seoul

Q. Beverly
Cambridgeshire and Peterborough NHS Foundation Trust, Cambridge CB21 5HH, UK

J. Lelli
Real-Time Systems Laboratory, Scuola Superiore Sant'Anna, 56124 Pisa, Italy

S. J. Kaar and E. Gago
OASIS Service, South London and Maudsley NHS Foundation Trust, London SE11, UK

J. Perez
Cambridgeshire and Peterborough NHS Foundation Trust, Cambridge CB21 5HH, UK
Department of Psychiatry, University of Cambridge, Cambridge CB2 0SZ, UK

P. McGuire
Institute of Psychiatry Psychology and Neuroscience (IoPPN), King's College London, London SE5 8AF, UK
OASIS Service, South London and Maudsley NHS Foundation Trust, London SE11, UK

Aureliano Crameri and Agnes von Wyl
Zurich University of Applied Sciences, Zurich, Switzerland

Christopher Schuetz and Andreas Andreae
Integrated Psychiatric ServicesWinterthur and Zurich Unterland (ipw),Winterthur, Switzerland

Margit Koemeda and Peter Schulthess
Swiss Charter of Psychotherapy, Stäfa, Switzerland

Volker Tschuschke
University Hospital of Cologne, Cologne, Germany
Sigmund FreudUniversity, Berlin, Germany

Hussain Ahmed Darraj
Jazan Health Affairs, Ministry of Health, Jazan 45911, Saudi Arabia

Mohamed Salih Mahfouz
Family and Community Medicine Department, Faculty of Medicine, Jazan University, P.O. Box 2531, Jazan 45142, Saudi Arabia

Rashad Mohamed Al Sanosi
Substance Abuse Research Centre (SARC), Jazan University, Jazan 45142, Saudi Arabia

Mohammed Badedi and Abdullah Sabai
Public Health Administration, Jazan Health Affairs, Ministry of Health, Jazan 82723, Saudi Arabia

Abdulrahman AL Refaei
Jazan General Directorate of Education, Ministry of Education, Jazan 82614, Saudi Arabia

Hussain Mutawm
Departments of English, Faculty of Languages and Translation, King Khalid University, Abha 62529, Saudi Arabia

Md. Hafizur Rahman Chowdhury, Mohammad S. I. Mullick, and S. M. Yasir Arafat
Department of Psychiatry, Bangabandhu SheikhMujib Medical University, Dhaka, Bangladesh

S. M. Yasir Arafat
Department of Public Health, ASA University Bangladesh, ASA Tower, 23/3 Bir Uttam ANM Nuruzzaman Sarak, Shyamoli,
Dhaka 1207, Bangladesh

Emmanuel Omamurhomu Olose
Department of Psychiatry, University of Calabar, Calabar, Nigeria

John Edet
Department of Clinical Services, Federal Neuropsychiatric Hospital, Calabar, Nigeria

Monday Nwite Igwe
3Department of Psychiatry, Ebonyi State University, Abakaliki, Nigeria

Donald Chidozie Chukwujekwu
Department of Psychiatry, University of Port Harcourt, Port Harcourt, Nigeria

Miriam Chinyere Aguocha
Department of Psychiatry, Imo State University, Orlu, Nigeria

Richard Uwakwe
Department of Psychiatry, Nnamdi Azikiwe University, Awka, Nigeria

Tariq M. Hassan
Providence Care Mental Health Services, 752 King StreetWest, Kingston, ON, Canada K7L 4X3

M. Selim Asmer, Nadeem Mazhar,Tariq Munshi and Dianne L. Groll
Department of Psychiatry, Queen's University at Kingston, ON, Canada

Tanya Tran
Queen's University at Kingston, ON, Canada

Index

O

P

S

T